ANNUAL REVIEW OF GERONTOLOGY AND GERIATRICS

VOLUME 35, 2015

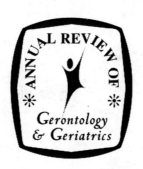

Annual Review of Gerontology and Geriatrics

Subjective Aging:
New Developments and Future Directions

VOLUME 35, 2015

Volume Editors

MANFRED DIEHL, PhD
HANS-WERNER WAHL, PhD

Series Editor

TONI C. ANTONUCCI, PhD

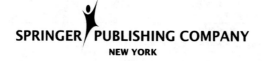

SPRINGER PUBLISHING COMPANY

NEW YORK

Springer Publishing Company, LLC
11 West 42nd Street
New York, NY 10036
www.springerpub.com

Acquisitions Editor: Sheri W. Sussman
Composition: Absolute Service, Inc.

ISBN: 978-0-8261-9649-1
E-book ISBN: 978-0-8261-9652-1
ISSN: 0198-8794
Online ISSN: 1944-4036

15 16 17/ 5 4 3 2 1

The author and the publisher of this Work have made every effort to use sources believed to be reliable to provide information that is accurate and compatible with the standards generally accepted at the time of publication. The author and publisher shall not be liable for any special, consequential, or exemplary damages resulting, in whole or in part, from the readers' use of, or reliance on, the information contained in this book. The publisher has no responsibility for the persistence or accuracy of URLs for external or third-party Internet websites referred to in this publication and does not guarantee that any content on such websites is, or will remain, accurate or appropriate.

Special discounts on bulk quantities of our books are available to corporations, professional associations, pharmaceutical companies, health care organizations, and other qualifying groups.

If you are interested in a custom book, including chapters from more than one of our titles, we can provide that service as well.

For details, please contact:
Special Sales Department, Springer Publishing Company, LLC
11 West 42nd Street, 15th Floor, New York, NY 10036-8002
Phone: 877-687-7476 or 212-431-4370; Fax: 212-941-7842
E-mail: sales@springerpub.com

Printed in the United States of America by Gasch Printing.

Contents

About the Volume Editors

Manfred Diehl, PhD, received his doctorate in Human Development and Family Studies, with a specialization in adult development and aging, from The Pennsylvania State University. Dr. Diehl is currently professor of Human Development and Family Studies at Colorado State University. His research program has two substantive foci: (a) adults' self-perceptions of aging and their associations with developmental outcomes and (b) social–emotional and self-concept development in adulthood. Dr. Diehl's research has been funded by the National Institute on Aging of the National Institutes of Health (NIH) and the Alexander von Humboldt Foundation (in collaboration with Hans-Werner Wahl), Bonn, Germany. Dr. Diehl has served as a member of a number of scientific review panels for NIH, including the special emphasis panel for the Roybal Centers for Translational Research on Aging, and he serves on several editorial boards. He also served a 3-year term on the Committee on Aging of the American Psychological Association (APA) and is currently a member of the Executive Committee of the Behavioral and Social Sciences Section of the Gerontological Society of America (GSA). Dr. Diehl is a fellow of Division 20: Adult Development and Aging of the APA and a fellow of the Behavioral and Social Sciences Section of the GSA. In 2011, he received the Scholarly Excellence Award of the College of Health and Human Sciences at Colorado State University and in 2012, the mentorship award of APA Division 20. Dr. Diehl is also the recipient of the Margret M. Baltes Early Career Award in Behavioral and Social Gerontology from the GSA.

Hans-Werner Wahl, PhD, is professor of Psychological Aging Research at the Institute of Psychology, Heidelberg University, Germany. He received his PhD in psychology from the Free University of Berlin in 1989. His research activities include the understanding of the role of physical–technological environments for aging well, adaptational processes in the context of age-related chronic functional loss, processes of awareness of aging in a life span perspective, and intervention research. He is the author or editor of more than 20 books and more than 200 scholarly journal articles and chapters related to the study of adult development and aging. He is co–editor-in-chief of the *European Journal of Ageing* and a member of the editorial board of *The Gerontologist*. Dr. Wahl is also a fellow of the GSA and has received the 2008 Social Gerontology Award (together with Manfred Diehl) and the 2009 M. Powell Lawton Award of the GSA. He has also been a fellow of the Marsilius-Kolleg of Heidelberg University.

Contributors

Anne E. Barrett, PhD, Associate Professor of Sociology, Department of Sociology, Florida State University, Tallahassee, FL

Allyson Brothers, MA, Doctoral Student, Department of Human Development and Family Studies, Colorado State University, Fort Collins, CO

Lindsey A. Cary, MA, Doctoral Student, Department of Psychology, University of Toronto, Ontario, Canada

Alison L. Chasteen, PhD, Associate Professor, Department of Psychology, University of Toronto, Ontario, Canada

Manfred Diehl, PhD, Professor of Human Development and Family Studies, Department of Human Development and Family Studies, Colorado State University, Fort Collins, CO

Gunhild O. Hagestad, PhD, Professor of Sociology, College of Applied Sciences, Norwegian Social Research, Oslo and Akershus University, Oslo, Norway

Mary Lee Hummert, PhD, Professor of Communication Studies, Vice Provost for Faculty Development, University of Kansas, Lawrence, KS

Anna E. Kornadt, PhD, Postdoctoral Research Associate, Faculty of Psychology and Sports Science/Department of Psychology, University of Bielefeld, Germany

Dana Kotter-Grühn, PhD, Assistant Professor, Department of Psychology & Neuroscience, Duke University, Durham, NC

Martina Miche, MSc, Doctoral Student, Department of Psychological Aging Research, Institute of Psychology, Ruprecht-Karls-University of Heidelberg, Germany

Joann M. Montepare, PhD, Professor of Psychology, Director, Fuss Center for Research on Aging and Intergenerational Studies, Lasell College, Newton, MA

Klaus Rothermund, PhD, Professor of Psychology, Institute of Psychology, Friedrich-Schiller-University of Jena, Germany

Richard A. Settersten, Jr., PhD, Professor of Social and Behavioral Health Sciences, College of Public Health & Human Sciences, Oregon State University, Corvallis, OR

Ursula M. Staudinger, PhD, Robert N. Butler Professor of Sociomedical Sciences and Professor of Psychology, Columbia Aging Center, Columbia University, New York, NY

Hans-Werner Wahl, PhD, Professor of Psychological Aging Research, Department of Psychological Aging Research, Institute of Psychology, Ruprecht-Karls-University of Heidelberg, Germany

Gerben J. Westerhof, PhD, Adjunct Professor of Psychology, Director, Dutch Life Story Lab, University of Twente, Enschede, The Netherlands

Susanne Wurm, PhD, Associate Professor of Psychology, Institute of Psychogerontology, Friedrich-Alexander-University of Erlangen-Nuremberg, Nuremberg, Germany

Previous Volumes in the Series

Forthcoming Volume in the Series

Volume 36, 2016

Optimizing Physical Activity and Function Across Settings

Table of Contents (tentative)

Preface

This volume of the *Annual Review of Gerontology and Geriatrics* represents the outcome of several years of collaboration and community building. The initial conversations about how adults may become aware of their own age and how they may perceive their own aging started between the two editors around 2005. Although at that time research on ageism and age stereotypes received a good deal of attention in the gerontological literature, the connection to the broader literature on phenomena of subjective aging was rather tentative. Thus, we perceived a need from a theoretical perspective to forge these connections and to develop a framework that would be capable of serving an integrating purpose. With this goal in mind, we started to work on a theoretical paper that proposed the concept of "awareness of age-related change" as an overarching construct. The resulting paper received the award for New Theoretical Developments in Social Gerontology from the Gerontological Society of America in 2008 and was subsequently published in *The Journals of Gerontology: Social Sciences* in 2010. Interestingly, while we were getting our paper ready for publication, several empirical articles were published reporting findings from longitudinal studies, such as the Berlin Aging Study, which showed that simple measures of subjective age predicted important developmental outcomes, such as functional health or mortality. We knew at that point that our interests were shared by other investigators and that our efforts were part of a larger community of aging researchers.

Because we wanted to formalize our collaboration and also address the topic of awareness of aging from a cross-cultural perspective, we applied for a grant through the TransCoop Program of the Alexander von Humboldt Foundation, Bonn, Germany. We were fortunate enough to receive the grant (funding period July 2010–June 2013), which not only allowed us to develop a multidimensional self-report questionnaire for our research but also provided us with the financial support to engage in systematic networking and community building. This networking and community building took place in the context of three workshops and a closing conference that included scholars from several countries. The primary objective of the workshops and the closing conference was to bring investigators who share an interest in subjective aging research or related topics together for an exchange of ideas and lively discussions. A secondary objective was to provide a forum for emerging scholars and investigators to take part in an ongoing discussion and to become part of a network of like-minded researchers. The closing conference was held in June 2013 at Heidelberg University, Germany, and provided a forum for lively interdisciplinary and cross-cultural exchange.

This volume builds on a selection of the presentations at the closing conference and expands on the lively discussions that occurred during this two-day event. Yet, it is important to note that all of the chapters move considerably beyond the conference presentations and incorporate additional theoretical propositions as well as findings from brand new studies—indeed, some of these studies were still in the process of being conducted at the time of the conference. In addition, all chapters were reviewed by two independent reviewers and went through a careful and rigorous "quality control." Thus, we hope that the resulting volume succeeds in presenting an up-to-date portrait of the overall field of subjective aging research, and we hope that the chapters will not only serve as a valuable source of information but that they will also inspire many new empirical studies. Overall, we believe that the research on subjective aging has entered a new and more advanced stage of development, and we hope that the current volume can serve as a building block for future theoretical and empirical work.

Because a project like this one always requires the support and involvement of many individuals, we would like to take this opportunity to thank all those individuals who have supported and encouraged our work in this area. In particular, Manfred Diehl would like to thank his department head, Dr. Lise Youngblade, and the vice provost for International Affairs at Colorado State University, Dr. Jim Cooney, for their unwavering support and encouragement. Hans-Werner Wahl would like to thank the former vice rector for Research and Structural Planning of Heidelberg University, Prof. Dr. Thomas Rausch, and the Heidelberg Center for American Studies for their generous support before and during the closing conference.

We both would like to thank Ms. Ursula König for her valuable help with formatting and finalizing the entire manuscript. We both would also like to thank the series editor, Dr. Toni C. Antonucci, and Ms. Sheri W. Sussman of Springer Publishing for being so receptive and supportive when we approached them about editing a volume of the *Annual Review of Gerontology and Geriatrics*. We are grateful for their encouragement and gentle guidance along the way. Finally, we would like to extend our gratitude to all of the contributors to this volume. We greatly appreciate your involvement and enthusiasm for this project.

Manfred Diehl and Hans-Werner Wahl
May 2014

ANNUAL REVIEW OF GERONTOLOGY AND GERIATRICS

VOLUME 35, 2015

CHAPTER 1

Subjective Aging and Awareness of Aging

Toward a New Understanding of the Aging Self

Manfred Diehl, Hans-Werner Wahl, Allyson Brothers, and Martina Miche

ABSTRACT

The objective of this chapter is to provide the overall background and framework for the remainder of the volume. Specifically, we will lay the foundation for the subsequent chapters by focusing on four major issues. First, we present a brief historical overview in part not only to pay homage to past contributions and accomplishments but in part also to delineate the reasons why research on subjective aging in the 1980s and for most part of the 1990s went through a period of skepticism and disinterest. Second, we discuss both theoretical as well as empirical reasons why we believe the field is making strides toward integration of new approaches and toward a new understanding of the role of subjective aging experiences. Third, we describe and explain what we see as the main components of this new understanding and how it is different from earlier approaches. Finally, we will discuss future challenges and directions for integrating the new developments with a new understanding of the aging self. In particular, we will advocate for a position that (a) views adult development and aging from a life span developmental perspective and (b) recognizes the bidirectional and dynamic interrelatedness of individual, social, and cultural factors in shaping adults' awareness and understanding of their own aging.

© 2015 Springer Publishing Company
http://dx.doi.org/10.1891/0198-8794.35.1

INTRODUCTION

Recent years have seen a renewed interest in conceptualizations of and empirical research on subjective aging and awareness of aging in the fields of social gerontology, life span psychology, and life course sociology.[1] The renewed interest in these constructs can be illustrated in various ways. From a conceptual perspective, for example, Levy (2009) proposed the stereotype embodiment theory as a psychological framework to better understand the individual and societal phenomena of age-related stereotyping, self-stereotyping, and ageism. Similarly, Montepare (2009) elaborated on fundamental theoretical issues related to subjective age and age identity, covering the age range from adolescence to old age. Diehl and Wahl (2010) proposed the construct of awareness of age-related change to address the self-reflective and multidimensional nature of the construct of subjective aging.

From the empirical perspective, several studies have been published since the late 1990s that reopened the discussion about phenomena of subjective aging and moved the field forward in significant ways. For example, based on data from old and very old adults in the Berlin Aging Study, Maier and Smith (1999) examined variables of subjective aging as predictors of mortality (see also the early study by Markides & Pappas, 1982). Similarly, using data from the Ohio Longitudinal Study, Levy, Slade, Kunkel, and Kasl (2002) showed that individuals who had positive self-perceptions of aging lived on average 7.5 years longer than individuals who had negative self-perceptions. Furthermore, the concept of subjective aging has increasingly gained importance as a predictor of health outcomes (e.g., Wurm, Tesch-Römer, & Tomasik, 2007) and as a viable psychological mechanism that may explain processes of adjustment to health challenges in old age (e.g., Wurm, Warner, Ziegelmann, Wolff, & Schüz, 2013). In addition, recent experimental work has started to address the plasticity of adults' subjective age judgments and whether experimental manipulations of individuals' awareness of aging are associated with positive outcomes (e.g., Stephan, Chalabaev, Kotter-Grühn, & Jaconelli, 2013). Furthermore, review chapters on attitudes toward aging (Hess, 2006) and age stereotypes (Hummert, 2011) were published in recent years in the highly respected *Handbook of the Psychology of Aging* (Birren & Schaie, 2006; Schaie & Willis, 2011).

This renewed interest comes after decades of research on subjective aging (see Kastenbaum, Derbin, Sabatini, & Artt, 1972) and raises the question whether we are simply dealing with an "old wine in new bottles" phenomenon or whether there is indeed a new momentum with the potential to move the field forward in significant and meaningful ways. This volume of the *Annual Review of Gerontology and Geriatrics* represents an attempt to answer this question. Specifically, the chapters in this volume are the products of a series of workshops and a conference that focused on several issues related to the broad area of subjective aging. These issues included, but were not limited to, topics related to (a) new theoretical developments and integrative efforts, (b) developments in terms of measurement and research methods, and (c) the assessment and critical evaluation of recent empirical findings.

The objective of this chapter is to provide the overall background and framework for the remainder of the volume. Specifically, we will lay the foundation for the subsequent chapters by focusing on four major issues. First, we present a brief historical overview in part not only to pay homage to past contributions and accomplishments but in part also to delineate the reasons why research on subjective aging in the 1980s and for most part of the 1990s went through a period of skepticism and disinterest. Second, we discuss both theoretical as well as empirical reasons why we believe the field is making strides toward integration of new approaches and toward a new understanding of the role of subjective aging experiences. Third, we describe and explain what we see as the main components of this new understanding and how it is different from earlier approaches. Finally, we will discuss future challenges and directions for integrating the new developments with a new understanding of the aging self. In particular, we will advocate for a position that (a) views adult development and aging from a life span developmental perspective and (b) recognizes the bidirectional and dynamic interrelatedness of individual, social, and cultural factors in shaping adults' awareness and understanding of their own aging.

THE TRADITION OF RESEARCH ON SUBJECTIVE AGING IN SOCIAL GERONTOLOGY, LIFE SPAN PSYCHOLOGY, AND LIFE COURSE SOCIOLOGY

Adults' subjective understanding of their own age and aging process has been a topic of theoretical and empirical inquiry in social gerontology, life span psychology, and life course sociology for over four decades (e.g., Bennett & Eckman, 1973; Kastenbaum et al., 1972; Montepare, 2009; Settersten, 1999). One of the originators of this area of research was Robert Kastenbaum who suggested that a person's subjective sense of age would, at a minimum, be represented by two major components: how old a person *looks* (i.e., physical or look age) and how old a person *feels* (i.e., social–emotional or feel age). Additional facets proposed by Kastenbaum et al. (1972) were "do age," "interest age," and "interpersonal age."

Overall, the emergence of subjective aging as a viable theoretical and empirical construct rests on the observation that individuals reflect on their own development and interpret their aging as they move across the life span.

Although chronological age is a reasonable proxy for developmental status early in life, this is definitely not the case in adulthood (see Chapter 9 by Staudinger, this volume). Therefore, subjective age (i.e., the discrepancy between felt age and actual age) has found substantial empirical interest. Specifically in adolescence, individuals start to perceive their age more in social and psychological terms and, indeed, frequently report feeling significantly older than their chronological age (Galambos, Turner, & Tilton-Weaver, 2005; Montepare, 2009). This process continues in early and middle adulthood, yet the subjective experience of age now starts to take the opposite direction and individuals report feeling younger than their chronological age. To illustrate this shift in subjective age, Rubin and Berntsen (2006) presented data from a Danish sample showing that from midlife on, individuals feel, on average, about 20% younger than their actual age (see also Montepare, 2009; Westerhof, Barrett, & Steverink, 2003). Moreover, feeling younger than one's chronological age tends to be associated with several positive outcomes, including better physical and cognitive health (Sargent-Cox, Anstey, & Luszcz, 2012; Wurm et al., 2007), greater life satisfaction (Wurm, Tomasik, & Tesch-Römer, 2008), more extended future time perspective (Weiss & Lang, 2012, Study 1), and lower morbidity and extended longevity (Kotter-Grühn, Kleinspehn-Ammerlahn, Gerstorf, & Smith, 2009; Uotinen, Rantanen, & Suutama, 2005). Although several different explanations (e.g., distancing from negative age stereotypes or a stigmatized group; see Chapter 5 by Chasteen & Cary, this volume) have been provided for the associations of a younger subjective age with outcomes, what has been so impressive is that these associations hold across diverse study samples and across different countries and cultures (Barak, 2009; Löckenhoff et al., 2009; Westerhof & Barrett, 2005). Moreover, the cross-sectional evidence is increasingly complemented by findings from longitudinal (Sargent-Cox et al., 2012; Spuling, Miche, Wurm, & Wahl, 2013; Westerhof et al., 2014; see also Chapter 7 by Westerhof & Wurm, this volume) and experimental studies (Miche & Wahl, 2014; Stephan et al., 2013) that permit the examination of the directionality and causality of effects. Thus, this body of evidence leaves no doubt that feeling younger than one's chronological age and holding positive views of aging (Wolff, Warner, Ziegelmann, & Wurm, 2014) have several beneficial effects, although at this point in time, we know fairly little about the exact pathways and mechanisms by which these effects are achieved (see Chapter 8 by Kotter-Grühn, this volume).

Aside from the traditional approach of assessing subjective age by asking a person the question, "How old do you feel?" several related concepts have been advanced in recent years. For example, the concepts of *self-perceptions of aging* and *attitudes toward own aging* have increasingly stimulated empirical research (Levy et al., 2002; Wurm et al., 2013; Miche, Elsässer, Schilling, & Wahl, in press), and concepts such as *awareness of age-related change* (Diehl & Wahl, 2010) or *awareness of aging* (Diehl et al., 2014) have been proposed to gain a better understanding of the experiences that underlie individuals' evaluations of subjective age (see the following texts for an in-depth discussion of these concepts). To illustrate the importance of self-perceptions of aging, for example, the study by Levy et al. (2002) provided longitudinal evidence for the association between positive self-perceptions of aging and survival. Other studies have shown substantial positive associations with adults' health and functional ability (Levy, Slade, Murphy, & Gill, 2012; Wurm et al., 2007), subjective well-being and life satisfaction (Kleinspehn-Ammerlahn, Kotter-Grühn, & Smith, 2008; Westerhof & Barrett, 2005; Wurm, Tomasik, Tesch-Römer, 2008), and preventive health behaviors (Levy & Myers, 2004; Wurm et al., 2010). In a similar vein, a large body of work documents the robust association between negative age stereotypes and older adults' maladaptive behavior (see Levy, 2003), such as lower memory performance, lower life satisfaction, and poorer functional health—behaviors that very much characterize the vulnerabilities of old and very old age (Hummert, 2011; Levy, 2003). Indeed, a recent study by Wurm et al. (2013) showed that negative self-perceptions of aging undermined older adults' compensatory behaviors while they coped with a serious health event.

In summary, there is a considerable body of cross-sectional and longitudinal evidence showing that measures of subjective aging have reliable and meaningful associations with developmental outcomes and with indicators of adaptive or maladaptive aging. These associations warrant a closer look at the different operationalizations of the subjective aging construct and the renewed theoretical (Diehl & Wahl, 2010; Diehl et al., 2014; Hess, 2006; Hummert, 2011) and empirical interest in the overall concept (Kleinspehn-Ammerlahn et al., 2008). Indeed, from an empirical perspective, it is not completely apparent why this construct in the late 1980s and for most parts of the 1990s was mostly dismissed in favor of measures of objective performance and that researchers, to a good extent, lost interest in the assessment of subjective aging. In the following text, we will briefly elaborate on what we view as the main *theoretical* and *empirical reasons* for this period of disinterest. In doing so, we intend to lay the foundation for our main argument in this chapter: that the time seems right to look at the construct of subjective aging from a new perspective and to view it as a key element for a new understanding of the aging self.

Theoretical Reasons for a Period of Disinterest

Although a comprehensive discussion of the diminished interest in the subjective aging construct in the 1980s and part of the 1990s is beyond the scope of this chapter, we believe that it is important to highlight several theoretical reasons for the lack of interest. First, aside from the early work of Kastenbaum et al. (1972) and some reasoning in the life course tradition of social gerontology (e.g., Settersten, 1999), there was not a great deal of theorizing on the construct of subjective age and aging during this period. Thus, the construct was theoretically underdeveloped, and its conceptual relevance was either taken as self-evident or as irrelevant. In part, this may also have been the reason for an inflation of additional terms, such as age identity, self-perceptions of aging, attitudes toward aging, age stereotyping, aging expectations, age anxiety, and so forth, that all referred to phenomena of subjective aging and that were often used interchangeably without explicating their unique and/or common elements (Diehl et al., 2014). Indeed, for most of these concepts, we have little more than short definitions and an (more or less) intuitive understanding of the phenomena they are supposed to capture. Given this situation, one may ask the question: Do all of these constructs basically measure the same phenomenon? That is, do these constructs all assess how adults interpret their own aging process, or do they differentiate between different facets of individuals' subjective aging experiences? Having a precise understanding of this issue was and still is crucial for significant advances in this area of inquiry.

Second, as we have discussed in more detail elsewhere (Diehl et al., 2014), no explicit connection was forged to *theoretical frameworks* of human development (e.g., Carstensen's [2006] socioemotional selectivity theory) or social–psychological theories of aging (e.g., identity theory, role theory). For example, although all major theories of human development—and especially theories of adult development—refer in one way or another to the subjective experiences and agentic motivations of the developing person (Baltes, Lindenberger, & Staudinger, 2006; Brandtstädter & Rothermund, 2002; Heckhausen & Schulz, 1995), with few exceptions (see Rothermund & Brandstädter, 2003; Teuscher, 2009), no systematic attempts were made to link the construct of subjective aging to these theories. This state of affairs has been rather unfortunate and resulted in a disconnection between theories of adult development and aging and the body of research on subjective aging.

Third, because theorizing in social gerontology often depends on synergies from different academic disciplines, such as life course sociology (MacMillan, 2005; Settersten, 2006) and life span developmental psychology (Baltes, 1987), another reason has been that such synergies have developed only very slowly and only fairly recently (Mayer, 2003; Settersten, 2009; see also Chapter 3 by Barrett & Montepare and Chapter 2 by Settersten & Hagestad, this volume). Given this lacking convergence among disciplines regarding subjective aging, several critical issues were overlooked. For example, the influences of societal and cultural images and stereotypes of aging or the effects of social norms and opportunity structures on individuals' personal development were only infrequently addressed, and, as a consequence, opportunities to better integrate macro- and microperspectives on subjective aging at a theoretical level were missed.

In summary, as this brief discussion shows, the construct of subjective aging was for a long time theoretically underdeveloped and not connected to any specific theoretical framework. Although there always has been the implicit assumption that the different operationalizations of subjective age reflect both personal experiences and societal and cultural influences, little systematic theorizing took place, hindering the advancement of the field. This situation on the theoretical side was mirrored by how the construct was implemented on the empirical side.

Empirical Reasons for a Period of Disinterest

On the empirical side, we believe that several reasons contributed to researchers' disinterest in the subjective aging construct at some point in time. First, despite some early calls for a multidimensional conceptualization (e.g., Kastenbaum et al., 1972), the operationalization of the construct was rather crude and relied on single items or unidimensional measures, such as the Attitudes Toward Own Aging Scale (Lawton, 1975). Although these measures were easy to administer and showed to some extent impressive predictive validity (Maier & Smith, 1999), not much effort was invested in more sophisticated multidimensional measures until the past decade and most recently (Kornadt & Rothermund, 2011; Laidlaw, Power, & Schmidt, 2007; Sarkisian, Hays, Berry, & Mangione, 2002; Steverink, Westerhof, Bode, & Dittmann-Kohli, 2001; Wahl, Konieczny, & Diehl, 2013). To what extent the lack of sophisticated measurement approaches was a consequence of the absence of more sophisticated theorizing is hard to determine.

Second, leaving aside the basic problems of single-item measures, questions were raised regarding the extent to which adults' answers to the question, "How old do you feel?" were potentially strongly influenced by tendencies to respond in socially desirable ways. In addition, critics raised the question to what extent adults' answers to such a general question reflected social norms and expectations rather than specific subjective experiences of growing older (Diehl et al., 2014).

Finally, gerontology as a field also (and for good reasons) gave performance-based, objective assessments of developmental and functional status, such as physical health or cognitive functioning, preference—often at the neglect of assessing subjective experiences of the aging process with greater sophistication. This was the case despite the fact that subjective measures in certain behavioral domains, such as subjective well-being or subjective health (see Idler

& Benyamini, 1997; Idler & Kasl, 1991; Kaplan & Camacho, 1983; Mossey & Shapiro, 1982), have consistently shown considerable predictive validity—often above and beyond the effects of objective measures.

In summary, as these examples illustrate, there were several reasons why the interest in the construct of subjective aging also waned from the empirical side and why researchers started to dismiss it as a viable construct. This dismissal or disinterest has been reversed only in the past few years, resulting in a renewed interest in the overall construct and in different facets of subjective aging and related constructs. We believe that this renewed interest is not just a short-lived revival but that the concept of subjective aging is entering a new and qualitatively different stage. Specifically, we argue that a closer conceptual and empirical connection between subjective aging and conceptualizations of the aging self, in particular action and self-theoretical conceptualizations, is crucial to stimulate and nurture such future development.

SUBJECTIVE AGING AS SPECIFIC SELF-KNOWLEDGE AND A NEW UNDERSTANDING OF THE AGING SELF

Our major objective in this section is to demonstrate that phenomena of subjective aging can be fruitfully construed as a specific form of self-knowledge. That is, we propose that experiences of subjective aging and a person's awareness of aging are integral psychological processes or conditions of the aging self (Ryff, 1984). As active producers of their development (Brandtstädter & Lerner, 1999; Brandtstädter & Rothermund, 2002), individuals construct, hold, and reconstruct awareness and knowledge of their own aging process. We propose that this awareness is a form of *self-awareness* and the resulting knowledge can be conceived as a form of *self-knowledge*, similar to other forms of self-knowledge, such as a person's self-representations (Diehl, 2006; Markus & Herzog, 1991; Ryff, 1984). For this reason, subjective aging becomes important for understanding the aging self and individuals' aging-related expectations, goals, actions, and identity processes (Brandtstädter & Greve, 1994; Greve & Wentura, 2003; Westerhof, Whitbourne, & Freeman, 2012).

To further elaborate linkages between subjective aging and the aging self, we proceed in two steps. First, building on key arguments put forward in Diehl et al. (2014), we consider the conceptual background of major subjective aging constructs as well as unidimensional versus multidimensional understandings (and assessments) emerging from different conceptualizations. We assume that such an analysis helps to explicate the kind of self-knowledge which subjective aging entails and which should be considered when it comes to assessment. Second, we provide a detailed explanation of the argument that there is a fundamental connection between phenomena of subjective aging and the understanding of the aging self. Indeed, we argue that the concept of subjective aging, if embedded into a broader conceptual framework and if grounded in multidimensional assessment, will infuse research on the aging self and will help to advance this area in the future.

A Closer Look at Subjective Aging Constructs

From a life span developmental perspective, multidimensionality and multidirectionality are postulated as fundamental characteristics of developmental constructs in general (Baltes, 1987) and of self-knowledge about age-related changes in particular (Brandtstädter & Greve, 1994; Diehl & Wahl, 2010; Greve & Wentura, 2003). However, there may also be cases in which a unidimensional conceptualization remains important and may be sufficient to make strong empirical predictions. The tension between simple unidimensional and more complex multidimensional conceptualizations seems to be particularly pronounced regarding key constructs of subjective aging. For this reason, a closer look at those key constructs seems to be warranted.

Subjective Age and Age Identity

The two most frequently used terms in the subjective aging literature are "subjective age" and "age identity."[2] These terms refer to the simple approach of asking individuals how old they feel or how old they view themselves or which age group they identify with. A multidimensional extension of this approach was first proposed by Kastenbaum et al. (1972). However, besides use in some recent experimental work (see Kotter-Grühn & Hess, 2012), Kastenbaum et al.'s multidimensional conception of subjective age/age identity did not become firmly established in the literature. This also applies to other multidimensional conceptions such as the differentiation between perceived "mental age" and perceived "physical age" (Uotinen et al., 2005) and "ideal age" (i.e., the age a person would like to be) as a facet of subjective age (Kaufman & Elder, 2002; Keyes & Westerhof, 2012).

Overall, although some data support differential associations of different subjective age dimensions with well-being and mental health (e.g., Keyes & Westerhof, 2012), the self-knowledge element mostly referred to in this approach remained the unidimensional self-evaluation of how old a person feels. Alternatively, adults' ratings may involve a unidimensional comparison between the own person and normative conceptions of aging.

Self-Perceptions of Aging

In recent years, the term "self-perceptions of aging" has been increasingly used to refer to adults' subjective aging experiences (Kleinspehn-Ammerlahn et al., 2008; Kotter-Grühn & Hess, 2012; Kotter-Grühn et al., 2009). The use of this term points to several recent developments. First, authors who use the term self-perceptions of aging—sometimes also called "self-views of aging"—acknowledge that subjective aging is a multidimensional construct. For example, Keller, Leventhal, and Larson (1989) conducted in-depth interviews with adults aged 50–80 years and identified five major dimensions of positive and negative aging experiences: (a) a natural and gradual process; (b) a period of life evaluation, philosophical reflection, or increased wisdom and maturity; (c) a period of increased freedom, new interests, and fewer demands; (d) a period of physical health difficulties and health concerns; and (e) a period of losses, including interpersonal and job-related losses (Keller et al., 1989). Similarly, factor analytic research by Steverink et al. (2001) on a nationally representative sample of German adults between the ages of 40 and 85 years identified three dimensions of personal experiences of aging. Two dimensions captured individuals' perceptions related to physical declines and social losses. The third dimension captured aspects of continued growth, reflecting adults' perceptions that their growing older was associated not only with losses but also with gains and further development. Thus, although these two studies employed quite different methods, their findings strongly support a multidimensional conceptualization of adults' self-perceptions of aging, including both positive and negative age-related experiences (see also Wurm et al., 2007).

Second, the use of the term self-perceptions of aging has also become more prevalent in the literature because research on the related constructs of aging expectations and aging stereotypes has shown that they are multidimensional. For example, Heckhausen, Dixon, and Baltes (1989) showed in a landmark study that young, middle-aged, and older adults had very similar expectations and beliefs regarding the occurrence of gains and losses in different behavioral domains throughout adulthood. Specifically, developmental gains and losses were expected to occur to some extent across the entire adult life span but in different ways in different behavioral domains. Moreover, gains were expected to be outnumbered by developmental losses in advanced old age (i.e., age 85 years and older). Similarly, research on aging stereotypes has shown that positive and negative stereotypes of old people coexist and vary by behavioral domain (Hummert, 2011; Kite, Stockdale, Whitley, & Johnson, 2005; Kornadt & Rothermund, 2011).

In summary, the term self-perceptions of aging focuses on the varied and predominantly multidimensional perceptions and experiences that create individuals' subjective aging experiences. Although many authors do not address this issue explicitly, the general assumption is that self-perceptions of aging are rooted in individuals' personal experiences and that they become part of their self-knowledge.

Attitudes Toward Aging and Age Stereotypes

A concept with a long-standing history in aging research is the construct of "atti-tudes toward aging" (Bennett & Eckman, 1973). The term attitudes toward aging refers to both societal as well as individual attitudes and includes affective, cogni-tive, and evaluative components of behavior toward older adults as an age group and toward the process of aging as a personal experience (Hess, 2006). Bennett and Eckman (1973) already pointed out in their review of the early literature that attitudes toward aging are considered critical for older people's adjustment and survival, contribute to their adaptive and maladaptive behaviors, and reinforce how individuals in younger age groups view and approach their own aging pro-cess. Empirical studies in this area have examined attitudes toward own aging mostly as a unidimensional construct, with the predominant measure being the Attitude Toward Own Aging subscale from the Philadelphia Geriatric Center Morale Scale (Lawton, 1975; see also Miche et al., in press). Research with the Attitude Toward Own Aging subscale has consistently shown that a negative atti-tude tends to be associated with poorer subjective health, lower life satisfaction, and other indicators of poorer functioning (see Levy et al., 2002).

Hess (2006) reiterated that negative attitudes toward older adults are quite pervasive and that older adults' views of their own behavior often reflect the societal beliefs and stereotypes about aging (see also Levy, 2009). Thus, attitudes toward aging are often linked to *age stereotypes* (Hummert, 2011) and, like age stereotypes, primarily convey the negative aspects of growing old (Hess, 2006; Kite et al., 2005). There is another important feature that aging-related attitudes and stereotypes have in common. This feature refers to the fact that over the course of the adult life span, both aging attitudes and age stereotypes become increasingly *self-relevant* (Kornadt & Rothermund, 2011; Levy, 2009). Thus, as individuals grow older, they may internalize attitudes toward and stereotypes about aging so that these attitudes and stereotypes increasingly affect (mostly unknowingly) their actual aging experiences and behavior. From this perspec-tive, aging attitudes and age stereotypes may exert similar effects on individuals' behaviors and may shape how they perceive and experience their own aging process (Kornadt & Rothermund, 2011; Mock & Eibach, 2011).

It is also important to note that age stereotypes do not necessarily have to be negative but can also focus on positive aspects of the aging process, such as personal growth, increase in experience, or personal accomplishments (see Hummert, 2011). Similar to our remarks on self-perceptions of aging, this reit-erates the need to consider gains *and* losses related to subjective aging. Such a multidimensional view implies that positive and negative stereotypes coexist and may also vary by behavioral domain (Kornadt & Rothermund, 2011; see Chapter 6 by Kornadt & Rothermund, this volume).

Awareness of Age-Related Change

A fairly recent contribution to the subjective aging literature is the concept of awareness of age-related change (AARC; Diehl & Wahl, 2010). Diehl and Wahl (2010) defined AARC as "all those experiences that make a person aware that his or her behavior, level of performance, or ways of experiencing his or her life have changed as a consequence of having grown older (i.e., increased chronological age)" (p. 340). Two aspects of this definition are noteworthy. First, Diehl and Wahl wanted to be explicit that a person's AARC is based on his or her *conscious perceptions* of changed behavior, performance, or reflected experiences. Second, in perceiving and reflecting about such changes, it is essential that the individual attributes them to his or her *increased chronological age* and not to any other conditions (e.g., changes in health status or living conditions). Diehl and Wahl proposed that AARC should be studied in five behavioral domains: (a) health and physical functioning, (b) cognitive functioning, (c) interpersonal relationships, (d) social–cognitive and social–emotional functioning, and (e) lifestyle and engagement. An additional essential feature of this approach is, as is the case with self-perceptions of aging and age stereotypes, that in each of these domains, losses as well as gains are considered, which may be seen as a kind of second-order factor of multidimensionality. Findings from a recently published diary study provide support for AARC's multidimensionality and the differential linkages of the proposed behavioral domains with developmental outcomes (Miche et al., 2014; Wahl et al., 2013).

FINDING A COMMON DENOMINATOR: SUBJECTIVE AGING AS A FORM OF SELF-KNOWLEDGE

Overall, we believe that the considerable empirical success of a mostly unidimensional understanding and assessment of subjective aging, particularly in the realm of subjective age, age identity, and attitudes toward aging, has been a mixed blessing for the field and has stifled further theoretical developments. In particular, such ratings tell us very little about (a) why individuals perceive their age and their place within the life course the way they do (Montepare, 2009) and (b) what specific age-related experiences may be reflected in their ratings. Furthermore, subjective age ratings are usually obtained in a completely decontextualized way and, therefore, ignore important developmental and personal reference points (Montepare, 2009). Given this critical view of unidimensional subjective age ratings, research in self-perceptions of aging, age stereotypes, and the recently proposed construct of AARC may be seen as new attempts to establish a more elaborated view of subjective aging as a key dimension of adults' self-knowledge and self-concept. Although differences between the various approaches remain, important foci of inquiry to better understand the nature of subjective aging and the associated self-knowledge are starting to emerge. In the following text, we highlight just three of these foci.

First, as a fundamental principle of life span developmental theory (e.g., Baltes et al., 2006; Heckhausen et al., 1989), the experience of *gains versus losses* related to individuals' own development and aging is an essential focus of perceptions and evaluations of subjective aging. This view is consistent with (a) empirical findings in the age stereotype literature showing that stereotypes can be negative as well as positive (Hummert, 2011), (b) findings related to self-perceived age-related growth and decline in adulthood and old age (Keller et al., 1989; Miche et al., 2014; Steverink et al., 2001), and (c) the theoretical propositions related to adults' AARCs (Diehl & Wahl, 2010). Specifically, Diehl and Wahl (2010) argued that the perception and awareness of age-related losses may impose developmental constraints on a person's behavior and experiences, whereas perceptions of age-related gains may foster an awareness of developmental opportunities and may motivate positive behaviors. Empirical support for this argument has been provided by several studies (see Levy et al., 2002; Wolff et al., 2014; Wurm et al., 2010).

A second important development has been the focus on investigating adults' age-related perceptions and experiences in specific *behavioral domains* such as the physical, cognitive, or interpersonal domain. This approach was strongly suggested by the empirical work of Steverink and colleagues (2001) and further advocated by Diehl and Wahl (2010). Specifically, based on a detailed review of the pertinent literature, Diehl and Wahl proposed that adults' AARCs could be fruitfully studied in five behavioral domains (e.g., healthy and physical functioning, cognitive functioning, interpersonal relations, social–cognitive and social–emotional functioning, and lifestyle and engagement). With their proposition, Diehl and Wahl wanted to build a stronger foundation for the argument that personal experiences of aging may be quite different in different behavioral domains and that such differences may affect the self-representations of an aging person in quite profound ways. For example, experiencing decline exclusively in one behavioral domain as compared to experiencing it simultaneously in multiple domains may strongly impact a person's self-image and may also affect that person's motivation to engage in any optimizing behaviors. In addition, interrelations among behavioral dimensions may tell us much about how events related to subjective aging are experienced and organized as self-knowledge (Miche et al., 2014).

Third, somewhat related to the second emerging focus, but taking more into account the social, societal, and cultural contexts in which individuals' aging occurs, are differentiations in terms of age stereotypes. The most advanced approach in this area is the work of Kornadt and Rothermund (2011; see also

Chapter 6 by these authors, this volume). These authors developed a measure to assess domain-specific age stereotypes, such as the domains of physical and mental fitness, work and employment, or family and partnership, and showed that old persons are evaluated differently in these life domains (Kornadt & Rothermund, 2011). In subsequent work, these authors also showed that the association between age stereotypes and current self-conceptions was mediated by adults' future self-views (Kornadt & Rothermund, 2012). Thus, this work not only showed that age stereotypes become increasingly self-relevant as individuals grow older, but it also suggested a psychological pathway by which age stereotypes become part of individuals' own self-concepts (i.e., through future self-views).

In summary, several recent developments go beyond simple ratings and unidimensional measures of subjective aging and instead focus on understanding the personal experiences and psychological processes that underlie adults' subjective age ratings. Based on these developments and a growing amount of empirical evidence, it is clear that individuals' judgments about their own age and aging represent a specific kind of self-knowledge. Importantly, this knowledge becomes increasingly self-relevant as individuals grow older and becomes part of individuals' *self-representations* (Diehl, 2006; Diehl et al., 2014). In the following text, we further describe what it means to take the construct of subjective aging seriously as a key element of the adult self.

SUBJECTIVE AGING AS A FUNDAMENTAL EXPERIENCE OF THE ADULT SELF

How do individuals develop an understanding of their own age and how do they incorporate their aging-related experiences into their overall self-representations? This is one of the key questions which is addressed in various ways in this volume. In the following text, we will outline some of the processes that we believe are involved in the formation of adults' awareness and understanding of their own age and aging. In addition, we will elaborate some of the characteristics of the self-knowledge that we believe underlies individuals' ratings and self-views of aging. We suggest, broadly speaking, that the self-focused and aging-related attention that results from a person's awareness of aging can be triggered by two major influences: (a) the age- and aging-related "feedback" a person receives or the reactions that a person elicits from his or her social environment or (b) the changes that a person perceives in his or her functioning and/or behavior as a consequence of getting older. We acknowledge that these two influences or sources of awareness of aging are not independent from each other and can operate conjointly or sequentially; yet for descriptive purposes, we will treat them here as if they would operate independent of each other.

The Role of the Social Environment

Although chronological age may not be of great value to determine a person's developmental status in adulthood (see Chapter 9 by Staudinger, this volume), it is nevertheless a critical *person characteristic* and *social category* (North & Fiske, 2012). Like other person characteristics and social categories, such as gender or race, signs of age and the aging process are outwardly visible and are salient cues for social judgments (Cuddy & Fiske, 2002). This is particularly the case in adulthood and old age.[3] In addition, chronological age is a category which is used by societies to assign positions, entitlements, and responsibilities within given social structures (George, 2007; see Chapter 2 by Settersten & Hagestad, this volume). Both the visible signs of age and aging as well as the age-related social categorizations that exist in a given society and which are adopted by others can serve as signals for a person that he or she has changed and that the observed changes are accompanied by altered expectations and beliefs in the social environment (e.g., in the family, the work place, the community). Indeed, this view is consistent with the proposition of symbolic interactionism (Wells & Stryker, 1988) that self-knowledge and self-representations are basically the reflected appraisals of others. Thus, we suggest that to the extent to which aging individuals react to and incorporate the aging-related messages of their social environment, including social comparisons with age peers, their reflected appraisals become part of their self-awareness and result in aging-related self-representations.

As described in earlier parts of this chapter, there is reasonable evidence to assume that the incorporation of aging-related feedback from social interactions differs by behavioral domain. That is, to what extent the aging-related messages of the social environment are incorporated by an individual into his or her self-representations very likely depends on the *personal salience* of a given behavioral domain (see also Levy, 2009). For example, one individual may be very sensitive to feedback regarding aging-related changes in physical appearance, whereas another person may be very sensitive to feedback in the cognitive or interpersonal domain. Depending on these domain-specific sensitivities, the feedback from the social environment will assume differential personal salience and will be incorporated into an individual's self-representations in different ways. Furthermore, the incorporation of aging-related feedback from social interactions also has to be seen in the context of other self-related processes, such as a person's needs for self-consistency (Swann, Rentfrow, & Guinn, 2003), self-enhancement and self-immunization (Greve & Wentura, 2003; Sedikides & Strube, 1995), and biographical continuity (Brandtstädter & Greve, 1994).

Chronological age, however, is not only important from a macrolevel perspective. From a microlevel view, it is equally important that chronological age gives individuals an understanding of their position within the life course (Macmillan,

2005; Settersten, 1999). For example, findings from numerous studies have shown that as individuals age, there is an increased tendency for them to become aware of their remaining lifetime, and this sense of remaining time has profound effects on basic psychological processes, including cognitive, motivational, and emotional functioning (Carstensen, 2006). Munnichs (1966) referred to this awareness as the "confrontation with the finitude of life" (p. 3). Although it is debatable to what extent the awareness of remaining lifetime is a conscious (explicit) or nonconscious (implicit) psychological process, it indicates that individuals become aware of how much time remains for them to live. In this sense, awareness of remaining lifetime has been examined as a motivational factor for different behaviors, including the selection of personal goals or the engagement in health-promoting behavior, and should be seen as a major contributing factor to individuals' awareness of aging.

Over the course of the adult life span, there are also numerous social *role transitions* (e.g., becoming a parent, transitioning to an empty nest or out of the work force, becoming a caregiver) that all serve as reminders of a person's age and position within the life course (see Chapter 2 by Settersten & Hagestad, this volume, and Chapter 3 by Barrett & Montepare, this volume). These role transitions, in combination with other influences, both on a personal as well as a societal level, contribute to the formation of a personal awareness of aging and shape (although not always knowingly) a person's understanding of what it means to grow old(er). Although this awareness of aging gains salience with age, it is important to note that its formation is a lifelong process, beginning before school age and continuing across the entire adult life span (see Levy, 2009).

In summary, social environments and social comparison processes are influential in shaping adults' awareness and understanding of their own aging. At the macrolevel, these influences result from societal and cultural age norms and the reliance on chronological age as a marker to assign social positions, responsibilities, and entitlements. Even if recent decades have seen a loosening of age norms and a "destandardization" of the life course (Settersten, 2006; Widmer & Ritschard, 2009), these social influences, in combination with the effects of societally accepted age stereotypes (Levy, 2009; Levy, Chung, Bedford, & Navrazhina, 2014), are real and have lasting effects on the individual. Indeed, these macrolevel influences combine with the feedback received in interpersonal interactions (see Chapter 5 by Chasteen & Cary, Chapter 4 by Hummert, and Chapter 10 by Miche, Brothers, Diehl, & Wahl, this volume) and the messages promoted in the mass media (Kessler, Rakoczy, & Staudinger, 2004) to create at the microlevel the awareness of aging that affects (more or less knowingly) a person's day-to-day behavior and experience. We postulate that this awareness leads to a specific kind of self-knowledge that plays an instrumental and lasting role in the way in which a person grows old(er).

The Role of Self-Perceptions

Although the social environment plays a crucial role in the development of a person's awareness of aging, we view the individual as being constructively involved in developing and shaping this awareness. This view of subjective aging draws on action-theoretical assumptions (Brandtstädter & Lerner, 1999) and propositions of life span developmental theory (Baltes, 1987). Specifically, these theoretical approaches emphasize the role of personal agency in ontogenetic development and conceive individuals—within the boundaries of the larger sociocontextual conditions—not only as products but also as producers of their own development. In the context of subjective aging, the role of the individual as an active producer of his or her development is demonstrated by the fact that individuals perceive and experience age-related changes and can make fairly accurate statements about them (see Diehl & Wahl, 2010; Hertzog & Hultsch, 2000; Miche et al., 2014; Schaie, Willis, & O'Hanlon, 1994). Thus, individuals' understanding of their own aging arises out of self-perceptive, self-reflective, and self-regulative processes (Brandtstädter & Greve, 1994; Brandtstädter & Rothermund, 2002; Greve & Wentura, 2003) and represents a form of self-awareness and self-knowledge that develops over the course of the adult years. We propose that this self-knowledge is (a) similar to other forms of self-knowledge and (b) as individuals grow older, this knowledge becomes part of their overall self-concept (Diehl, 2006; Markus & Herzog, 1991). Thus, processes that contribute to adults' awareness of aging become fundamentally important for understanding the aging self and its expectations, goals, actions, and identity processes (Brandtstädter & Greve, 1994; Brandtstädter & Rothermund, 2002; Greve & Wentura, 2003; Westerhof, Whitbourne, & Freeman, 2012). In the following text, we highlight several key features of a *self-theoretical perspective* on subjective aging.[4]

First, a self-theoretical perspective of awareness of aging assumes that aging-related experiences initially lay the foundation for a kind of *tacit knowledge* (Cianciolo, Matthew, Sternberg, & Wagner, 2006) that over time will become *metacognitive knowledge* (Hertzog & Hultsch, 2000) and eventually becomes part of a person's self-representation. Thus, we postulate that individuals' aging-related self-perceptions will be incorporated into the multidimensional, contextualized, and dynamic structure of their self-concept and will serve the same self-regulatory functions as other self-related knowledge (Brandtstädter & Greve, 1994; Higgins, 1996; Markus & Wurf, 1987).

Indeed, as a kind of self-knowledge, a person's aging-related self-understanding is in many ways similar to other kinds of self-knowledge, including its order of development, structural organization, and cognitive complexity (for a review of self-concept development in adulthood, see Diehl, 2006). For example, in the same way as research has documented a specific order in which children's self-understanding develops (Damon & Hart, 1988; Diehl, Youngblade, Hay, & Chui, 2011; Harter, 2012), it can be speculated that aging-related self-knowledge follows a similar developmental order. Specifically, similar to the markers of children's self-understanding in early and middle childhood (Damon & Hart, 1988; Harter, 2012), aging-related self-knowledge may first result from perceptions of changes in *physical characteristics,* such as physical appearance (e.g., graying of hair, wrinkling of skin, changes in posture and mobility), physical functioning (e.g., reduced stamina, longer recovery after strenuous exercise), or physical health (e.g., onset of age-related illnesses). These self-perceived changes in physical characteristics may then be increasingly reinforced by aging-related self-perceptions in the *social/interpersonal domain* (e.g., age-related remarks in the work place, experience of age discrimination) and the *psychological domain* (e.g., changes in cognitive, motivational, and emotional functioning). In combination, these experiences, which are embedded in adults' everyday lives (see Miche et al., 2014), will make up the self-knowledge that will become part of a person's self-concept of what it means to be a "middle-aged adult" or an "older adult." Also, the self-relevance of aging-related information will increase with advancing calendar age and will increasingly become self-defining (see Levy, 2009). Thus, the main point here is that a self-theoretical view of awareness of aging represents a new way of studying the mechanisms and pathways by which adults form an understanding of their own aging. Having a more detailed understanding of the mechanisms and pathways, in turn, will be important for the development of potential intervention and training programs because adults will be increasingly encouraged to take responsibility for the way in which they grow old(er) (National Institute on Aging, 2011; see also Chapter 8 by Kotter-Grühn and Chapter 10 by Miche et al., this volume).

In summary, we postulate that the awareness and knowledge of a person's own aging is a fundamental process of adult development and an important part of what Brandtstädter (1999) called "intentional self-development" (p. 37). Thus, understanding how this awareness develops and how it translates into judgments of subjective aging (i.e., ratings of felt age) and, more importantly, into attitudes and behaviors that may obstruct or promote optimal aging is of fundamental importance for gerontology, life course sociology, and life span psychology. We propose that an action- and self-theoretical understanding of how individuals perceive and reflect on their age and aging can contribute to a better and more fundamental understanding of the aging self.

OUTLOOK: NEW BEGINNINGS AND A PROMISING FUTURE

We started this chapter with the following question: Is the renewed interest in the concept of subjective aging simply an old wine in new bottles phenomenon or is the field witnessing a qualitatively different development with the potential to move the scientific inquiry forward in significant and meaningful ways? We believe that we are indeed witnessing a new beginning and that the current interest in conceptions of subjective aging are qualitatively different from the early beginnings. Several indications support this view.

First, we suggest that the current developments in this area of scientific inquiry represent a second phase that is characterized by (a) greater theoretical diversity and sophistication (see Diehl & Wahl, 2010; Diehl et al., 2014; Hess, 2006; Hummert, 2011; Levy, 2009), (b) a clear and strong commitment to multidimensional approaches, and (c) a commitment to diversity in research approaches and designs. The commitment to diversity in research approaches and designs includes the entire range from experimental (Miche & Wahl, 2014; Stephan et al., 2013) to longitudinal (Kleinspehn-Ammerlahn et al., 2008; Kotter-Grühn et al., 2009; Levy et al., 2002; Sargent-Cox et al., 2012, 2014; Spuling et al., 2013) to intervention studies (Wolff et al., 2014) and meta-analyses (Westerhof et al., in press). Such diversity suggests that the first phase, which was characterized by unidimensional approaches and by establishing the predictive relevance of simple ratings of subjective age, may have come to an end and may have paved the way for where we currently are and where we are heading in the future.

Second, recent years have also seen several theoretical advances and an overall increase in theoretical sophistication in the field as indicated by several review chapters in well-respected handbooks (Hess, 2006; Hummert, 2011). This suggests a renewed interest in issues of subjective aging. In addition, there have been several publications that have outlined new theoretical frameworks (Diehl & Wahl, 2010; Diehl et al., 2014; Levy, 2009) and have served as attempts to integrate different traditions and directions in the field (see also Chapter 9 by Staudinger, this volume). A particular emphasis in these papers has been the focus on identifying plausible social and psychological mechanisms and pathways by which self-perceptions of aging affect long-term developmental outcomes.

Third, analyses of subjective aging data in several longitudinal studies (Kleinspehn-Ammerlahn et al., 2008; Kotter-Grühn et al., 2009; Levy et al., 2002; Sargent-Cox et al., 2012, 2014; Spuling et al., 2013), although still often relying on single-item or unidimensional measures, have shown that subjective age ratings have considerable predictive validity, including relevance in terms of health status and mortality. This predictive relevance is significant above and beyond the effects of potential confounding variables, such as level of education, socioeconomic status, and objective measures of physical and mental health.

Finally, we believe that the renewed focus on issues of subjective aging is to some extent also related to the overall phenomenon of *population aging* and to questions of resource allocation and entitlements (Kotlikoff & Burns, 2005). In terms of the societal implications, it has become obvious that the aging of the baby boom cohorts (birth cohorts 1946–1964) poses several challenges that are unprecedented in human history. We predict, for example, that policy and public health debates will increasingly focus on questions such as, "How can we motivate individuals already at a younger age to adopt and cultivate health-promoting behaviors that will improve their chances to grow old in a healthy way?"—and these questions and debates will increasingly call for evidence-based intervention and training programs that can address exactly this issue. We believe that based on existing research (Levy et al., 2002; Levy et al., 2012), intervention programs targeting middle-aged and older adults' negative self-perceptions of aging hold great promise as a major avenue to promote successful aging (see also Chapter 8 by Kotter-Grühn and Chapter 10 by Miche et al., this volume). Specifically, such programs should focus on middle-aged and older adults' age stereotypes and personal awareness of aging and should change the mostly negative age stereotypes (Meisner, 2012) through psychoeducational and behavioral interventions (Sarkisian, Prohaska, Davis, & Weiner, 2007; Wolff et al., 2014). We also believe that such programs would potentially complement and strengthen other intervention approaches, such as programs that focus on increasing adults' level of physical activity (King, 2001) or level of cognitive engagement (Willis et al., 2006). In conclusion, we believe that this area of inquiry has a promising future ahead, and we hope that the chapters in this volume will stimulate many new research efforts.

NOTES

1. In this introductory chapter, we use the terms "subjective aging" and "awareness of aging" as interchangeable superordinate constructs to subsume several related concepts, such as subjective age, age identity, self-perceptions of aging, attitudes toward aging and age stereotypes, and awareness of age-related change.

2. It needs to be noted that both terms are frequently used interchangeably, although there are differences in their theoretical origin and their operationalizations. Details of these differences are discussed in Diehl et al. (2014).

3. Indeed, several authors have pointed out that age is the only social category which everyone eventually joins, provided that they live long enough (see North & Fiske, 2012).

4. We would like to state explicitly that we are not presenting a comprehensive theory. For example, we are not addressing processes of within-person temporal comparisons that may impact an individual's aging-related self-perceptions.

ACKNOWLEDGMENTS

The preparation of this work was supported by a grant from the Alexander von Humboldt Foundation awarded to Manfred Diehl and Hans-Werner Wahl. Martina Miche's work on this chapter was supported by a fellowship from the German National Academic Foundation. Manfred Diehl and Allyson Brothers's work was supported in part by grant R21 AG041379 from the National Institute of Aging, National Institutes of Health.

REFERENCES

Baltes, P. B. (1987). Theoretical propositions of life-span developmental psychology: On the dynamics between growth and decline. *Developmental Psychology, 23*, 611–626. http://dx.doi.org/10.1037/0012-1649.23.5.611

Baltes, P. B., Lindenberger, U., & Staudinger, U. M. (2006). Life-span theory in developmental psychology. In W. Damon (Series Ed.) & R. M. Lerner (Vol. Ed.), *Handbook of child psychology: Theoretical models of development* (6th ed., Vol. 1, pp. 569–664). Hoboken, NJ: Wiley.

Barak, B. (2009). Age identity: A cross-cultural global approach. *International Journal of Behavioral Development, 33*, 2–11. http://dx.doi.org/10.1177/0165025408099485

Bennett, R., & Eckman, J. (1973). Attitudes toward aging: A critical examination of recent literature and implications for future research. In C. Eisdorfer & M. P. Lawton (Eds.), *The psychology of adult development and aging* (pp. 575–597). Washington, DC: American Psychological Association.

Birren, J. E., & Schaie, K. W. (Eds.). (2006). *Handbook of the psychology of aging* (6th ed.). San Diego, CA: Academic Press.

Brandtstädter, J. (1999). The self in action and development: Cultural, biosocial, and ontogenetic bases of intentional self-development. In J. Brandtstädter & R. M. Lerner. (Eds.), *Action and development: Theory and research through the life span* (pp. 37–65). Thousand Oaks, CA: Sage.

Brandtstädter, J., & Greve, W. (1994). The aging self: Stabilizing and protective processes. *Developmental Review, 14*, 52–80.

Brandtstädter, J., & Lerner, R. M. (Eds.). (1999). *Action and development: Theory and research through the life span.* Thousand Oaks, CA: Sage.

Brandtstädter, J., & Rothermund, K. (2002). Intentional self-development: Exploring the interfaces between development, intentionality, and the self. In L. J. Crockett (Ed.), *Nebraska symposium on motivation: Agency, motivation, and the life course* (Vol. 48, pp. 31–75). Lincoln, NE: University of Nebraska Press.

Carstensen, L. L. (2006). The influence of a sense of time on human development. *Science, 312*, 1913–1915.

Cianciolo, A. T., Matthew, C., Sternberg, R. J., & Wagner, R. K. (2006). Tacit knowledge, practical intelligence, and expertise. In K. A. Ericsson, N. Charness, P. J. Feltovich, & R. R. Hoffman (Eds.), *The Cambridge handbook of expertise and expert performance* (pp. 613–632). New York, NY: Cambridge University Press.

Cuddy, A. J. C., & Fiske, S. T. (2002). Doddering but dear: Process, content, and function in stereotyping of older persons. In T. D. Nelson (Ed.), *Ageism: Stereotyping and prejudice against older persons* (pp. 3–26). Cambridge, MA: MIT Press.

Damon, W., & Hart, D. (1988). *Self-understanding in childhood and adolescence.* New York, NY: Cambridge University Press.

Diehl, M. (2006). Development of self-representations in adulthood. In D. K. Morczek & T. D. Little (Eds.), *Handbook of personality development* (pp. 373–398). Mahwah, NJ: Lawrence Erlbaum Associates.

Diehl, M. K., & Wahl, H. W. (2010). Awareness of age-related change: Examination of a (mostly) unexplored concept. *The Journals of Gerontology. Series B, Psychological Sciences and Social Sciences, 65,* 340–350. http://dx.doi.org/10.1093/geronb/gbp110

Diehl, M., Wahl, H. W., Barrett, A. E., Brothers, A. F., Miche, M., Montepare, J. M., . . . Wurm, S. (2014). Awareness of aging: Theoretical considerations on an emerging concept. *Developmental Review, 34,* 93–113. http://dx.doi.org/10.1016/j.dr.2014.01.001

Diehl, M., Youngblade, L. M., Hay, E. L., & Chui, H. (2011). The development of self-representations across the life span. In K. L. Fingerman, C. A. Berg, J. Smith, & T. C. Antonucci (Eds.), *Handbook of life-span development* (pp. 611–646). New York, NY: Springer Publishing.

Galambos, N. L., Turner, P. K., & Tilton-Weaver, L. C. (2005). Chronological and subjective age in emerging adulthood: The crossover effect. *Journal of Adolescent Research, 20,* 538–556. http://dx.doi.org/10.1177/0743558405274876

George, L. K. (2007). Age structures, aging, and the life course. In J. M. Wilmoth & K. F. Ferraro (Eds.), *Gerontology: Perspectives and issues* (3rd ed., pp. 203–222). New York, NY: Springer Publishing.

Greve, W., & Wentura, D. (2003). Immunizing the self: Self-concept stabilization through reality-adaptive self-definitions. *Personality and Social Psychology Bulletin, 29,* 39–50. http://dx.doi.org/10.1177/0146167202238370

Harter, S. (2012). *The construction of the self: Developmental and sociocultural foundations* (2nd ed.). New York, NY: Guilford Press.

Heckhausen, J., Dixon, R. A., & Baltes, P. B. (1989). Gains and losses in development throughout adulthood as perceived by different adult age groups. *Developmental Psychology, 25,* 109–121. http://dx.doi.org/10.1037/0012-1649.25.1.109

Heckhausen, J., & Schulz, R. (1995). A life-span theory of control. *Psychological Review, 102,* 284–304. http://dx.doi.org/10.1037/0033-295X.102.2.284

Hertzog, C., & Hultsch, D. F. (2000). Metacognition in adulthood and old age. In F. I. M. Craik & T. A. Salthouse (Eds.), *The handbook of aging and cognition* (2nd ed., pp. 417–466). Mahwah, NJ: Lawrence Erlbaum Associates.

Hess, T. M. (2006). Attitudes toward aging and their effects on behavior. In J. E. Birren & K. W. Schaie (Eds.), *Handbook of the psychology of aging* (6th ed., pp. 379–406). San Diego, CA: Academic Press.

Higgins, E. T. (1996). The "self-digest": Self-knowledge serving self-regulatory functions. *Journal of Personality and Social Psychology, 71,* 1062–1083. http://dx.doi.org/10.1037/0022-3514.71.6.1062

Hummert, M. L. (2011). Age stereotypes and aging. In K. W. Schaie & S. L. Willis (Eds.), *Handbook of the psychology of aging* (7th ed., pp. 249–262). San Diego, CA: Academic Press.

Idler, E. L., & Benyamini, Y. (1997). Self-rated health and mortality: A review of twenty-seven community studies. *Journal of Health and Social Behavior, 38,* 21–37.

Idler, E. L., & Kasl, S. (1991). Health perceptions and survival: Do global evaluations of health status really predict mortality? *The Journals of Gerontology. Series B, Psychological Sciences and Social Sciences, 46,* S55–S65.

Kaplan, G. A., & Camacho, T. (1983). Perceived health and mortality: A nine-year follow-up of the human population laboratory cohort. *American Journal of Epidemiology, 117,* 292–304.

Kastenbaum, R., Derbin, V., Sabatini, P., & Artt, S. (1972). "The ages of me": Toward personal and interpersonal definitions of functional aging. *Aging and Human Development, 3,* 197–211.

Kaufman, G., & Elder, G. H., Jr. (2002). Revisiting age identity: A research note. *Journal of Aging Studies, 16,* 169–176.

Keller, M. L., Leventhal, E. A., & Larson, B. (1989). Aging: The lived experience. *International Journal of Aging and Human Development, 29,* 67–82.

Kessler, E. M., Rakoczy, K., & Staudinger, U. M. (2004). The portrayal of older people in prime time television series: The match with gerontological evidence. *Ageing & Society, 24,* 531–552. http://dx.doi.org/10.1017/S0144686X04002338

Keyes, C. L. M., & Westerhof, G. J. (2012). Chronological and subjective age differences in flourishing mental health and major depressive episode. *Aging & Mental Health, 16,* 67–74. http://dx.doi.org/10.1080/13607863.2011.596811

King, A. C. (2001). Interventions to promote physical activity by older adults [Special issue 2]. *The Journals of Gerontology. Series A, Biological Sciences and Medical Sciences, 56,* 36–46. http://dx.doi.org/10.1093/Gerona/56.suppl_2.36

Kite, M. E., Stockdale, G. D., Whitley, E. B., & Johnson, B. T. (2005). Attitudes toward younger and older adults: An updated meta-analytic review. *Journal of Social Issues, 61,* 241–266. http://dx.doi.org/10.1111/j.1540-4560.2005.00404.x

Kleinspehn-Ammerlahn, A., Kotter-Grühn, D., & Smith, J. (2008). Self-perceptions of aging: Do subjective age and satisfaction with aging change during old age? *The Journals of Gerontology. Series B, Psychological Sciences and Social Sciences, 63,* P377–P385. http://dx.doi.org/10.1093/geronb/63.6.P377

Kornadt, A. E., & Rothermund, K. (2011). Contexts of aging: Assessing evaluative age stereotypes in different life domains. *The Journals of Gerontology. Series B, Psychological Sciences and Social Sciences, 66,* 547–556. http://dx.doi.org/10.1093/geronb/gbr036

Kornadt, A. E., & Rothermund, K. (2012). Internalization of age stereotypes into the self-concept via future self-views: A general model and domain-specific differences. *Psychology and Aging, 27,* 164–172. http://dx.doi.org/10.1037/a0025110

Kotlikoff, L. J., & Burns, S. (2005). *The coming generational storm.* Boston, MA: MIT Press.

Kotter-Grühn, D., & Hess, T. M. (2012). The impact of age stereotypes on self-perceptions of aging across the adult lifespan. *The Journals of Gerontology. Series B,*

Psychological Sciences and Social Sciences, 67, 563–571. http://dx.doi.org/10.1093/geronb/gbr153

Kotter-Grühn, D., Kleinspehn-Ammerlahn, A., Gerstorf, D., & Smith, J. (2009). Self-perceptions of aging predict mortality and change with approaching death: 16-year longitudinal results from the Berlin Aging Study. *Psychology and Aging, 24*, 654–667. http://dx.doi.org/10.1037/a0016510

Laidlaw, K., Power, M. J., & Schmidt, S. (2007). The attitudes to ageing questionnaire (AAQ): Development and psychometric properties. *International Journal of Geriatric Psychiatry, 22*, 367–379. http://dx.doi.org/10.1002/gps.1683

Lawton, M. P. (1975). The Philadelphia Geriatric Center Morale Scale: A revision. *Journal of Gerontology, 30*, 85–89.

Levy, B. R. (2003). Mind matters: Cognitive and physical effects of aging self-stereotypes. *The Journals of Gerontology. Series B, Psychological Sciences and Social Sciences, 58*, P203–P211. http://dx.doi.org/10.1093/geronb/58.4.P203

Levy, B. R. (2009). Stereotype embodiment: A psychosocial approach to aging. *Current Directions in Psychological Science, 18*, 332–336. http://dx.doi.org/10.1111/j.1467-8721.2009,01662.x

Levy, B. R., Chung, P. H., Bedford, T., & Navrazhina, K. (2014). Facebook as a site for negative age stereotypes. *The Gerontologist, 54*, 172–176. http://dx.doi.org/10.1093/geront/gns194

Levy, B. R., & Myers, L. M. (2004). Preventive health behaviors influenced by self-perceptions of aging. *Preventive Medicine, 39*, 625–629. http://dx.doi.org/10.1016/j.ypmed.2004.02.029

Levy, B. R., Slade, M. D., Kunkel, S. R., & Kasl, S. V. (2002). Longevity increased by positive self-perceptions of aging. *Journal of Personality and Social Psychology, 83*, 261–270. http://dx.doi.org/10.1037/0022-3514.83.2.261

Levy, B. R., Slade, M. D., Murphy, T. E., & Gill, T. M. (2012). Association between positive age stereotypes and recovery from disability in older persons. *JAMA: Journal of the American Medical Association, 308*, 1972–1973.

Löckenhoff, C. E., De Fruyt, F., Terracciano, A., McCrae, R. R., De Bolle, M., Costa, P. T., Jr., . . . Yik, M. (2009). Perceptions of aging across 26 cultures and their culture-level associates. *Psychology and Aging, 24*, 941–954. http://dx.doi.org/10.1037/a0016901

Macmillan, R. (2005). The structure of the life course: Classic issues and current controversies. In R. Macmillan (Ed.), *Advances in life course research: The structure of the life course: Standardized? Individualized? Differentiated?* (Vol. 9, pp. 3–24). Amsterdam, The Netherlands: Elsevier.

Maier, H., & Smith, J. (1999). Psychological predictors of mortality in old age. *The Journals of Gerontology. Series B, Psychological Sciences and Social Sciences, 54*, P44–P54. http://dx.doi.org/10.1093/geronb/54B.1.P44

Markides, K. S., & Pappas, C. (1982). Subjective age, health, and survivorship in old age. *Research on Aging, 4*, 87–96. http://dx.doi.org/10.1177/016402758241004.

Markus, H. R., & Herzog, R. (1991). The role of the self-concept in aging. In K. W. Schaie (Ed.), *Annual review of gerontology and geriatrics* (Vol. 11, pp. 110–143). New York, NY: Springer Publishing.

Markus, H. R., & Wurf, E. (1987). The dynamic self-concept: A social psychological perspective. *Annual Review of Psychology, 38,* 299–337. http://dx.doi.org/10.1146/annurev.ps.38.020187.001503

Mayer, K. U. (2003). The sociology of the life course and lifespan psychology: Diverging or converging pathways? In U. M. Staudinger & U. Lindenberger (Eds.), *Understanding human development: Dialogues with lifespan psychology* (pp. 463–481). Norwell, MA: Kluwer Academic.

Meisner, B. A. (2012). A meta-analysis of positive and negative age stereotype priming effects on behavior among older adults. *The Journals of Gerontology. Series B, Psychological Sciences and Social Sciences, 67,* 13–17. http://dx.doi.org/10.1093/geronb/gbr062

Miche, M., Elsässer, V. C., Schilling, O. K., & Wahl, H. W. (in press). Attitude toward own aging in midlife and early old age over a 12-year period: Examination of measurement equivalence and developmental trajectories. *Psychology and Aging.*

Miche, M., & Wahl, H. W. (2014). *"Slow but more accurate—that's due to my age": Effects of induced age attributions of cognitive performance on awareness of aging.* Manuscript submitted for publication.

Miche, M., Wahl, H. W., Diehl, M., Oswald, F., Kaspar, R., & Kolb, M. (2014). Natural occurrence of subjective aging experiences in community-dwelling older adults. *The Journals of Gerontology. Series B, Psychological Sciences and Social Sciences, 69,* 174–187. http://dx.doi.org/10.1093/geronb/gbs164

Mock, S. E., & Eibach, R. P. (2011). Aging attitudes moderate the effect of subjective age on psychological well-being: Evidence from a 10-year longitudinal study. *Psychology and Aging, 26,* 979–986. http://dx.doi.org/10.1037/a0023877.

Montepare, J. M. (2009). Subjective age: Toward a guiding lifespan framework. *International Journal of Behavioral Development, 33,* 42–46. http://dx.doi.org/10.1177/0165025408095551

Mossey, J. M., & Shapiro, E. (1982). Self-rated health: A predictor of mortality among the elderly. *American Journal of Public Health, 72,* 800–808.

Munnichs, J. M. A. (1966). *Old age and finitude: A contribution to psychogerontology.* Basel, Switzerland: Karger.

National Institute on Aging. (2011). *Global health and aging* (NIH Publication No. 11-7737). Bethesda, MD: Author.

North, M. S., & Fiske, S. T. (2012). An inconvenienced youth? Ageism and its potential intergenerational roots. *Psychological Bulletin, 138,* 982–997. http://dx.doi.org/10.1037/a0027843

Rothermund, K., & Brandstädter, J. (2003). Age stereotypes and self-views in later life: Evaluating rival assumptions. *International Journal of Behavioral Development, 27,* 549–554. http://dx.doi.org/10.1080/01650250344000208

Rubin, D. C., & Berntsen, D. (2006). People over forty feel 20% younger than their age: Subjective age across the lifespan. *Psychonomic Bulletin & Review, 13,* 776–780. http://dx.doi.org/10.3758?BF03193996.

Ryff, C. D. (1984). Personality development from the inside: The subjective experience of change in adulthood and aging. In P. B. Baltes & O. G. Brim, Jr. (Eds.), *Life-span development and behavior* (Vol. 6, pp. 243–279). Orlando, FL: Academic Press.

Sargent-Cox, K. A., Anstey, K. J., & Luszcz, M. A. (2012). Change in health and self-perceptions of aging over 16 years: The role of psychological resources. *Health Psychology*, 31, 423–432. http://dx.doi.org/10.1037/a0027464

Sargent-Cox, K. A., Anstey, K. J., & Luszcz, M. A. (2014). Longitudinal change of self-perceptions of aging and mortality. *The Journals of Gerontology. Series B, Psychological Sciences and Social Sciences*, 69, 168–173. http://dx.doi.org/10.1093/geronb/gbt005

Sarkisian, C. A., Hays, R. D., Berry, S., & Mangione, C. M. (2002). Development, reliability, and validity of the Expectations Regarding Aging (ERA-38) survey. *The Gerontologist*, 42, 534–542. http://dx.doi.org/10.1093/geront/42.4.534

Sarkisian, C. A., Prohaska, T. R., Davis, C., & Weiner, B. (2007). Pilot test of an attribution retraining intervention to raise walking levels in sedentary older adults. *Journal of the American Geriatrics Society*, 55, 1842–1846. http://dx.doi.org/10.1111/j.1532-5415.2007.01427.x

Schaie, K. W., & Willis, S. L. (Eds.). (2011). *Handbook of the psychology of aging* (7th ed.). San Diego, CA: Academic Press.

Schaie, K. W., Willis, S. L., & O'Hanlon, A. M. (1994). Perceived intellectual performance change over seven years. *Journal of Gerontology*, 49, P108–P118.

Sedikides, C., & Strube, M. J. (1995). "The multiply motivated self". *Personality and Social Psychology Bulletin*, 21, 1330–1335. http://dx.doi.org/10.1177/0146167295211201

Settersten, R. A. (1999). *Lives in time and place: The problems and promises of developmental science*. Amityville, NY: Baywood.

Settersten, R. A. (2006). Aging and the life course. In R. H. Binstock & L. K. George (Eds.), *Handbook of aging and the social sciences* (6th ed., pp. 3–19). San Diego, CA: Academic Press.

Settersten, R. A. (2009). It takes two to tango: The (un)easy dance between life-course sociology and life-span psychology. *Advances in Life Course Research*, 14, 74–81. http://dx.doi.org/10.1016/j.alcr.2009.05.002

Spuling, S. M., Miche, M., Wurm, S., & Wahl, H. W. (2013). Exploring the causal interplay of subjective age and health dimensions in the second half of life: A cross-lagged panel analysis. *Zeitschrift für Gesundheitspsychologie*, 21, 5–15.

Stephan, Y., Chalabaev, A., Kotter-Grühn, D., & Jaconelli, A. (2013). "Feeling younger, being stronger": An experimental study of subjective age and physical functioning among older adults. *The Journals of Gerontology. Series B, Psychological Sciences and Social Sciences*, 68, 1–7. http://dx.doi.org/10.1093/geronb/gbs037

Steverink, N., Westerhof, G. J., Bode, C., & Dittmann-Kohli, F. (2001). The personal experience of aging, individual resources, and subjective well-being. *The Journals of Gerontology, Series B: Psychological and Social Sciences*, 56, 364–373. http://dx.doi.org/10.1093/geronb/56.6.P364.

Swann, W. R., Rentfrow, P. J., & Guinn, J. S. (2003). Self-verification: The search for coherence. In M. R. Leary & J. P. Tangney (Eds.), *Handbook of self and identity* (pp. 367–383). New York, NY: Guilford Press.

Teuscher, U. (2009). Subjective age bias: A motivational and information processing approach. *International Journal of Behavioral Development*, *33*, 22–31. http://dx.doi.org/10.1177/0165025408099487

Uotinen, V., Rantanen, T., & Suutama, T. (2005). Perceived age as a predictor of old age mortality: A 13-year prospective study. *Age and Ageing*, *34*, 368–372. http://dx.doi.org/10.1093/ageing/afi091

Wahl, H. W., Konieczny, C., & Diehl, M. K. (2013). Zum Erleben von altersbezogenen Veränderungen im Erwachsenenalter: Eine explorative Studie auf der Grundlage des Konzepts "awareness of age-related change" (AARC) [Experiencing age-related changes in adulthood: An exploratory study focusing on the concept of awareness of age-related change (AARC)]. *Zeitschrift für Entwicklungspsychologie und Pädagogische Psychologie*, *45*, 66–76. http://dx.doi.org/10.1026/0049-8637/a00008

Weiss, D., & Lang, F. R. (2012). "They" are old but "I" feel younger: Age-group dissociation as a self-protective strategy in old age. *Psychology and Aging*, *27*, 153–163. http://dx.doi.org/10.1037/a0024887

Wells, L. E., & Stryker, S. (1988). Stability and change in self over the life course. In P. B. Baltes, D. L. Featherman, & R. M. Lerner (Eds.), *Life-span development and behavior* (Vol. 8, pp. 191–229). Hillsdale, NJ: Lawrence Erlbaum Associates.

Westerhof, G. J., & Barrett, A. E. (2005). Age identity and subjective well-being: A comparison of the United States and Germany. *The Journals of Gerontology. Series B, Psychological Sciences and Social Sciences*, *60*, S129–S136. http://dx.doi.org/10.1093/geronb/60.3.S129

Westerhof, G. J., Barrett, A. E., & Steverink, N. (2003). Forever young? A comparison of age identities in the United States and Germany. *Research on Aging*, *25*, 366–383. http://dx.doi.org/10.1177/0164027503025004002

Westerhof, G. J., Miche, M., Brothers, A. F., Barrett, A. E., Diehl, M., Montepare, J. M., Wahl, H.-W., & Wurm, S. (in press). The influence of subjective aging on psychophysical functioning and longevity: A meta-analysis of longitudinal data. *Psychology and Aging*.

Westerhof, G. J., Whitbourne, S., & Freeman, G. P. (2012). The aging self in a cultural context: The relation of conceptions of aging to identity processes and self-esteem in the United States and the Netherlands. *The Journals of Gerontology, Series B: Psychological Sciences and Social Sciences*, *67*, 52–60. http://dx.doi.org/10.1093/geronb/gbr075

Widmer, E. D., & Ritschard, G. (2009). The de-standardization of the life course: Are men and women equal? *Advances in Life Course Research*, *14*, 28–39. http://dx.doi.org/10.1016/j.alcr.2009.04.001

Willis, S. L., Tennstedt, S. L., Marsiske, M., Ball, K., Elias, J., Koepke, K. M., . . . Wright, E. (2006). Long-term effects of cognitive training on everyday functional outcomes in older adults. *Journal of the American Medical Association*, *296*, 2805–2814.

Wolff, J. K., Warner, L. M., Ziegelmann, J. P., & Wurm, S. (2014). What do targeting positive views on ageing add to a physical activity intervention in older adults?

Results from a randomised controlled trial. *Psychology & Health, 29*, 915–932. http://dx.doi.org/10.1080/08870446.2014.896464

Wurm, S., Tesch-Römer, C., & Tomasik, M. J. (2007). Longitudinal findings on aging-related cognitions, control beliefs, and health in later life. *The Journals of Gerontology. Series B, Psychological Sciences and Social Sciences, 62*, P156–P164.

Wurm, S., Tomasik, M. J., & Tesch-Römer, C. (2008). Serious health events and their impact on changes in subjective health and life satisfaction: The role of age and a positive view on ageing. *European Journal of Ageing, 5*, 117–127. http://dx.doi.org/10.1007/s10433-008-0077-5

Wurm, S., Tomasik, M. J., & Tesch-Römer, C. (2010). On the importance of a positive view on ageing for physical exercise among middle-aged and older adults: Cross-sectional and longitudinal findings. *Psychology & Health, 25*, 25–42. http://dx.doi.org/10.1080/08870440802311314

Wurm, S., Warner, L. M., Ziegelmann, J. P., Wolff, J. K., & Schüz, B. (2013). How do negative self-perceptions of aging become a self-fulfilling prophecy? *Psychology and Aging, 28*, 1088–1097. http://dx.doi.org/10.1037/a0032845

CHAPTER 2

Subjective Aging and New Complexities of the Life Course

Richard A. Settersten, Jr. and Gunhild O. Hagestad

ABSTRACT

How individuals evaluate their aging must be understood within a context of structural and cultural forces that transformed the human life course over the last century. This chapter applies social science perspectives to explore how structural and cultural dynamics shape the contour and content of aging and affect individual expectations and evaluations. The starting assumption is that subjective aging is largely intersubjective: How human beings experience aging is shaped by shared meanings, accumulated through lifelong socialization and feedback from persons around them. The chapter examines how subjective aging is connected to societal change in demographic and epidemiological conditions, the cultural shift toward individualization, and complex contingencies related to social relationships in contemporary life. It examines markers of becoming and being old and the degree to which subjective aging is similar or different for women and men. It closes with a discussion of how social factors can better be brought into research on subjective aging, and of how gerontologists are resistant participant observers in their own aging process and their communication about aging.

INTRODUCTION

Questions about how individuals understand and evaluate their aging present researchers with difficult conceptual and empirical challenges. These individual

http://dx.doi.org/10.1891/0198-8794.35.29

experiences must be understood within a context of structural and cultural forces that transformed the human life course over the last century. In this chapter, we apply social science perspectives, mostly from life course sociology, to explore how structural and cultural dynamics shape the contour and content of aging and affect individual expectations and evaluations. We hope to offer an important complement to the psychological perspectives that have been central to the evolution of inquiry into subjective aging since the 1960s.

Our starting assumption is that subjective aging is largely *intersubjective*: It is shaped by shared meanings, accumulated through lifelong socialization and feedback from other persons and interpreted in the particular social contexts in which we exist. Put simply, lives are embedded in social experiences. Our perspective builds, in part, on the "symbolic interaction" tradition in sociology and social psychology with central concepts such as Charles Horton Cooley's (1902) "looking glass self" or George Herbert Mead's (1913) concepts of the "I," "me," and the "generalized other," among other classical theorists and ideas associated with this tradition.

We begin by considering how subjective aging is connected to societal change in demographic and epidemiological conditions, the cultural shift toward individualization, and complicated contingencies related to social relationships in contemporary life. We entertain some markers of becoming and being old and the degree to which subjective aging is gendered. We end with a discussion of how social factors can better be brought into research on subjective aging, and why gerontologists need to be "reflexive," to use Bourdieu's (1992) term, about their own experiences with and communication about subjective aging.

THE IMPACT OF DEMOGRAPHIC AND EPIDEMIOLOGICAL CONDITIONS ON SUBJECTIVE AGING

The last century saw significant declines in mortality, morbidity, and fertility. These demographic changes created aging societies and transformed the aging experiences of individuals and families. Demographic change initially gave rise to the very concept of the life course when it became statistically normal to survive to a mature age (Kohli, 2007). Subsequently, demographic shifts permitted the reorganization of the life course and the reconfiguration of education, work, and family. Individuals can now generally count on surviving eight decades, with much of this time lived jointly with others. The unprecedented duration of relationships today is particularly striking in the family realm.

Demographic changes have in many countries created a more extensive and healthier context for old age, making it possible for individuals to become and be old in new ways. However, it is important to remember that there are also many countries in which general life expectancy is younger than the age of 80 years, especially for men, and in which there are widespread concerns about the future longevity and health of contemporary cohorts of children and young adults and the plateauing or reversal of gains that have come to older cohorts. In some regions of the world, and even for subpopulations in seemingly well-positioned nations such as the United States, a long life cannot be counted on—whether because of political and economic upheaval, war, and violence, or because of high rates of infant and child mortality.

Nonetheless, old age now spans multiple decades and is composed of early and late phases that are often markedly different from one another—a "third age" of great potential, often facilitated by good health; and a "fourth age" of significant challenge and hardship, often triggered and punctuated by chronic and acute health conditions that seriously limit functional capacity (e.g., Baltes & Smith, 2003).

Dramatic shifts in life expectancy present a form of paradox: Human beings now live longer and generally healthier lives, yet death and old age are more strongly coupled than was the case in earlier times, when early childhood was the life phase characterized by the most severe danger of dying. The shift from infectious disease to "wear-and-tear" lifestyle-related disease, known as the "epidemiological transition" (Omran, 2005), has also brought important and sometimes sharp contrasts between the length and health of men's and women's lives.

Increased stability in survival brings a risk of overestimating the predictability of death for oneself and others, producing a sense that we have more time than we do—a kind of illusion that our lives and relationships have an infinite duration. This is nicely reflected in a scene from the 1981 film *On Golden Pond*, in which the old mother (Katherine Hepburn) is having a conversation with her middle-aged daughter (Jane Fonda) about her father (Henry Fonda). The daughter says that *at some time*, she will have an honest talk with her father, and the mother replies, "Just how much time do you think you have?" Today, the death of one's parents has become a predictable marker of a child's middle age, and the question, "Are your parents still living?" is often raised among midlife peers in social conversation.

Individuals' evaluations of how old they feel, where they are in the aging process, and how they fare relative to others are grounded in the demographic realities around them. As societies age, both the process and markers of subjective aging will continue to be shaped by the growth and visibility of an older population. Two aspects of population must be heeded: First, given women's higher life expectancy, to be very old, especially, is to be female and to be a long-lived society is to have a "feminized" aged population. For example, in 2010, the ratio of American men to women aged 65–69 years was 85 to 100; for older than 80 years, it was 57 to 100 (U.S. Census Bureau, 2011). The differential life expectancy of men and women affects subjective aging through the composition of social networks and the presence of a partner. For example, it is more typical for old women to experience widowhood; the aging (and death) of men is normally experienced alongside a partner, whereas the aging of women often includes a final phase of life without a partner.

Second, there are fewer children and youth in social settings of everyday life, given low fertility, and these proportions are especially striking when they are understood in relation to the old. For example, in Italy today, there are 14 old persons (aged 65 years and older) for every child (younger than age 15 years); by 2025, this ratio is projected to be 24 to 1 (United Nations Demographic Statistics Division, 2012). The major storylines of what it means to live in aging societies are to be found not only in what it means for the old but also in what it means for the young (for illustrations, see Hagestad, 2008; Uhlenberg, 2008). For example, being a child or being aged in a high-longevity context—surrounded by many aged men and (especially) women, and embedded in families that span several generations—is far different from being a child or aged in a low-longevity context without these characteristics.

THE IMPACT OF INDIVIDUALIZATION ON SUBJECTIVE AGING

In addition to discussing dramatic demographic shifts, writers on social change and human lives have devoted a good deal of attention to the cultural shift toward individualization in "postmodern" societies. Many of these authors focus on youth and the transition to adulthood in discussing how individuals are the architects of their own lives, making their own life choices and taking pathways that are unique and variable. Several authors warn of serious risks associated with individualization (Bauman, 2006; Beck, 2000; Furlong, Cartmel, Biggart, Sweeting, & West, 2006). To our knowledge, however, few of these discussions have considered older persons. Many of today's older adults grew up in a society characterized by strong class differences in life course options and opportunities. During their adult years, society has undergone dramatic structural and cultural shifts, creating new possibilities for choice. These changes have produced some strong contrasts and discontinuities within and between generations, both on a societal and a family level. Norwegian anthropologist Gullestad (1996) provides a nice example of these tensions in her analysis of the life plans and histories of individuals in different family generations: A maternal grandmother is trying to understand her teenage granddaughter. The granddaughter is struggling to find her own "niche" in life, and no matter how hard she tries, she feels as if she cannot create it. The grandmother, who is not part of a cohort with a worldview that emphasizes "human agency" (having direct control over one's life) to the same degree, says, "Why not make the best of the niche where you have been put?" Her response is typical of the mentalities of older cohorts, which take for granted that we must make the most of the situations we are dealt, situations which reflect our location in society and over which we have little or no control. Such accounts raise thought-provoking questions about policies and services for older persons. Do we find situations in which policymakers and professionals, who are members of "individualized" cohorts, operate from premises that are alien to the very people they target or serve?

The individualization of the life course has opened opportunities for people of all ages, including those who are old, to live their lives in ways that are congruent with their personal interests and wishes. But new freedoms also bring new risks. This is particularly true of "liberal market" states, such as the United States or the United Kingdom, where the responsibility for managing risk is to be assumed by individuals and families, using whatever resources they have or can marshal, rather than by governments, markets, or other entities (Esping-Andersen, 2002; Hacker, 2006; Mayer, 2004). ("Liberal market states" are given this label not because they are generous, but because they reflect a free market economy and emphasize personal liberty.) The challenges of managing choices and risks in these environments seem particularly great for individuals in late life: The future is unpredictable and a short time horizon means there is less time to recover from negative outcomes.

Conditions of individualization affect subjective aging because the implication is that understandings and evaluations of aging also become highly individualized, as are the responses for managing aging processes. Even though some of the markers or triggers of subjective aging may be widely shared, many are likely to be highly individualized and or uniquely experienced. When the expanse of old age is understood to be highly variable and shifting, the task of evaluating our own aging, and that of others, becomes difficult because there are few standards on which to base our judgments. Which experiences are understood to be common to most people as they grow older, and which experiences distinguish people in one period of life from another, whether old age from midlife or the fourth age from the third? What happens to the mental health of individuals if there is no shared framework within which to assess personal aging and the aging of others? In this scenario, the things that happen to individuals—positive or negative—are interpreted as being of their own doing. When aging experiences are positive, they are ours to celebrate, and when aging experiences are negative, they are ours to own as personal shortcomings or failures. These risks are accentuated by models of successful aging, as we will later discuss.

SUBJECTIVE AGING AND THE CONTINGENCIES OF LATE LIFE

The individualization of the life course may also lead us to overestimate the role of personal choice and control in determining the course of our aging. Being able to count on an old age is not the same as being able to count on *how* those years will be experienced or *whether* the balance of experiences will be positive. Indeed, the later years have a highly contingent quality. They are embodied with so much possibility, yet their potentials, if they are to be realized, depend on some important factors that cannot necessarily be predicted or controlled.

These contingencies especially relate to health and resources: *If* I am (or we are) still alive, *if* I am (or we are) healthy, *if* I (or we) can manage financially, *if* I (or we) can live independently, *if* my (or our) children are able or willing to help, and so on. Most individuals, we suspect, have physical health as the dominant dimension in their appraisals: Aging goes well when you are healthy, it falls apart when you get sick, and death eventually comes from disease or a body that gives up. After having your life and your health, other factors—such as finances, social support, or the ability to maintain independence—change the parameters on how the later years are experienced.

The repeated "we" and "our" alongside the "I" in the sentences earlier reveal the interwoven nature of human lives and the contingencies created by social relationships. These are strongly emphasized in one of the core principles of a life course perspective: "linked" or "interdependent" lives (e.g., Elder, Shanahan, & Jennings, in press; Settersten, 2009). Aging, including subjective aging, is often treated as an individual process, but it is never completely one's own. Our aging makes claims on others, just as their aging makes claims on us—creating risks, protections, constraints, and opportunities. The aging of others is also likely to trigger awareness of our own aging. Many aspects of an individual's aging are also partially beyond her or his control. This seems especially true of health and resources, which are heavily tied to genetics (and epigenetics) and to fortunes or misfortunes of one's birth family or cohort, the latter of which creates structural conditions that shape collective aging via changing historical circumstances or opportunities (e.g., for marriage, education, jobs, and housing). Subjective aging is surely affected by these resources and opportunities, and altered by changes in them.

Demographic changes have altered the structure of families and the nature of relationships, both of which affect subjective aging. Reduced mortality and fertility mean that aging occurs in taller and narrower family structures (or "bean-pole" families, to use Bengtson, Rosenthal, & Burton's [1990] phrase), with more generations alive at once and fewer in each one. This shape brings the potential for family relationships to become more important, active, and intense because there are fewer relationships in which to invest, they are of longer duration, and they exist across several generations. At the same time, the "second demographic transition" (van de Kaa, 1987) has reshaped families through multiple divorces and remarriages across generations, multipartner fertility and nonmarital fertility, nontraditional partnerships, geographic dispersion, and mobility of immediate family members. These pose new challenges to the maintenance of intimate relationships.

An important aspect of the contingencies of social relationships in old age is the loss of what Plath (1980) calls "consociates"—central fellow life travelers. The older we are, the more likely it is that we have lost key others who know and have shared our histories and understand our frames of reference. These "co-biographers," to use Bertaux's (1981) term, can help in a process of assessing and editing our life stories and foster a sense of continuity between present and past selves. This is a key aspect of subjective aging and of Erikson's (1986) task of creating integrity in old age.

Part of what Neugarten (1995) called "the costs of survivorship" is the loss of these co-biographers. In some populations (e.g., migrants or refugees), the lack of such persons in old age may be extremely painful. These losses are especially prevalent and painful for women, given their longer life expectancy and the cultivation of family and other social relationships over a lifetime. Discontinuities are extreme when individuals have migrated across national and cultural divides, but they also emerge within a given cultural context because of social change. As Margaret Mead (1970) so poignantly formulated it: In societies characterized by rapid social change, the old, in having begun their lives in an earlier era, become "immigrants in time" because they are confronted with a world so different from what they once knew. Although the old may convey to the young a sense of tradition and appreciation of the past, it is the young who are at home in the new world and become teachers to the old.

MARKERS OF SUBJECTIVE AGING
Chronological Age, Life Phases, and Social Systems

Chronological age is not only a property of individuals, but it also is embedded in social systems (Dannefer & Settersten, 2010), including age-homogeneous social institutions (e.g., schools, residential facilities), age-based policies (e.g., compulsory schooling, adult rights and duties that come at 18 and 21 years, retirement and pension rules), public discourse, and face-to-face social interactions. These social institutions, policies, and interactions all frame subjective aging.

Subjective aging is also framed by the social construction of broader life phases and the age-based social norms associated with them. These affect subjective aging by guiding expectations and goal setting and by shaping identity (see also Heckhausen, 1999). In the last century, distinct phases of the life course emerged and became increasingly differentiated as knowledge about human development grew alongside gains in life expectancy. Childhood was segmented into "early childhood," "middle childhood," "youth and adolescence"; adulthood was segmented into "early adulthood," "midlife," and "old age"; and old age was segmented into "young-old," "old-old," and "advanced old age" (or "oldest-old") phases.

The social and legal regulation of the two ends of life—childhood and old age—has been heaviest. In the case of childhood, there was growing recognition of the need to protect children based on their dependence—and, in recent years, awareness that young adults also experience an extended period of risk as "dependents" (e.g., parental support is prolonged with floundering in higher education or with unemployment, low wages, or no benefits). In the case of old age, there was growing recognition of the need to protect older adults not only based on risks associated with aging (including the risk of *becoming* dependent) but also framed as a reward for their prior contributions to society (Skocpol, 2000).

As individuals move out of one life period and into another, social rituals may heighten subjective aging. Early anthropological studies of age grading emphasized the change in social identities that came as individuals passed from one age class to another. "Rites of passage" marked this movement and prompted what van Gennep (1908/1960) called "ceasings and becomings." Individuals ceased being what they were and became something new in crossing the threshold, and social rites helped both individuals and members of their community to adjust perceptions and expectations. Such rites, which were separate for men and women, were most typical of transitions associated with becoming an adult, particularly sexual maturation. It is not just that individuals think about themselves differently; it is that others see and acknowledge changes in the individual's social status. Today, rites of passage accompany transitions such as graduations, marriages and births, landmark birthdays or anniversaries, retirements, and funerals. To the extent that such markers carry important social meanings and are recognized publicly, they would seem important in increasing the subjective awareness of aging both of and for oneself and others.

Anthropological accounts highlight the fact that most, but not all, cultures and societies have their own frameworks for understanding age, age periods, and the life course as a whole. The anthropological research of Project AGE (Keith et al., 1994), for example, revealed that age was a meaningful concept in five of the seven sites in which they conducted fieldwork (in Hong Kong; Momence, Illinois and Swarthmore, Pennsylvania; suburban Blessington, Ireland; and among the Herero of Botswana), although there was variation in the exact meanings of age, the number of life periods perceived, and the ages at which different periods of life begin and end. In contrast, age was largely irrelevant in two of the seven communities (among the !Kung bushmen and in Clifden, Ireland). For example, in response to questions about people of different ages, the !Kung say things such as, "Oh, they have all kinds of names. There's John, Sue, Jane, George . . ." The !Kung actually define all life transitions in terms of physical capability or functionality rather than chronological age. In fact, the !Kung do not use numbers, and questions about chronological age are meaningless.

Entry into adulthood is often associated with an array of clear legal rights and responsibilities which are assumed to remain intact thereafter. In old age, concerns do sometimes emerge about the conditions under which those cherished rights and responsibilities (including the ability to make independent decisions) can be taken away—particularly in the face of cognitive decline or physical frailty. Apart from eligibility ages for aging programs, such as Social Security and Medicare, which traditionally served as institutional markers of old age, there are no clear legal markers of old age. And although eligibility ages have inched upward with gains in life expectancy, few people who pass these thresholds are likely to self-classify as old. The same seems true of eligibility ages for other "senior" benefits, which may come even earlier, such as the AARP membership at age 50. And yet, a consumption-oriented culture may also prompt individuals to embrace or claim the benefits which come with advancing age.

Discrepancies Between Chronological Age and Subjective Ages

Research on subjective age identity has consistently revealed discrepancies between how old individuals actually are (chronological age) and how old they report feeling, looking, and acting (Barrett, Redmond, & Rohr, 2012; Daatland, 2007; Diehl & Wahl, 2010; Rubin & Berntsen, 2006; Settersten & Mayer, 1997). In the second half of life, individuals begin to report younger subjective ages than their chronological age. One Danish study, by Rubin and Berntsen (2006), suggests that this process may begin as early as 40 years, when individuals start to feel about 20% younger than their actual chrono-logical age.

Consistent with Benjamin Franklin's quote that "everybody wants to have a long life, but nobody wants to be old," evidence suggests that there is particu-larly great resistance to labeling oneself as old at later ages, even among people who would be classified as old based on ages that exceed eligibility criteria for old-age policies and programs. Old also seems to be a label that is much easier to apply to others, even (or especially) to create social distance between other old people and oneself (e.g., the resistance of individuals to move to an assisted living facility or nursing home because they do not seem themselves as anything like those residents).

Adopting and fostering a "youthful" identity can serve as a mechanism of individual and social self-protection or enhancement, especially in youth-oriented cultures such as the United States. But at what point does the main-tenance of a youthful identity become limited in its effectiveness—and even problematic if individuals are unable to experience old age for all that it is? Old age has been described as a "leveler" (Dowd & Bengtson, 1978) of inequalities because normal declines in physical and cognitive health can be delayed but not escaped for anybody. When individuals' expectations of aging are unrealistic, or when individuals blame themselves or others for negative but natural outcomes of aging, (positive) subjective aging would seem threatened. This seems espe-cially likely in the transition to the fourth age because losses in functional capac-ity demand that individuals "face their limits" and wrestle with human dignity (Baltes, 2006).

Beyond Chronological Age: Alternative Markers of Subjective Aging

Apart from chronological age and its connection to life phases and social poli-cies, what experiences might signal to individuals that they are aging? Little is known about the specific markers on which individuals rely, how they judge and apply these markers to themselves and others, and what these markers mean to different kinds of people in diverse life circumstances (for a recent illustration, see Miche et al., 2014).

In Table 2.1 we offer some good candidates to be explored in the case of old age, many of which can be extracted from existing literature. These relate to health, time, meaning, family, and social relationships.

This list is by no means exhaustive, but it does contain some of the experi-ences we imagine to be the most poignant markers or triggers of subjective aging in the second half of life. Many of these experiences are inherently social; all of them take place within social environments which will condition their larger meanings and personal applications.

TABLE 2.1

Markers or Triggers of Subjective Aging in the Second Half of Life: Examples

Time

Dwindling time horizon and the need to come to terms with one's finitude

Increasing focus on time left to live

Increasing premium on how time is spent, reprioritizing of goals

Growing sense that the pace of time has quickened

Growing concern about one's future and those of others

Increasing reminiscence, resurgence of early memories, search for continuity

Meaning and generativity

Increasing search for meaning in life

Growing concern for younger generations

Concerns and acts related to generativity, ensuring one's legacy

Family experiences

Experiencing the illness or death of parents, moving up the family "ladder"

Crossing the ages at which parents died

Experiencing the illness or death of siblings, friends

Becoming a widow or widower

Becoming a grandparent or great-grandparent

Seeing one's children reach middle age

Seeing one's grandchildren reach adulthood

Social experiences

Being treated by others in ageist ways (positive or negative)

Experiencing age discrimination

Becoming dependent on others

Shrinking social networks

Feeling invisible

Body and health

Changing physical appearance of the body

Changing sleep

Losing balance

Feeling fatigue

(Continued)

TABLE 2.1

Markers or Triggers of Subjective Aging in Second Half of Life: Examples   *(Continued)*

Decreasing libido

Emerging chronic, even multiple, health problems

Onset of acute health conditions

Changing memory or cognitive processing

Decreasing mobility

Growing salience of health concerns in individuals' self-definitions

Challenges associated with activities of daily living

Housing

Needing to adapt one's living environment to accommodate health changes

Moving to an assisted living or long-term care community

Policy

Drawing a pension—Social Security or Medicare

Eligibility for other "senior" benefits or discounts

SUBJECTIVE AGING: A GRADUAL PROCESS?

It seems unlikely that any single marker will render someone old in his or her own mind or in the minds of others—especially in cultures or populations in which the category old is one that is not embraced but rather resisted, as noted earlier. Achieving an identity as old, like that of an "adult" earlier in the life course (Settersten, 2011), seems likely to happen slowly and be punctuated by notable moments that signal to individuals and those around them that they are changing. Some of these markers may be more significant than others, depending on their qualities (e.g., whether or not they are anticipated, controllable, typical, desirable, or acute). Like the ages of 18 or 21 years, which are encrypted in policies that mark adulthood, the age of 65 years, which traditionally brought eligibility for Social Security and pensions, might also trigger this process.

Some of these experiences may accumulate with little awareness, reflected in the commonly expressed sentiment that age "creeps up" on us, that old age is here "before we know it," or that life passes "in the blink of an eye." These sentiments need not mean that the course to feeling older or becoming old is entirely gradual. On one hand, it seems plausible to imagine that old age can be reached without fanfare or recognition. This might be especially likely if the process of aging is met with resistance or denial, such that signals may be dismissed or explained away to the contrary. On the other hand, the expressions noted earlier more often seem to evoke the sense that, even if a process has been gradual, some things happen to penetrate our consciousness or leave us suddenly aware of our aging—"old age moments" or a "jolt" of some kind. These may even be small unexpected interpersonal encounters: when the Transportation Security Administration agent at the airport shouts out that "the shoes belong to the old woman!" and the second author (GOH) does not realize he is talking about her; when a friend who epitomizes successful aging dies suddenly of a heart attack; or when the doctor says in response to new physical ailments, "Well, what do you expect at your age?" These signs of aging, whatever they may be, must ultimately be confronted by and incorporated into the identities of individuals and the views of others.

Much like the transition to adulthood, in which young people do not feel fully adult until well into their 30s, if then (Settersten, 2011), it seems likely that most older people, even those who would fit the category old in policy terms, do not feel old or fully old. Feeling old is likely to be multifaceted and sensitive to social contexts: In some ways, with some people, and in some places, individuals may feel old, and in other ways, with other people, and in other places, they do not. In young adulthood, *feeling* adult and *doing* adult things are reciprocally important in establishing an adult identity. One wonders about the corollary in later life—whether there are costs or benefits to building an identity as old (i.e., allowing oneself to feel old and do things that old people do) and whether there are costs or benefits to rejecting such an identity.

For example, a quest to stay active and healthy in old age may be undertaken with the goal of feeling younger, but if individuals feel younger, they may also strive to be active and healthy. (The sentiment that being young is completely "in the mind" is probably only uttered by people who are active and healthy!) Subjective aging is inherently connected to aging bodies. Indeed, medical and consumer efforts to slow human aging are meant to change both bodies and minds—but often with the assumption that improving physical aging is the key to improving subjective aging (Fishman, Settersten, & Flatt, 2010).

Similarly, the early timing of many of the potential markers of old age proposed earlier probably accelerate a subjective sense of being older, whereas delays in these experiences would seem to slow it. For example, the second author (GOH) has described her experience with cancer in middle age as creating a sense that she had fallen "out of time"—disrupting expected rhythms of work and family life, losing the comfort of schedules and predictability, and feeling uncertain about her future and the futures of loved ones (Hagestad, 1996). These experiences triggered her awareness, and the awareness of others, that a situation so often associated with late life had come well before its time.

The things that prompt us to fall "off the line"—experiences that come early, late, or never at all, or experiences that have never been in our mind as possibilities—will likely heighten subjective aging because they catch us off guard and shatter our assumptions about what constitutes a "normal, expectable life," to use Neugarten's (1969) phrase.

In these circumstances, how the experience is framed matters for how it is evaluated. An experience that is perceived as something that happened *to* an individual will be quite different from one that is perceived as something that was actively chosen *by* an individual. Of course, falling off the line may also bring silver linings—such as the reprioritizing of time, goals, relationships, and quality of life—things that may positively affect future aging and subjective aging.

The alternative markers raised earlier were described as being "beyond chronological age," but it would be naïve to suggest that they are wholly unrelated to age. They seem to be an integral part of a process of a growing "awareness of age-related change," to use Diehl and Wahl's (2010) phrase. Although they do not occur in lockstep at fixed ages, they are nonetheless experiences that many old people share, even if they are experienced differently and are an essential part of what it means to be human.

SUBJECTIVE AGING: GENDERED LIVES, GENDERED BODIES

There is a long tradition in sociology, dating back to Linton's (1942) and Parsons' (1942) classic articles, to regard age and sex as "twin statuses." Together, age and sex categories were the "building blocks" of society. "Her" life and "his" life were highly differentiated by social roles (especially family and work, respectively) and subject to different expectations.

There are no generic old *people*; there are old *men* and old *women*. Much research on aging today, including subjective aging, is, in direct contrast, theorized or conducted as if there is a unisex model of aging. There may be some universal experiences related to subjective aging that are shared by women and men, but there are probably many more experiences that are distinct for each gender. As we touched on earlier, there are objectively different parameters for the aging of women and men around morbidities and mortality (reflected in the saying that "women are sicker and men die quicker," although the story is more complicated than this). But subjective aging processes are also likely to reflect gender-based cultural ideas about the course of aging and its markers (e.g., Calasanti, 2010; Canetto, Kaminski, & Felicio, 1995).

These cultural ideas are clearly related to the differential valuation of gendered aging bodies. First made visible in cultural essays by Inge Powell Bell (1970) and Susan Sontag (1972), the notion of the "double standard" of aging for men and women is surely a particularly important part of subjective aging: the physical signs of aging affect men and women differently, with wrinkled skin and grey hair making a man look distinguished and the very same characteristics making a woman look over the hill—leading to harsher evaluation of women's aging, not only by men but also potentially by women, and to a sense of becoming invisible. Indeed, antiaging medical practices are focused on women (e.g., hormone replacement therapies, injections, and plastic surgeries), and the patients who consume these (generally out-of-pocket) services are largely middle-aged women with ample financial resources (Fishman, Settersten, & Flatt, 2010; Mykytyn, 2006). There is also the massive over-the-counter cosmetic market, focused on "regenerative" antiaging products, which caters to women. However, there seems to be a growing premium on men's bodies as well: medical treatments and industries aimed at helping men maintain sex and virility in old age (e.g., Viagra and testosterone therapies, hair replacement, plastic surgery, and cosmetic lines). These things surely factor into the judgments men and women make about themselves and each other with respect to aging and aging bodies.

In a revealing study, Siders (2010) probed the conditions under which old persons in long-term care facilities feel that they are cared for. When female residents were asked what it would take for them to feel cared for, most responded that they themselves would have an opportunity to provide care for *others*. Men did not express the need to *give* care as part of a definition of being cared *for*. Men, in contrast, were more likely to cite the need to be cared for by a woman with whom they are in an intimate relationship. (For this generation of women, providing care has been central to their identities; for this generation of men, the primary close relationships they have had are with the women who have cared for them. Both men and women had women as confidants.) One wonders whether this situation will differ much for cohorts of men and women now on the cusp of old age, or for cohorts who are now young adults, when they become old. But this example offers a good illustration of how cohort membership and intimate relationships differentially shape the subjective aging of men and women.

At the same time, there is also evidence that some of the long-standing differentiation between women's and men's social roles is eroding—although women have moved closer to (and are even surpassing) men in educational and occupational attainments more than men have moved closer to women in shouldering responsibility for the care and rearing of children (Gerson 2009; Levy & Widmer, 2013; Widmer & Ritschard, 2009). Some markers of subjective aging (e.g., related to work and retirement, income, and social security) may therefore in the future become more equivalent for men and women, whereas others (e.g., related to family relationships, caretaking, widowhood, social networks, or physical aging) might remain more central to women.

Although age and sex are two prominent dimensions of social organization and differentiation, there are others. Every society classifies its members in several different ways simultaneously. In the United States, for example, social class is crucial to take into account because the different kinds of capital that come with it (such as cultural, social, material) lead to different life-course outcomes, which will have both direct and indirect effects on subjective aging. Because these kinds of capital are important determinants of health and many dimensions of well-being, they are especially likely to have strong indirect effects on subjective aging *through* health and well-being. In the United States, racial and ethnic differences similarly create different meanings and markers of aging. Intersections between gender, social class, race, and ethnicity offer important niches for probing differences and similarities in subjective aging across social groups.

DISCUSSION

Consistent with social processes emphasized in the tradition of symbolic interactionism, we argue that subjective aging is inherently social because it is intersubjective. It rests on (a) how individuals see themselves—not only relative to their younger selves and to the older selves they imagine, but also relative to other people who are younger, older, or of a similar age; (b) how others see the individual and respond to his or her aging; and (c) how individuals see and respond to the aging of others.

Subjective aging is also rooted in social processes that extend beyond interpersonal relationships. Although social ties are especially important, appraisals of aging are shaped by opportunities and constraints presented by demographic, epidemiological, and historical contexts; the welfare state and social policies; cultural ideas about the phases of life and the transitions that punctuate them; and cultural ideas related to age, aging, and gender. Age, as we have seen, is a property of social systems, not just people. Yet, social forces do not simply or only push down on people. Much of the relevant action for understanding subjective aging is to be found in the transactions that are forged between people and systems. That is, age is not only co-constructed by characteristics of the social and cultural environment, but it is also a personal characteristic that is shaped by individual behaviors, attitudes, and perceptions.

Gerontologists and geriatricians may negatively affect subjective aging via the images they promote, the theories they develop, and the research they conduct. For example, many aging professionals reject terms such as "old person," "old people," and old age, instead preferring softer language such as "older adults" or "later life." In doing so, they may promote an ideology of agelessness, itself a kind of ageism, in which aging and old age are viewed as things that should be transcended (see also Andrews, 1999). In this scenario, gerontology is in the awkward position of wanting to overcome one of the central dimensions that has traditionally been at its core: chronological age.

In Europe, 2012 was the "International Year of Active Aging and Solidarity Among Generations." Most of the international meetings and materials of the year were dominated by models and images of successful, and especially "active" aging. The message was clear: Individuals are responsible for their own aging. This focus is well-aligned with the neoliberal emphasis on personal responsibility (e.g., Hacker, 2006), but it does a disservice to elders who cannot or will not meet these criteria or live up to these ideals. Some of these calls are reasonable to the extent that scientists and professionals are trying to convince people to pursue heart-healthy lifestyles or to refrain from tobacco smoking or excessive alcohol consumption. We know from health economics that these create significant health risks for individuals and have taken great tolls in the United States and in European and Asian countries. We cannot change our genetic makeup, but research on the effects of lifestyle factors (such as physical activity, healthy nutrition, or cognitive stimulation) suggest opportunities for individuals to—at least to some extent—make active efforts to improve the course of his or her aging.

However, gerontologists have an obligation to make visible the full spectrum of aging experiences, balancing positive alongside negative ones; to recognize that sometimes negative experiences are not of individuals' own doing; and to give people the means to do the best they can, given their circumstances. Messages about successful aging, and especially antiaging, end up restricting rather than expanding the range of possible models of aging for public consumption because they communicate that *defying* aging is the primary way to *go about* aging (for other critiques of successful aging, see Dillaway & Byrnes, 2009; Flatt, Settersten, Ponsaran, & Fishman, 2013; Katz & Calasanti, 2014). In this sense, the preoccupation with being age*less* itself becomes a marker of old age, for agelessness is something that seems largely sought by and marketed to people who *are* chronologically old—or *not quite old*—rather than to the young.

Gerontologists would also do well to more clearly address the relationship between age and aging (and therefore between subjective age and aging as well). As noted earlier, age is a feature of social structure as well as of individuals. As both a dynamic and structural feature of social life, age operates in ways that transcend and frame individual aging. Age encompasses larger social phenomena in areas such as social policy, age discrimination and ageism, age integration and segregation, age relations, and so on.

In this regard, it may be useful to consider the analogy between aging/age on one hand and sex/gender on the other. In each case, the former term refers to a specific characteristic anchored in the body (in biological sex and biological age), whereas the latter not only includes such individual characteristics but also includes social constructs that have varied significance and meaning in different contexts (Dannefer & Settersten, 2013). These social constructs must be better explicated in research on subjective aging, for they play crucial roles in framing individual appraisals and, for that matter, may not even enter individual consciousness. Research on subjective aging will become more powerful if it is able to unveil forces at work that are not immediately visible.

Finally, there is a need to more systematically examine the social sources and social consequences of subjective aging, from micro- to macrolevels of analysis. We must study subjective aging in relation to the many and varied social environments that shape it and determine its consequences. Some will say there is little value in understanding subjective states alone; that is, what people do and how they function matter more than what they think or feel. To strengthen the broader case for subjective aging, research should continue to link subjective aging to meaningful behavior that has meaningful consequences (recent examples of research in these directions include Spuling, Miche, Wurm, & Wahl, 2013; Stephan, Chalabaev, Kotter-Grühn, & Jaconelli, 2013; Weiss & Lang, 2012; Wurm, Warner, Ziegelmann, Wolff, & Schüz, 2013) but move outward into other social sources and consequences of the kinds highlighted in this chapter.

Advances in theory and research on subjective aging are to be found in understanding the predictive, mediating, or moderating influence of subjective aging *on* the health and well-being outcomes of individuals, families, and societies. To the extent that subjective aging is viewed as a mechanism for improving health and well-being, it is then important to know which factors produce it— and which of these factors can actually be altered if they are to be effective levers for improving subjective aging. In addition, a stronger case will need to be made that interventions into subjective aging are more effective at improving health and well-being across these levels than other interventions that operate through other levers. In the process, we also cannot statistically control the very dimensions that are central to understanding subjective aging—including chronological age and gender.

POSTSCRIPT: GERONTOLOGISTS AS RESISTANT PARTICIPANT OBSERVERS OF SUBJECTIVE AGING

We have touched on the role of gerontologists in shaping views on subjective aging. One aspect of this role has to do with ontology: What *is* aging? What is the range of "normal" aging? We have suggested that too exclusive an emphasis on active or successful aging may create gaps in individuals' awareness of the full complexity of aging experiences and have adverse effects on their evaluations of themselves and others. When aging processes are framed in a limited way, individuals may feel inadequate, even though the decline and limitations they experience are, statistically, within the normal range. Thus, researchers face a potential moral dilemma in that our priorities and messages may bring negative and unintended consequences for the health and well-being of the very population we may be hoping to affect. Conversely, some might argue that ever-present images of active or successful aging will increase optimism about aging and "raise the bar" by prompting individuals to strive for things that they might otherwise not see as within their reach.

There is also an epistemological aspect to the question of how we can know and understand aging. For all other phases of life, it is common for social and behavioral scientists to use personal experience as a basis for questions, hypotheses, and understanding. Is gerontology different from the study of other life periods in this regard? In 1922, Stanley Hall, the psychologist who coined the term adolescence, made an interesting observation in the book *Senescence*, commenting that old age is unique among life phases in that researchers do not have personal retrospective knowledge and understanding on which to draw.

One could argue that it is exactly for this reason that it is extremely important for gerontologists to be open and honest about their own aging, and to leave detailed records of their last phase of life. Few gerontologists have done so. Most appear to participate in two separate and distinct discourses on aging: a public, scholarly one and a private one. Often, there are sharp contrasts between these sets of accounts.

In a symposium at a recent meeting of the Gerontological Society of America, the second author (GOH; Hagestad, 2013) argued that gerontologists are engaging in what Said (1979) called "othering"—in this case, of old people. Researchers in their 60s and 70s, even 80s, refer to old people as "them" or "they," as if the old are members of a strange tribe of which the researchers are not part: the geronts. It is rare to find first-person accounts of aging by gerontologists. An exception is Hendricks (2008, p. 113), who pointed to an interesting state of affairs:

> Those of us who study aging have the unique opportunity to live their subject matter. As social gerontologists, we have been quick to assert that broad social currents carry persons to the doorstep of old age and beyond, but we have been far less reflective about our own journey.

B. F. Skinner, a well-known psychologist, but not a gerontologist, may have provided the most honest accounts of his own aging. At the annual meeting of the American Psychological Association (APA) in 1982, and in an interview with Jennes (1983), Skinner used himself as a case study, saying,

> [At the age of 79 years] I am very careful as to how much time I work, and I schedule relaxing activities so I won't try to get in an extra hour of hard thinking, which is too tiring. . . . It is also important to get plenty of rest. . . . If you tried to do something very serious in every waking hour, you wouldn't last a year!

At the same APA meeting, Bernice Neugarten, then aged 68 years, spoke on "successful aging," arguing that the United States was becoming an "age-irrelevant society" in which people remain vigorous and do things at 70 or 80 years that would not have been possible even 30 years earlier and suggesting that the term old ought to be dropped. But only a few years later, she would privately quote Bette Davis: "This aging stuff, it ain't for sissies!"

Nearly three decades after the APA session on aging, gerontologist Elaine Brody (2010, p. 5) used considerable humor to describe her own experience of being an aging researcher:

> My present perspective . . . is that of an 86-year-old woman who, I suppose, was prepared for old age intellectually but not emotionally. Even my children are growing into the stages of life I studied. Common experiences of old age, such as illness and losses, were unexpected, even though expectable. I do not remember becoming old.

In the examples earlier, researchers have openly addressed the limitations and problems presented by aging. Austrian gerontologist Leopold Rosenmayr has pointed to the new social freedoms that come in old age. At the age of 58 years, he published *Die Späte Freiheit* (*The Late Freedom*; Rosenmayr, 1983). Twenty-four years later, he published *Schöpferisch Altern* (*Creative Aging*) with the subtitle *Eine Philosophie des Lebens* (*A Philosophy of Life*; Rosenmayr, 2007). Rosenmayr's perspective is much needed. Old age can bring a newfound sense of personal liberation, especially from social conventions.

An application of this idea can be found in a recent *New York Times* article with the headline "How to Get Spontaneity? Practice" (Tommasini, 2014). The piece focused on old musicians, among them Arthur Rubinstein, who completed a series of Chopin recordings at the age of 78 years. The journalist concluded, "The most exciting spontaneity often comes from mature artists with decades of experience" (p. AR9). In a documentary about his life and career, Rubinstein spoke of how old age gave him permission to focus on emotion, not technique. Among retired academics, it is not uncommon to hear joyful accounts of having the freedom to say what they did not dare express earlier for fear of possible career consequences.

We must also probe the factors which bring us to our subject matter. David Gutmann (1997) once commented that he sees two groups of people who are drawn to gerontology for quite different reasons: *gerophiles* and *gerophobes*. Many recruits to the field of gerontology, Gutmann said, are gerophiles who "were once rescued by their grandparents and now they want to repay the favor" (p. xviii). Gerophiles want to do good to old people. However, an "underground community of gerophobes" exists. Gerophobes are attracted to the field of gerontology, consciously or unconsciously, because they fear, and want to be protected from, growing old. These selection processes shape the questions we ask, the methods we use, and the assumptions we make about the nature and meaning of aging.

There are few examples of gerontologists who have been reflexive about their own aging and the insights generated in the process. This creates a state of affairs that limits understanding and theoretical advances. Hendricks (2008), building on the phenomenologist Schütz (1932/1967), emphasizes the need to build theory in ways that incorporate "subjective meanings for real actors in real situations" (p. 110). Perhaps nowhere is this perspective needed more in gerontology than the subfield devoted to *subjective* aging. Our work will not only be better for it, but it will also be more honest.

REFERENCES

Andrews, M. (1999). The seductiveness of agelessness. *Ageing and Society, 19,* 301–318.

Baltes, P. B. (2006). Facing our limits: Human dignity in the very old. *Daedalus, 135,* 32–39. http://dx.doi.org/10.1162/001152606775321086

Baltes, P. B., & Smith, J. (2003). New frontiers in the future of aging: From successful aging of the young old to the dilemmas of the fourth age. *Gerontology, 49,* 123–135.

Barrett, A., Redmond, R., & Rohr, C. (2012). Avoiding aging? Social psychology's treatment of age. *American Sociologist, 43,* 328–347. http://dx.doi.org/10.1007/s12108-012-9157-2

Bauman, Z. (2006). *Liquid times: Living in an age of uncertainty.* Cambridge, MA: Polity Press.

Beck, U. (2000). Living your own life in a runaway world: Individualisation, globalisation, and politics. In W. Hutton & A. Giddens (Eds.), *Global capitalism* (pp. 164–174). New York, NY: The New Press.

Bell, I. P. (1970). The double standard. *Transaction/Society, 8,* 75–80.

Bengtson, V. L., Rosenthal, C. J., & Burton, L. M. (1990). Families and ageing: Diversity and heterogeneity. In R. H. Binstock & L. K. George (Eds.), *Handbook of aging and the social sciences* (pp. 263–287). New York, NY: Academic Press.

Bertaux, D. (Ed.). (1981). *Biography and society: The life history approach in the social sciences.* Beverly Hills, CA: Sage.

Bourdieu, P. (1992). *Invitation to a reflexive sociology*. Chicago, IL: University of Chicago Press.

Brody, E. (2010). On being very, very old: An insider's perspective. *The Gerontologist, 50*, 2–10. http://dx.doi.org/10.1093/geront/gnp143

Calasanti, T. (2010). Gender relations and applied research on aging. *The Gerontologist, 50*, 720–734. http://dx.doi.org/10.1093/geront/gnq085

Canetto, S. S., Kaminski, P. L., & Felicio, D. M. (1995). Typical and optimal aging in women and men: Is there a double standard? *The International Journal of Aging & Human Development, 40*, 187–207.

Cooley, C. H. (1902). *Human nature and the social order*. New York, NY: Scribner.

Daatland, S. O. (2007). Age identifications. In R. Fernández-Ballesteros (Ed.), *Geropsychology: European perspectives for an aging world* (pp. 31–48). Göttingen, Germany: Hogrefe & Huber.

Dannefer, W. D., & Settersten, R. A., Jr. (2010). The study of the life course: Implications for social gerontology. In W. D. Dannefer & C. Phillipson (Eds.), *International handbook of social gerontology* (pp. 3–19). London, United Kingdom: Sage.

Dannefer, W. D., & Settersten, R. A., Jr. (2013, Summer). Section name change: Continuing discussion and recommendation. *Newsletter of the Section on the Sociology of Aging and the Life Course*, (Summer), 4.

Diehl, M., & Wahl, H. W. (2010). Awareness of age-related change: Examination of a (mostly) unexplored concept. *The Journals of Gerontology. Series B, Psychological Sciences and Social Sciences, 65*, 340–350. http://dx.doi.org/10.1093/geronb/gbp110

Dillaway, H. D., & Byrnes, M. (2009). Reconsidering successful aging: A call for renewed and expanded academic critiques and conceptualizations. *Journal of Applied Gerontology, 28*, 702–722. http://dx.doi.org/10.1177/0733464809333882

Dowd, J. J., & Bengtson, V. L. (1978). Aging in minority populations: An examination of the double jeopardy hypothesis. *Journal of Gerontology, 33*, 427–436.

Elder, G. H., Jr., Shanahan, M. J., & Jennings, J. A. (in press). Human development in time and place. In T. Leventhal & M. Bornstein (Eds.), *Handbook of child psychology and developmental science: Ecological settings and processes in developmental systems* (7th ed., Vol. 4). Hoboken, NJ: Wiley.

Erikson, E. H. (1986). *The life cycle completed*. New York, NY: Norton.

Esping-Andersen, G. (2002). Towards the good society, once again? In G. Esping-Andersen (with D. Gallie, A. Hemerijck, & J. Myles) (Ed.), *Why we need a new welfare state* (pp. 1–25). Oxford, United Kingdom: Oxford University Press.

Fishman, J. R., Settersten, R. A., Jr., & Flatt, M. A. (2010). In the vanguard of biomedicine? The curious and contradictory case of anti-aging medicine. *Sociology of Health & Illness, 32*, 197–210. http://dx.doi.org/10.1111/j.1467-9566.2009.01212.x

Flatt, M. A., Settersten, R. A., Jr., Ponsaran, R., & Fishman, J. R. (2013). Are "anti-aging medicine" and "successful aging" two sides of the same coin? Views of anti-aging practitioners. *The Journals of Gerontology. Series B, Psychological Sciences and Social Sciences, 68*, 944–955. http://dx.doi.org/10.1093/geronb/gbt086

Furlong, A., Cartmel, F., Biggart, A., Sweeting, H., & West, P. (2006). Social class in an "individualized" society. *Sociology Review, 15*, 28–32.

Gerson, K. (2009). *The unfinished revolution: How a new generation is reshaping family, work, and gender in America.* New York, NY: Oxford University Press.

Gullestad, M. (1996). *Everyday life philosophers: Modernity, morality and autobiography in Norway.* Oslo: Universitetsforlaget.

Gutmann, D. (1997). *The human elder in nature, culture, and society.* Boulder, CO: Westview Press.

Hacker, J. (2006). *The great risk shift.* New York, NY: Oxford University Press.

Hagestad, G. O. (1996). On-time, off-time, out of time? Reflections on continuity and discontinuity from an illness process. In V. L. Bengtson (Ed.), *Adulthood and aging: Research on continuities and discontinuities* (pp. 204–221). New York, NY: Springer Publishing.

Hagestad, G. O. (2008). The book-ends: Emerging perspectives on children and old people. In C. Saraceno (Ed.), *Families, ageing and social policy: Intergenerational solidarity in European welfare states* (pp. 20–37). Cheltenham, United Kingdom: Edward Elgar.

Hagestad, G. O. (2013, November). *Optimization or othering? Thoughts on how gerontologists deal with their own aging.* Paper presented at the Annual Scientific Meeting of the Gerontological Society of America, New Orleans, LA.

Hall, G. S. (1922). *Senescence: The last half of life.* New York, NY: Appleton.

Heckhausen, J. (1999). *Developmental regulation in adulthood: Age-normative and sociocultural constraints as adaptive challenges.* Cambridge, United Kingdom: Cambridge University Press.

Hendricks, J. (2008). Coming of age. *Journal of Aging Studies, 22*, 109–114. http://dx.doi.org/10.1016/j.jaging.2007.12.015

Jennes, G. (1983, November 28). Growing old gracefully, says psychologist BF Skinner, means tailoring your life to fit your infirmities. *People Magazine, 20*(22). Retrieved from http://www.people.com/people/article/0,,20086422,00.html

Katz, S., & Calasanti, T. (2014). Critical perspectives on successful aging: Does it "appeal more than it illuminates"? *The Gerontologist.* Advance online publication. http://dx.doi.org/10.1093/geront/gnu027

Keith, J., Fry, C. L., Glascock, A. P., Ikels, C., Dickerson-Putnam, J., Harpending, H. C., & Draper, P. (1994). *The aging experience: Diversity and commonality across cultures.* Newbury Park, CA: Sage.

Kohli, M. (2007). The institutionalization of the life course: Looking back to look ahead. *Research in Human Development, 4*, 253–271. http://dx.doi.org/10.1080/15427600701663122

Levy, R., & Widmer, E. D. (Eds.). (2013). *Gendered life courses: Between standardization and individualization.* Zürich, Switzerland: Lit Verlag.

Linton, R. A. (1942). Age and sex categories. *American Sociological Review, 7*, 589–603.

Mayer, K. U. (2004). Whose lives? How history, societies, and institutions define and shape life courses. *Research in Human Development, 1*, 161–187. http://dx.doi.org/10.1207/s15427617rhd0103_3

Mead, G. H. (1913). The social self. *Journal of Philosophy, Psychology and Scientific Methods*, *10*, 374–380.

Mead, M. (1970). *Culture and commitment: A study of the generation gap*. Garden City, NY: Natural History Press.

Miche, M., Wahl, H. W., Diehl, M., Oswald, F., Kaspar, R., & Kolb, M. (2014). Natural occurrence of subjective aging experiences in community-dwelling older adults. *The Journals of Gerontology. Series B, Psychological Sciences and Social Sciences, 69*, 174–187. http://dx.doi.org/10.1093/geronb/gbs164

Mykytyn, C. E. (2006). Anti-aging medicine: A patient/practitioner movement to redefine aging. *Social Science and Medicine, 62*, 643–653. http://dx.doi.org/10.1016/j.socscimed.2005.06.021

Neugarten, B. L. (1969). Continuities and discontinuities of psychological issues into adult life. *Human Development, 12*, 121–130. http://dx.doi.org/10.1159/000270858

Neugarten, B. L. (1995). The costs of survivorship. *Center on Aging Newsletter*, 11.

Omran, A. R. (2005). The epidemiological transition: A theory of the epidemiology of population change. *The Milbank Quarterly, 83*, 731–757.

Parsons, T. (1942). Age and sex in the social structure of the United States. *American Sociological Review, 7*, 604–616.

Plath, D. W. (1980). Contours of consociation: Lessons from a Japanese narrative. In P. B. Baltes & O. G. Brim, Jr. (Eds.), *Life-span development and behavior* (Vol. 3, pp. 287–305). New York, NY: Academic Press.

Rosenmayr, L. (1983). *Die Späte Freiheit: Das Alter, ein Stück bewusst gelebten Lebens* [The late freedom: Old age—A piece of consciously experienced life]. Berlin, Germany: Severin and Siedler.

Rosenmayr, L. (2007). *Schöpferisch Altern: Eine Philosophie des Lebens* [Creative aging: A philosophy of life]. Münster, Germany: LIT-Verlag.

Rubin, D. C., & Berntsen, D. (2006). People over forty feel 20% younger than their age: Subjective age across the lifespan. *Psychonomic Bulletin and Review, 13*, 776–780. http://dx.doi.org/10.3758/BF03193996

Said, E. (1979). *Orientalism*. New York, NY: Vintage Books.

Schütz, A. (1967). *The phenomenology of the social world*. Evanston, IL: Northwestern University Press. (Original work published 1932)

Settersten, R. A., Jr. (2009). It takes two to tango: The (un)easy dance between life-course sociology and life-span psychology. *Advances in Life Course Research, 14*, 74–81.

Settersten, R. A., Jr. (2011). Becoming adult: Meanings and markers for young Americans. In M. Waters, P. Carr, M. Kefalas, & J. Holdaway (Eds.), *Coming of age in America: The transition to adulthood in the twenty-first century* (pp. 169–190). Berkeley, CA: University of California Press.

Settersten, R. A., Jr., & Mayer, K. U. (1997). The measurement of age, age structuring, and the life course. *Annual Review of Sociology, 23*, 233–261.

Siders, R. A. (2010, November). *Meanings of care: A gendered perspective*. Paper presented at the Annual Scientific Meeting of the Gerontological Society of America, New Orleans, LA.

Skocpol, T. (2000). How Americans forgot the formula for successful social policy. In *The missing middle: Working families and the future of American social policy* (pp. 22–58). New York, NY: Norton.

Sontag, S. (1972, September 23). The double standard of aging. *The Saturday Review, 55,* 29–38.

Spuling, S. M., Miche, M., Wurm, S., & Wahl, H. W. (2013). Exploring the causal interplay of subjective age and health dimensions in the second half of life. *Zeitschrift für Gesundheitspsychologie, 21,* 5–15. http://dx.doi.org/10.1026/0943-8149/a000084

Stephan, Y., Chalabaev, A., Kotter-Grühn, D., & Jaconelli, A. (2013). "Feeling younger, being stronger": An experimental study of subjective age and physical functioning among older adults. *The Journals of Gerontology. Series B, Psychological Sciences and Social Sciences, 68,* 1–7. http://dx.doi.org/10.1093/geronb/gbs037

Tommasini, A. (2014, March 14). How to get spontaneity? Practice. *The New York Times,* pp. AR9.

Uhlenberg, P. (2008). Children in an aging society. *The Journals of Gerontology. Series B, Psychological Sciences and Social Sciences, 64,* 489–496. http://dx.doi.org/10.1093/geronb/gbp001

United Nations Demographic Statistics Division. (2012). *Demographic yearbook 2012.* Retrieved from http://unstats.un.org/UNSD/Demographic/products/dyb/dyb2012.htm

U.S. Census Bureau. (2011, May). *Age and sex composition: 2010* (Census Publication No. C2010BR-03). Washington, DC: U.S. Department of Commerce, Economic and Statistics Administration.

van de Kaa, D. J. (1987). Europe's second demographic transition. *Population Bulletin, 42.*

van Gennep, A. (1960). *The rites of passage* (M. B. Vizedom & S. T. Kimball, Trans.). Chicago, IL: University of Chicago Press. (Original work published 1908)

Weiss, D., & Lang, F. R. (2012). "They" are old but "I" feel younger: Age-group dissociation as a self-protective strategy in old age. *Psychology and Aging, 27,* 153–163. http://dx.doi.org/10.1037/a0024887

Widmer, E., & Ritschard, G. (2009). The de-standardization of the life course: Are men and women equal? *Advances in Life Course Research, 14,* 28–39. http://dx.doi.org/10.1016/j.alcr.2009.04.001

Wurm, S., Warner, L. M., Ziegelmann, J. P., Wolff, J. K., & Schüz, B. (2013). How do negative self-perceptions of aging become a self-fulfilling prophecy? *Psychology and Aging, 28,* 1088–1097. http://dx.doi.org/10.1037/a0032845

CHAPTER 3

"It's About Time"

Applying Life Span and Life Course
Perspectives to the Study of Subjective Age

Anne E. Barrett and Joann M. Montepare

ABSTRACT

Subjective age, a component of subjective aging, has received growing empirical attention locally and globally. Reflecting the age individuals perceive themselves to be, subjective age involves the experience of time along multiple dimensions—including lifetime, marked by movement through developmental life stages and socially structured, historically contextualized life course transitions. However, issues of temporality have received limited attention in studies of subjective age. We address this limitation by considering subjective age through the lens of two theoretical perspectives that center on temporality: the life span and life course perspectives. The life span perspective illuminates variation across and within life stages by pointing to developmental processes and age triggers that drive age identity. The life course perspective highlights other temporal issues that shape age-related patterns in subjective age, pointing to social, cultural, and historical factors that impact developmental processes. We employ these perspectives to organize what is known about subjective age and to suggest new contexts and connections for further research. Our analysis calls attention to the importance of considering the multidimensionality of subjective age across broad spans of time as well as the need to explore intersections among developmental processes, life course trajectories, and historical contexts.

© 2015 Springer Publishing Company
http://dx.doi.org/10.1891/0198-8794.35.55

INTRODUCTION

Subjective aging entails a constellation of age-related constructs, one of which is *subjective age*, or the age an individual feels (Diehl et al., 2014). Also referred to as "age identity," subjective age has been the focus of growing empirical interest, as illustrated by the inclusion of subjective age measures in large-scale national and international surveys of aging and adult development (e.g., Midlife in the United States [MIDUS], Health and Retirement Survey, Berlin Aging Study, German Aging Survey). This interest has sparked discussions about the components and measurement of subjective age, along with investigations of diverse demographic and psychological correlates in an attempt to pin down factors fueling age identity. Although informative, existing research has not fully exploited two prominent theoretical frameworks that consider temporal processes: life span developmental and life course perspectives. Our chapter shows the use of these frameworks for organizing what is known about subjective age and suggesting new connections and contexts for future explorations.

Both perspectives address the unfolding of human lives across time, but they have different vantage points. The life span developmental perspective focuses on the psychological processes generating change and continuity among individuals across their lives (Baltes, 1987). Although this perspective takes the individual as the starting point, the more sociologically oriented life course perspective begins with the age-related structuring of social life across intersecting domains, such as paid work, family, and education (Elder, Johnson, & Crosnoe, 2003). Life span and life course perspectives can inform the study of subjective age, given its link to the experience of time across multiple levels. At the individual level, subjective age is shaped by the passage of lifetime, marked by movement through life stages with unique developmental challenges as well as socially structured transitions constituting the life course. Subjective age also has a transient temporal dimension influenced by fleeting, everyday experiences—for example, the momentary, situation-specific feeling of being "old." In addition to reflecting the passage of individual lifetime and daily temporal rhythms, subjective age operates at a social level, entailing sociocultural and structural dimensions. It is influenced by social meanings of age that often are embedded within social institutions—for example, views of 65 as the start of old age, deriving from Social Security criteria. Subjective age also relates to historical time, as perceptions of one's own age are shaped by multiple contexts present at a particular point in time, including age-related demographics, social valuations of different age groups, and the relative importance of age in structuring social life.

In this chapter, we begin with a brief overview of early research on subjective age. Then, we use a life span perspective to examine what research suggests about the psychological factors shaping differences in subjective age across life stages, as well as variations in age identity within particular life stages. Next, we use a life course perspective to examine structural factors that further moderate variations in subjective age. We close with recommendations for new avenues of research that draw on both perspectives.

A LIFE SPAN DEVELOPMENTAL PERSPECTIVE ON SUBJECTIVE AGE

Seminal gerontological research on subjective age explored the age individuals perceived themselves to be, look, and act, documenting surprising, yet common, discrepancies between older adults' chronological and subjective ages. In general, older adults perceived themselves to be many years younger than their age (Baum & Boxley, 1983; Bultena & Powers, 1978; Kastenbaum, Derbin, Sabatini, & Artt, 1972). The dominant explanation in early research given for older adults' perceptions was that youthful identities were a response to an aging-biased culture and reflected a way aging adults could reduce their fears of aging and disassociate themselves from the stigma of old age (Bultena & Powers, 1978; Peters, 1971). However, empirical support for this age denial explanation was weak insofar as little or no relationship was found between older adults' age identities and their personal fears of aging or the negativity of their age stereotypes (Keith, 1977; Montepare & Lachman, 1989; Ward, 1977).

Since these early ventures, subjective age research has burgeoned locally and globally, providing a wealth of information about its biological, psychological, cognitive, and social correlates (Diehl et al., 2014; Montepare, 2009; Settersten & Mayer, 1997). Moreover, research with younger individuals found that they also experience discrepancies between their chronological and subjective ages—with children, adolescents, and adults in their early 20s perceiving themselves as slightly older than their age. As individuals approach the age of 30, they view themselves as slightly younger than their actual age, a discrepancy that expands with advancing age (Galambos, Kolaric, Sears, & Maggs, 1999; Goldsmith & Heiens, 1992; Montepare, 1991, 1996a; Montepare & Lachman, 1989). At the same time, individual variations in subjective age have been evident within age groups.

What accounts for across-age and within-stage variations in subjective age? Drawing on the life span developmental premise that behavior reflects a multidirectional and multidetermined process of change and constancy from youth through old age (Baltes, 1987), one answer is that subjective age identification reflects a process of anchoring, adjusting, and adapting one's age across developmental stages to internal models and external markers (Montepare, 2009;

Westerhof, Whitbourne, & Freeman, 2012). The outcomes of this dynamic process are differences in how old or young individuals experience themselves to be from one developmental stage to the next as well as variations they experience within particular stages.

Variations in Subjective Age Across Life Stages

Social developmental research has revealed that age is a major touchstone by which people organize information about themselves. From an early developmental stage, age is one of the basic attributes people use to differentiate themselves from others and come to understand themselves as members of social categories (Lewis & Brooks-Gunn, 1979; Montepare & Zebrowitz, 1998). Although age continues to be a core personal attribute, people often maintain age identities that deviate from their actual age, resulting in the young feeling old and the old feeling young. However, it has yet to be determined what accounts for this distinctive life span pattern.

As individuals mature, knowledge and experiences derived from an age-differentiated world form the basis for internalized conceptions of the life course that include beliefs and expectations about past, present, and future age–related behaviors and events against which people evaluate themselves (Whitbourne, 1985). Moreover, such implicit conceptions are thought to contribute to perceptions of the self through time by shaping how people interpret stability and change in themselves (Ross, 1989). These intrinsic models may provide a reference against which individuals evaluate their developmental movement and position in the life span (Montepare, 2009). That is, individuals may compare where they are in their lives to personal models denoting where they are expected to be. Moreover, these models are presumed to take on a curvilinear shape with gains anticipated in the future and losses expected thereafter, as suggested by research exploring individuals' experiences and expectations about paths of development across the adult years (Heckhausen, Dixon, & Baltes, 1989; McFarland, Ross, & Giltrow, 1992; Ross, 1989). In other words, whereas intrinsic models of early development emphasize growth and advancement, models of later development turn the course toward decline with advancing age. As such, Montepare (2009) has proposed that these personal models possess midpoints reflecting peak stages of self-perceived developmental functioning—the point of being a "full-blown" adult. Consequently, earlier in the life span, individuals often assert older identities consistent with perceptions of their progressing, goal-oriented move toward adulthood. Across the later years, individuals assert younger identities, reflecting the developmental achievement of having "grown up" and reached adulthood. And they continue to experience themselves at this state despite growing chronologically older—to the extent that age cues do not signal that a salient change has occurred. Feeling younger with advancing age may further reflect what life span theorists describe as identity assimilation, whereby adults attempt to maintain self-continuity by integrating ongoing experiences in terms of previously established self-schemata (Westerhof et al., 2012).

Evidence that individuals hold such developmental models is gleaned from research showing that adults hold systematic beliefs about how attributes change with age and how they evaluate age-related changes in light of these beliefs (Heckhausen et al., 1989; McFarland et al., 1992; Ross, 1989; Ross, McFarland, & Fletcher, 1981). Other work has found that when young adults were asked to "draw their lives," they most often depicted their development as a steady "coming of age" progression marked by movements through age-graded contexts (e.g., reaching milestones such as completing school, leaving home) that promote "growing up" and achieving sustained maturity at adulthood (Montepare & Petrov, 2012). Like adults, adolescents have implicit developmental models that entail expectations about paths toward maturity. Facilitated by the growth of abstract thinking and an emerging future orientation, adolescents envision adulthood as a goal-oriented state reached by achieving autonomy and responsibility (Barker & Galambos, 2005).

This life span characterization is consistent with the rise of older subjective ages and the fall to younger identities occurring around the transition to adulthood found by Galambos, Turner, and Tilton-Weaver (2005), as well as the persistence in subjective age discrepancies across adulthood observed by other researchers (Uotinen, Rantanen, Suutama, & Ruoppila, 2006; Ward, 2013). Galambos and colleagues speculated that the curvilinear crossover observed in emerging adults happens when younger individuals transition out of adolescence and experience a shift in their reference group from younger to older peers. This *bottom dog* phenomenon leads younger individuals to no longer see themselves at the top of their age reference group but rather as part of an older age group characterized by behaviors more normative for adults than adolescents. Referencing this older group then results in a younger subjective age. In their study of subjective age across the adult years, Rubin and Berntsen (2006) found a similar crossover point at 25 years, where age identities shifted from older to younger. Moreover, when the discrepancy between subjective and chronological age was computed as a proportion of chronological age, no increase was seen after age 40. With advancing age, all age groups felt about 20% younger than their actual age. Consistent with the perspective offered here, Rubin and Bernsten argued that "although the dominant view in the study of subjective age has been age denial, we believe that a life span developmental view is needed. Such a view better describes the data, which should facilitate theoretical advancement" (p. 780).

Although more work is needed to elucidate how developmental models drive life span patterns of age identity, research showing cross-cultural universality in subjective age is consistent with the proposition that individuals possess such models against which age is evaluated. A review by Barak (2009) of studies conducted in 18 nations finds that the pattern of older adults holding younger identities holds across diverse cultures. Moreover, consistent with work in more modernized Western and non-Western societies, a study of older adults in Senegal found that they perceived themselves as somewhat younger than their chronological age (Macia, Duboz, Montepare, & Gueye, 2012). Consistency also is revealed in research examining a wider age range, as illustrated by Sato, Shimonaka, Nakazato, and Kawaai's (1997) study of Japanese individuals between the ages of 8 and 92 years that revealed a shift from older to younger subjective ages similar to that observed in American samples. Additional support is found in research showing similarities in subjective age across groups that are the same age, but differ with respect to other distinctive features. For instance, Galambos, Darrah, and Magill-Evans (2007) found that young adults with and without motor disabilities reported similar age identities, suggesting that they hold similar implicit developmental models against which they evaluate their age.

Although intrinsic developmental models may very well shape general patterns in subjective age across the life span, the role of personal views should also be considered. Although links between older adults' youthful age identities and fears of aging or negative age attitudes have been found to be weak, other indicators point to age-related attitudes at work in age identification. For example, Heckhausen (1997) found that middle-aged and older adults evaluated their personal hopes, plans, and goals for the next few years as more consistent with the goals of younger than same-aged peers, presumably because comparisons to a non–elderly adult, nonstigmatized reference group reduces feared losses and elevates aging adults' self-image. Relatedly, when older adults were asked to respond to questions about losses versus gains associated with aging, Weiss and Lang (2012) found that those who responded to questions about losses were more likely to dissociate themselves from their peer age group and report younger age identities.

Just as older adults may "deny their age," younger individuals may "deny their youth" by aspiring to goals and responsibilities typically associated with older, more mature individuals who hold a more desirable social status. Consistent with this possibility, adolescents and young adults with older identities hold a strong desire to abandon their present age group status and achieve an older one expected to carry greater responsibility, freedom, and independence (Barker & Galambos, 2005; Montepare & Clements, 1995). It is also possible that aging attitudes may be better cast as moderators than mediators of subjective age relationships, as demonstrated by Mock and Eibach (2011). These authors found that adults' older identities predicted lower life satisfaction and higher negative affect when aging attitudes were favorable but not when attitudes were unfavorable. New work examining the role of aging attitudes in the process of age identification is needed to pinpoint how aging attitudes fuel age perceptions at different life stages.

Other age-related psychological variables may likewise play a role shaping subjective age across life stages, although they have been studied in less detail. For instance, the extent to which individuals consider age to be a salient attribute may moderate how age is evaluated, and this salience may vary across the life span (Montepare, 1996b; Montepare & Clements, 2001). Recent work exploring personality correlates of age identity also finds that extraversion predicts younger subjective ages in older adults, whereas conscientiousness predicts older identities in younger adults (Stephan, Demulier, & Terracciano, 2012). Achieving a fuller understanding of age-related variations in subjective age will surely need to consider the intervening role of such age-related variables.

Variations in Subjective Age Within Life Stages

In addition to understanding processes shaping patterns of age identity across the life span, it is important to examine the considerable variation across individuals and the factors producing it. For example, Westerhof (2008) noted that although 75% of American middle-aged adults held younger identities, 15% felt their actual age, and 10% felt older. Variation also is reported in older (Ward, 2013) and younger samples (Galambos et al., 1999; Galambos et al., 2007). What factors might yield these variations within age groups? A life span perspective suggests that proximal age-symbolic events, experiences, and encounters within particular life stages trigger the salience of age and shape age identities (Giles, McIlrath, Mulac, & McCann, 2010; Lowe, Dillon, Rhodes, & Zwiebach, 2013; Montepare, 2009; Ward, 2013). For example, celebrated developmental life events, such as birthdays, weddings, anniversaries, reunions, and memorials are likely to call attention to one's position in the life span and prompt an evaluation of discrepancies between subjective and chronological age. Consistent with this proposition, older adults experience age identities closer to their actual age the nearer their birthdays and see themselves as younger the more distant their birthdays (Montepare, 1996b).

Other triggers include social interactions with others who either differ in age or hold expectations about age-related behaviors. For example, the composition of and communications within adults' social networks strongly affect age identities (Giles, Fox, Harwood, & Williams, 1994; Montepare & Birchander,

1994). Older adults who interact with individuals from various age groups, particularly children, have subjective ages that are significantly younger than those whose social networks are more age-restricted (Montepare & Birchander, 1994). Adolescents' social relationships also impact their age identities, as evidenced by older identities held by those who date older partners (Arbeau, Galambos, & Jansson, 2007). As well, communication scholars suggest that age-biased language in social exchanges impacts subjective age (Harwood, 2007).

Age-related physical events, such as health-related events (e.g., heart attacks, strokes, or memory loss), reproductive-related events (e.g., becoming a grandparent or the onset of menopause or balding), and death-related events (e.g., the passing of a partner or friend) also may shift subjective age. Similarly, normative, age-graded practices, such as achieving the status of "senior citizen," retiring, or becoming eligible for Social Security, may produce variations in subjective age. Along these lines, general declines in health not only are significant predictors of older subjective ages in aging adults but also explain a sizable portion of the variance in age identities (Barrett, 2003; Hubley & Russell, 2009; Markides & Boldt, 1983). Moreover, the adoption of older identities has been associated with the experience of distinctive events viewed as transitional age markers in adulthood, such as balding in men (Girman et al., 1998) and menopause in women (Ballard, Kuh, & Wadsworth, 2001). However, although some researchers have found that adults who have recently retired or become widowed adopt older subjective ages (Barak & Stern, 1986), others have not found this to be the case (Ward, 2013). Clearly, more work needs to be done to understand the link between particular age-symbolic experiences and subjective age. One issue worth considering is the meaning surrounding particular experiences. For instance, Kaufman and Elder (2003) found that becoming a grandparent impacted age identity, with some qualifications. That is, adults who became grandparents at a younger age felt older in comparison to those who entered the role at a later life stage, which they considered to be more "on time." And although the effect of birthday nearness held for older adults, it was not significant for younger adults, possibly reflecting differences within life stages in the meaning or salience of birthdays (Montepare, 1996b). Although annual birthdays may hold significance in later adult years, distinct milestone birthdays (18th, 21st) may be more potent age triggers in earlier years.

Individual differences in adolescents' age identities also have been linked to age-related physical, social, and normative cues. Reactions to physical triggers can be seen in taller, heavier, and postmenarcheal adolescent girls' holding older subjective ages than their less physically mature peers (Montepare, Reirdan, Koff, & Stubbs, 1989). Adolescents engaging in behaviors that youth associate with an older age status (e.g., engaging in sex, smoking, drinking) also maintain older subjective ages (Arbeau et al., 2007). Moreover, longitudinal analysis has shown that engaging in these behaviors *precedes* and *predicts* changes in adolescents' subjective age, supporting the premise that individual variations in subjective age reflect reactions to age-symbolic proximal cues (Galambos, Albrecht, & Jansson, 2009).

Further insights about the dynamics of subjective age triggers are provided by Giles and colleagues (2010) who asked young, middle-aged, and older adults what made them feel their age, feel younger, and feel older. A few similar triggers emerged across all age groups—for example, all groups identified recreational pursuits as youthful age triggers. However, the pursuits varied across the groups, reflecting different developmental emphases. For younger adults, these triggers included activities like watching cartoons or young TV shows, partying irresponsibly, and having lively friends. However, for middle-aged and older adults, they included physical, creative, and travel activities. Age variation also was found in older identity triggers. Whereas middle-aged and older adults frequently reported physical and mental decrements as triggers, younger adults made little mention of them, likely reflecting differences in both the salience and meaning of such changes experienced by older groups. Younger adults' older identity triggers included new responsibilities, such as working, voting, and living on one's own—age cues not reported by other groups. Younger adults also cited media as an age trigger, an unsurprising finding given their time spent with new media technology.

In addition to taking into account the meaning associated with triggers at different developmental stages, it is important to consider the transient or episodic nature of age cues. For example, age-symbolic events, such as being asked for proof of one's age, concluding a last day at work, attending a friend's funeral, or receiving a senior citizen discount, may elicit momentary shifts in subjective age but not a lasting change in age identity. When and how temporary versus sustained effects occur in people's daily lives are important questions for future research. As well, a life span approach calls for the need to consider accumulated effects across developmental time that shape age identities. Indeed, Schafer and Shippee (2010) found that increased levels of turmoil within intimate social networks occupied by spouses, parents, and children predicted increases in adults' age identities over time and that chronic health conditions hastened changes in less youthful age identities over the adult life span. It was argued that the stress produced by these experiences diminishes adults' psychosocial resources, which in turn generates age identity change, akin to the "graying" effect researchers have described in reaction to prolonged personal uncertainty (Foster, Hagan, & Brooks-Gunn, 2008). Research at younger stages also shows accumulated effects, with hardships during childhood and adolescence (e.g., living in unsafe environments, experience of violence, limited economic resources, turbulent family structures) being associated with older subjective ages and the identification of oneself as an adult in the late teens and 20s (Johnson & Mollborn, 2009).

It is interesting to note that Giles et al. (2010) found distinct differences in the value associated with "feeling younger" versus "feeling older" within age groups. Consistent with the notion that being younger places them in a less desirable age group with respect to their perceived developmental status, younger adults viewed feeling younger more negatively than feeling older or even same-aged. In contrast, middle-aged and older adults viewed feeling younger as the most positive identity, consistent with the more favorable developmental status of younger individuals, who are seen as attractive, strong, active, and healthy. Along similar lines, exploring the phenomenological experience of age in adults from 85–96 years, Nilsson, Sarvimäki, and Ekman (2000) found that "feeling old" was associated with a greater sense of distance from one's former self, consistent with self-referencing implicit models. At the same time feeling old entailed fears of helplessness and dependency, suggesting that aging attitudes are a psychological component of subjective age. In addition, adolescents who associated achieving adulthood as a marker of desired freedom versus responsibility were more likely to ascribe to feeling older and participate in problem behaviors (Barker & Galambos, 2005). Taken together, these findings suggest that the positive value ascribed to an older age identity by younger adults, and the appeal of a younger age identity to older adults, may be intervening factors impacting individuals' willingness to assume particular age identities at particular life stages.

A LIFE COURSE PERSPECTIVE ON SUBJECTIVE AGE

Another theoretical perspective focusing on temporal processes—the life course perspective—has been exploited to a limited degree in the study of subjective age. This perspective has a goal of linking historical and biographical contexts through a focus on the age-related structuring of social life. However, it has more often been employed to examine the objective patterning of lives—for example, the timing of transitions in and out of social roles, along with their long-range social, economic, and psychological implications—than the subjective experience of growing older, as it relates to movement within and across age-related social structures. The neglect of the subjective dimension of the life course, noted over the years by many scholars of aging and the life course (e.g., Elder, 1975; Elder & Johnson, 2002; George, 1996; Han & Moen, 1999; Hitlin & Elder, 2007; Settersten, 1999), remains relevant: "A subjective perspective is one of the oldest approaches to the study of lives, and yet it is undeveloped relative to its potential" (Elder & Johnson, 2002, p. 72). Illustrating its potential, we explore how five principles connect with and extend research on subjective age: (a) life-long development, (b) agency, (c) time and place, (d) timing, and (e) linked lives (Elder, 1975; Elder, Johnson, & Crosnoe, 2003).

Consistent with the life span developmental perspective, the life-long development principle suggests that a long-range view is needed to understand human development and aging (Elder et al., 2003). For life course sociology, this approach derives from the observation that events and transitions in one period of life often have consequences for those occurring in later periods. Reflecting this awareness, studies of subjective age have increasingly employed panel rather than cross-sectional data (e.g., Bowling, See-Tai, Ebrahim, Gabriel, & Solanki, 2005; Kleinspehn-Ammerlahn, Kotter-Grühn, & Smith, 2008; Schafer & Shippee, 2010). Providing an illustration, Kleinspehn-Ammerlahn and colleagues (2008) examined the subjective age of individuals aged 70–104 years in the Berlin Aging Study over four waves spanning 6 years. These older adults felt about 13 years younger than their actual ages, with no significant change over time in average subjective age. However, baseline level and change in subjective age were associated with chronological age: Older adults had more youthful identities and adopted more youthful identities over time than did their younger peers. Using a younger sample, Schafer and Shippee (2010) examined change in subjective age across two waves of the MIDUS study, a nationally representative sample of adults 25–74 years of age at the first wave. Consistent with the older adults in the Berlin study, these midlife adults felt younger than their actual ages; however, they felt only about 7 years younger at Wave 1 and held subjective ages that were, on average, 7 years older at Wave 2 than Wave 1. Taken together, these findings illustrate how subjective age varies in initial levels and changes at different rates across the life span, underscoring the use of examining these processes across broad spans of time.

The second principle—agency—emphasizes how individuals are active agents making choices about their lives (Elder et al., 2003). Agency is reflected in the very construction of age identity—a self-perception that can diverge from chronological age and the age others perceive one to be. However, the life course perspective emphasizes the interplay of agency and structure, defined as the enduring social patterns emerging from and shaping social life. Elements of structure include systems of inequality (e.g., age, gender, race and ethnicity), social institutions (e.g., marriage, work, media), and social networks (e.g., ties among family members).

Research points to relationships between elements of social structure and subjective age. However, less is known about either the specific ways that structure constrains age identity or the age identification processes of individuals within particular structural contexts. Social structural influences on subjective age are revealed by studies finding relationships with gender, race and ethnicity, and socioeconomic status (SES). Examinations of gender tend to find that women report younger identities than men (Pinquart & Sörensen, 2001), perhaps reflecting their efforts to avoid the stigma of old age that is particularly strong for women (Barrett, 2005). But this explanation is speculative and warrants a direct test tapping both agency and structure. Similarly, studies have noted race and ethnic differences, although less consistently. Some find that non-Whites hold older identities than Whites (Markides, 1980), whereas others report either the opposite (Barrett, 2003; Schafer, 2009) or no differences (Barak & Stern, 1986; Henderson, Goldsmith, & Flynn, 1995; Markides & Boldt, 1983). Variation also is found across groups of non-Whites, with African American young adults reporting older identities and Asian and Hispanic young adults reporting younger identities compared with White peers (Johnson, Berg, & Sirotzki, 2007). More consistent patterns are found for SES, with lower SES individuals reporting older identities (Barrett, 2003; Schafer & Shippee, 2010). Although cross-sectional work finds that their worse health, including lower perceived control over health, contributes to the explanation (Barrett, 2003), the processes would be illuminated by research focused on unpacking the interplay between structure and agency in the construction of subjective age.

A third life course principle highlights the importance of historical time and place in shaping individuals' lives (Elder et al., 2003). Regarding time, individuals' lives unfold within particular historical contexts that influence them in numerous ways having relevance for subjective age. Historical timing influences objective features of the life course, such as its overall length and the likelihood and timing of transitions like marriage and grandparenthood that denote life course progression. Dramatic shifts in objective features of the life course, particularly over the past century, point to the importance of considering historical shifts in subjective age. As illustrations, the extension of life expectancy, postponement of disability, and later transitions to marriage and parenthood may have generated conceptions of a more elongated life course and, by extension, more youthful identities among recent cohorts. A historical analysis by Chudacoff (1989) provides support for the argument that changes in the age-related structuring of the life course have implications for subjective aging. He found evidence of an increase over the 20th century in the extent to which age organized social life—for example, the timing of individuals' attachments to institutions like education, marriage, and work. This more widespread role of chronological age in structuring lives increased in its salience to individuals. Related to these shifts in the structuring and timing of lives, subjective features of the life course, such as conceptions of the timing and markers of life stages, are likely to change over time and have implications for subjective age. Similarly, generational distinctions (e.g., Baby Boomers, Millennials) are cultural constructions illustrating another historical contingency of individuals' subjective age. However, these historical questions have received limited research attention. For example, potential cohort differences in subjective age remain underexamined, although they may represent an alternative explanation for the observed age patterns or may reveal shifts over time in developmental processes.

Research also points to variation in subjective age by geographic place. The cross-national review by Barak (2009) revealed a consistent pattern of youthful identities in middle and later adulthood, suggesting an underlying developmental process at play; however, statistical comparisons across nations were not made, leaving unanswered questions about the relative magnitude of the youthful bias. Differences are suggested in studies reporting that some cultures, particularly more individually oriented ones, may promote more youthful identities (Uotinen, 1998; Westerhof, Barrett, & Steverink, 2003). For example, a comparison of the United States and Germany found significantly more youthful identities and a stronger association between youthful identities and psychological well-being among Americans (Westerhof & Barrett, 2005; Westerhof et al., 2003). Further evidence of cross-national variation is found in studies of other components of subjective aging. A study of 28 nations finds conceptions of the beginning of old age ranging from 55 years in Turkey to 68 years in Greece, with later ages found in countries with higher education and greater income inequality (Ayalon, Doron, Bodner, & Inbar, 2014). Also revealing variation, a study comparing 5 nations found that approximately 25% of respondents in the United Kingdom viewed retirement as a marker of old age, compared with only 9% of Americans; between 13% and 15% of participants from France, Japan, and the Dominican Republic held this view (O'Brien-Suric, 2013). However, little is known about the mechanisms generating cross-national variation in subjective age. Further, limited attention has been given to differences within nations, particularly across regions varying widely in age demographics, as well as health, economic inequality, and other factors shaping subjective age.

The fourth life course principle emphasizes timing, referring to the fact that the consequences of events and transitions vary depending on when they occur in the life course. Events and transitions, or changes in role statuses, derive meaning from the trajectories in which they are embedded—that is, the sequences of transitions occurring within particular social institutions or life domains, such as paid work, marriage, and family (Elder et al., 2003). The principle of timing points to the importance of considering how characteristics of trajectories shape subjective age, including timing and number of transitions and duration within statuses. It also highlights the intertwining of trajectories spanning different life domains, which influence one another and could have interactive effects on subjective age.

Studies of subjective age have tended to focus on individual transitions, such as retirement, rather than characteristics of the trajectories in which they are embedded. For example, as described before, studies have examined retirement and found mixed results. Although some found that retired people felt older than their employed peers (Kaufman & Elder, 2003), including a panel study examining entry into retirement (Schafer & Shippee, 2010), others reported no difference (Logan, Ward, & Spitze, 1992). A few studies also have examined the timing of transitions (Barrett, 2005; Kaufman & Elder, 2003; Schafer, 2009). Although Barrett (2005) found no association between subjective age and timing of marriage, parenthood, or retirement, others found significant associations for other transitions. As an illustration, Schafer (2009) found that maternal death in childhood was associated with having older identities, but no association with age identity was observed for parental loss in adulthood.

The fifth life course principle—"linked lives"—highlights the interdependence of the life paths of social network members (Elder et al., 2003). Several studies illustrate this principle. Using panel data spanning a decade, Schafer and Shippee (2010) found that family adversity (e.g., financial problems or illness experienced by spouses/partners, children, or parents) produced older age identities over time. Other studies have focused on parents and children, the most frequently examined social ties in this literature. For example, having a parent in poor health predicted feeling older (Barrett, 2003), but parental death was not associated with subjective age (Barrett, 2003; Kaufman & Elder, 2003)—unless it occurred in childhood (Schafer, 2009). Findings on parenthood are mixed. Although some research found that having more children was associated with an older subjective age (Kaufman & Elder, 2003), other work reported the opposite relationship (Barrett, 2005) or no effect of parenthood (Schafer & Shippee, 2010). However, Schafer and Shippee (2010) found that the death of a child predicted the adoption of an older subjective age over time. A qualitative study by Sherman (1994) provided further evidence of the role of family relationship in shaping subjective age, as respondents reported feeling older when younger family members experienced transitions such as marriage and parenthood.

NEW RESEARCH DIRECTIONS

In addition to organizing existing research, our consideration of subjective age through the lens of both life span and life course perspectives illustrates the use of giving greater attention to issues of time in future research. The life span perspective illuminates variation across and within life stages by pointing to developmental processes that may underlie them. The life course perspective brings to light other temporal issues, raising alternative explanations for age-related patterns in subjective age, as well as pointing to social, cultural, and historical factors that may intervene in developmental processes. We point to questions raised by each perspective, along with those suggested by their collective consideration.

Beyond raising questions about the nature of underlying personal models, the salience and meaning of particular age cues, and the intervening role of related age attitudes, a life span perspective calls for closer attention to the multidimensional nature of subjective age. Although several researchers have found that individual measures of subjective age (e.g., felt age, look age, act age) described initially by Kastenbaum et al. (1972) are intercorrelated and operate statistically as a unidimensional construct (e.g., Hubley & Russell, 2007; Teuscher, 2007), others have argued that subjective age should be treated as multidimensional. For example, Montepare (1996a, 1996c) has found that although multidimensional measures of psychological, physical, and social subjective age may show similar patterns across age groups, they show different associations with other personal variables at various ages (e.g., self-esteem, aspects of body image, personality attributes). Other researchers have also called for more differentiated measures of subjective age. For example, Weiss and Lang (2012) proposed that age perceptions entail generational identity and that subjective age and generational identity involve different cognitive representations of age and have different social psychological implications. Thus, more work is needed to examine the components and consequences of dimensions of age identity.

Although the literature provides some insight into the unfolding of subjective age over time, studies have not yet fully appreciated the principle of lifelong development—likely a result of both data limitations and social science orientations toward the study of human lives within, rather than across, life stages. Studies of subjective age tend to focus on specific life stages—typically adolescence (e.g., Galambos et al., 2005) or later adulthood (e.g., Bowling et al., 2005). As a result, we know little about how subjective age changes across wide swathes of human lives, a void begging questions for future research. For example, how do subjective ages in childhood or adolescence relate to those observed across stages of adulthood? It is plausible that an older identity at a relatively young age in adolescence or early adulthood foreshadows a trajectory of less youthful identities over middle and later life; however, other patterns are possible as well. Longitudinal studies are needed that provide not only descriptions of how subjective age changes over multiple life decades but also estimates of variability around the general patterns and social and psychological factors producing it. Studying subjective age over longer spans of time also permits a closer examination of the interplay of biography and history by providing a larger window within which social change can occur and can be detected. For example, data spanning the past four decades would allow an examination of how average patterns and variation in subjective age have been affected by a wide range of social changes, such as those related to SES conditions, health patterns, and age-related demographic trends.

Further research is needed to explore trajectories within which events or transitions are embedded. For example, one of the strongest and most consistent predictors of subjective age is health (e.g., Barrett, 2003; Bowling et al., 2005; Hubley & Russell, 2009; Kaufman & Elder, 2003); however, studies have primarily examined current health rather than sequences of health ratings or events. Illustrating an exception, Schafer and Shippee (2010) examined the decade-long effect of number of illnesses and change in illnesses and found that higher initial levels and greater increases in illness predicted older age identities. However, the life course principle of timing, along with lifelong development, highlights the use of examining such changes within the context of health trajectories that span the life course. One question raised by this consideration is how health status and behaviors in early life influence subjective age in later life, including its direction and rate of change over time.

Application of the life course principle of linked lives highlights the importance of not only considering a wider range of social relationships but also taking a longer range view of them. Social relationships receiving less attention include those with significant others and friends. However, some research points to their importance. For example, Barrett (2005) reported that having an older or less healthy spouse or partner not only predicted feeling older but also suppressed the effect of gender on subjective age. The study also found that perceived control over intimate relationships was associated with subjective age, with greater control being associated with feeling younger. Studies are needed examining characteristics of other relationships, such as those with friends who are likely to be age peers and may serve as reference groups for one's own aging. Studies also should attend to changes in relationships across long time spans, as underscored by the principles of linked lives and lifelong development. Although some research has looked at the effect of change in family roles and relationships across waves on subjective age (Schafer & Shippee, 2010), this work did not examine family trajectories and their characteristics, such as duration in statuses or number of transitions, that could have implications for subjective age.

Taken together, life span and life course perspectives beg additional questions for future research. For example, combining the life course perspective's focus on elements of social structure with the life span perspective's emphasis on developmental contexts within particular life stages raises the question of whether (and how) the influence of particular social institutions (e.g., media, education, work) or dimensions of inequality (e.g., race and ethnicity, gender) on subjective age varies across life stages. Another question centers on unpacking the mechanisms that link broad sociohistorical shifts—including changes in not only the age structuring of the life course but also the definitions and evaluations of various life stages—to individual-level perceptions, such as subjective age. A possible bridge across these levels of analysis involves research examining how subjective age is influenced by mesolevel social structures, including workplaces and family and friend networks, as they represent likely information sources and frames of reference about aging. Another avenue for further research raised by these perspectives focuses on examining the extent to which typical life span patterns of subjective age might vary along social structural dimensions, such as gender, class, or race and ethnicity. Research in this vein would provide a more nuanced understanding of systematic variation in how people navigate the developmental challenges they face at different life stages.

Our life span and life course consideration of subjective age also lays the groundwork for intervention studies. Interest in interventions is driven by the unprecedented rise in the aging population that calls for new ways to promote physical and psychological well-being. A promising avenue for intervention research centers on leveraging older adults' age identities, as feeling youthful has been associated with lower mortality and better health (Boehmer, 2007; Demakakos, Gjonca, & Nazroo, 2007; Kotter-Grühn, Kleinspehn-Ammerlahn, Gerstorf, & Smith, 2009; Uotinen, Rantanen, & Suutama, 2005). Interventions addressing younger individuals' age identities also are of interest, given that feeling older has been linked to riskier behaviors in adolescents and greater self-confidence and social potency in young adults (Galambos et al., 2007; Montepare, 1991). Although recent research has successfully shown that changes in subjective age can be experimentally manipulated (e.g., Stephan, Chalabaev, Kotter-Grühn, & Jaconelli, 2013), researchers interested in more long-lasting interventions should consider that different age identities have different values and implications at different points in the life span. Similarly, the methods or triggers needed to prompt shifts in subjective age that, in turn, are expected to induce positive behavioral or psychological outcomes, are likely to vary across the life span. Designing such interventions will be aided by the further exploration of the temporal dimensions of subjective age, an undertaking we hope will be facilitated by our application of life span and life course perspectives to the study of subjective age.

REFERENCES

Arbeau, K. J., Galambos, N. J., & Jansson, S. K. (2007). Dating, sex, and substance use as correlated of adolescents' subjective experience of age. *Journal of Adolescence, 30*, 435–447. http://dx.doi.org/10.1016/j.adolescence.2006.04.006

Ayalon, L., Doron, I., Bodner, E., & Inbar, N. (2014). Macro- and micro-level predictors of age categorization: Results from the European Social Survey. *European Journal of Ageing, 11*, 5–18. http://dx.doi.org/10.1007/s10433-013-0282-8

Ballard, K., Kuh, D., & Wadsworth, M. (2001). The role of the menopause in women's experiences of the "change of life." *Sociology of Health and Illness, 23*, 397–424. http://dx.doi.org/10.1111/1467-9566.00258

Baltes, P. B. (1987). Theoretical propositions of life span developmental psychology: On the dynamics between growth and decline. *Developmental Psychology, 23*, 611–626. http://dx.doi.org/10.1037/0012-1649.23.5.611

Barak, B. (2009). Age identity: A cross-cultural global approach. *International Journal of Behavioral Development, 33*, 2–11. http://dx.doi.org/10.1177/0165025408099485

Barak, B., & Stern, B. (1986). Subjective age correlates: A research note. *The Gerontologist, 5*, 571–578. http://dx.doi.org/10.1093/geront/26.5.571

Barker, E. T., & Galambos, N. L. (2005). Adolescents' implicit theories of maturity: Ages of adulthood, freedom, and fun. *Journal of Adolescent Research, 20*, 557–578. http://dx.doi.org/10.1177/0743558405274872

Barrett, A. E. (2003). Socioeconomic status and age identity: The role of dimensions of health in the subjective construction of age. *The Journals of Gerontology. Series B, Psychological and Social Sciences, 58*, S101–S109. http://dx.doi.org/10.1093/geronb/58.2.S101

Barrett, A. E. (2005). Gendered experiences in midlife: Implications for age identity. *Journal of Aging Studies, 19*, 163–183. http://dx.doi.org/ 10.1016/j.jaging.2004.05.002

Baum, S. K., & Boxley, R. L. (1983). Age identification in the elderly. *The Gerontologist, 23*, 532–537. http://dx.doi.org/10.1093/geront/23.5.532

Boehmer, S. (2007). Relationships between felt age and perceived disability, satisfaction with recovery, self-efficacy beliefs and coping strategies. *Journal of Health Psychology, 12*, 895–906. http://dx.doi.org/10.1177/1359105307082453

Bowling, A., See-Tai, S., Ebrahim, S., Gabriel, Z., & Solanki, P. (2005). Attributes of age-identity. *Ageing & Society, 2*, 479–500. http://dx.doi.org/10.1017/S0144686X05003818

Bultena, G. L., & Powers, E. A. (1978). Denial of aging: Age identification and reference group orientations. *Journal of Gerontology, 33*, 748–754. http://dx.doi.org/10.1093/geronj/33.5.748

Chudacoff, H. P. (1989). *How old are you? Age consciousness in American culture.* Princeton, NJ: Princeton University Press.

Demakakos, P., Gjonca, E., & Nazroo, J. (2007). Age identity, age perceptions, and health: Evidence from the English Longitudinal Study of Aging. *Annals of the New York Academy of Sciences, 1114*, 279–287. http://dx.doi.org/10.1196/annals.1396.021

Diehl, M., Wahl, H. W., Barrett, A. E., Brothers, A. F., Miche, M., Montepare, J. A., . . . Wurm, S. (2014). Awareness of aging: Theoretical considerations on an emerging concept. *Developmental Review, 34*, 93–113. http://dx.doi.org/10.1016/j.dr.2014.01.001

Elder, G. H., Jr. (1975). Age differentiation and the life course. *Annual Review of Sociology*, *1*, 165–190. http://dx.doi.org/10.1146/annurev.so.01.080175.001121

Elder, G. H., Jr., & Johnson, M. K. (2002). The life course and aging: Challenges, lessons, and new directions. In R. A. Settersten, Jr. (Ed.), *Invitation to the life course: Toward new understandings of later life* (pp. 49–81). Amityville, NY: Baywood.

Elder, G. H., Jr., Johnson, M. K., & Crosnoe, R. (2003). The emergence and development of life course theory. In J. T. Mortimer & M. J. Shanahan (Eds.), *Handbook of the life course* (pp. 3–19). New York, NY: Plenum Press. http://dx.doi.org/10.1007/978-0-306-48247-2_1

Foster, H., Hagan, J., & Brooks-Gunn, J. (2008). Growing up fast: Stress exposure and subjective "weathering" in emerging adulthood. *Journal of Health and Social Behavior*, *49*, 162–77. http://dx.doi.org/10.1177/002214650804900204

Galambos, N. L., Albrecht, A. K., & Jansson, S. M. (2009). Dating, sex, and substance use predict increases in adolescents' subjective age across two years. *International Journal of Behavioral Development*, *33*, 32–41. http://dx.doi.org/10.1177/0165025408095552

Galambos, N. L., Darrah, J., & Magill-Evans, J. (2007). Subjective age in the transition to adulthood for persons with and without motor disabilities. *Journal of Youth and Adolescence*, *36*, 825–834. http://dx.doi.org/10.1007/s10964-007-9190-6

Galambos, N. L., Kolaric, G. C., Sears, H. A., & Maggs, J. L. (1999). Adolescents' subjective age: An indicator of perceived maturity. *Journal of Research on Adolescence*, *9*, 309–337. http://dx.doi.org/10.1207/s15327795jra0903_4

Galambos, N. L., Turner, P. K., & Tilton-Weaver, L. C. (2005). Chronological and subjective age in emerging adulthood: The crossover effect. *Journal of Adolescent Research*, *20*, 538–556. http://dx.doi.org/10.1177/0743558405274876

George, L. K. (1996). Missing links: The case for a social psychology of the life course. *The Gerontologist*, *36*, 248–255. http://dx.doi.org/10.1093/geront/36.2.248

Giles, H., Fox, S., Harwood, J., & Williams, A. (1994). Talking age and aging talk: Communicating through the life span. In M. Hummert, J. M. Wiemann, & J. F. Nussbaum (Eds.), *Interpersonal communication in older adulthood: Interdisciplinary theory and research* (pp. 130–161). Thousand Oaks, CA: Sage.

Giles, H., McIlrath, M., Mulac, A., & McCann, R. M. (2010). Expressing age salience: Three generations' reported events, frequencies, and valences. *International Journal of the Sociology of Language*, *206*, 73–91.

Girman, C. J., Rhodes, T., Lilly, F. R. W., Guo, S. S., Siervogel, R. M., Patrick, D. L., & Chumlea, W. C. (1998). Effects of self-perceived hair loss in a community sample of men. *Dermatology*, *197*, 223–229. http://dx.doi.org/10.1159/000018001

Goldsmith, R. E., & Heiens, R. A. (1992). Subjective age: A test of five hypotheses. *The Gerontologist*, *32*, 312–317. http://dx.doi.org/10.1093/geront/32.3.312

Han, S., & Moen, P. (1999). Clocking out: Temporal patterning of retirement. *American Journal of Sociology*, *105*, 191–236. http://dx.doi.org/10.1086/210271

Harwood, J. (2007). *Understanding communication and aging: Developing knowledge and awareness*. Thousand Oaks, CA: Sage.

Heckhausen, J. (1997). Developmental regulation across adulthood: Primary and secondary control of age-related challenges. *Developmental Psychology, 33,* 176–187. http://dx.doi.org/10.1037/0012-1649.33.1.176

Heckhausen, J., Dixon, R. A., & Baltes, P. B. (1989). Gains and losses in development throughout adulthood as perceived by different adult age groups. *Developmental Psychology, 25,* 109–121. http://dx.doi.org/10.1037/0012-1649.25.1.109

Henderson, K. V., Goldsmith, R. E., & Flynn, L. R. (1995). Demographic characteristics of subjective age. *Journal of Social Psychology, 135,* 447–457. http://dx.doi.org/10.1080/00224545.1995.9712214

Hitlin, S., & Elder, G. H., Jr. (2007). Time, self, and the curiously abstract concept of agency. *Sociological Theory, 25,* 170–191. http://dx.doi.org/10.1111/j.1467-9558.2007.00303.x

Hubley, A. M., & Russell, L. B. (2007). Prediction of subjective age, desired age, and age satisfaction in older adults: Do some health dimensions contribute more than others? *International Journal of Behavioral Development, 33,* 12–21. http://dx.doi.org/10.1177/0165025408099486

Hubley, A. M., & Russell, L. B. (2009). Prediction of subjective age, desired age, and age satisfaction in older adults: Do some health dimensions contribute more than others? *International Journal of Behavioral Development, 33,* 12–21. http://dx.doi.org/10.1177/0165025408099486

Johnson, M. K., Berg, J. A., & Sirotzki, T. (2007). Differentiation in self-perceived adulthood: Extending the confluence model of subjective age identity. *Social Psychology Quarterly, 70,* 243–261. http://dx.doi.org/10.1177/019027250707000304

Johnson, M. K., & Mollborn, S. (2009). Growing up faster, feeling older: Hardship in childhood and adolescence. *Social Psychology Quarterly, 72,* 39–60. http://dx.doi.org/10.1177/019027250907200105

Kastenbaum, R., Derbin, V., Sabatini, P., & Artt, S. (1972). The ages of me: Toward personal and interpersonal definitions of functional aging. *Aging and Human Development, 3,* 197–211. http://dx.doi.org/10.2190/TUJR-WTXK-866Q-8QU7

Kaufman, G., & Elder, G. H., Jr. (2003). Grandparenting and age identity. *Journal of Aging Studies, 17,* 269–282. http://dx.doi.org/10.1016/S0890-4065(03)00030-6

Keith, P. M. (1977). Life changes, stereotyping, and age identification. *Psychological Reports, 41,* 661–666. http://dx.doi.org/10.2466/pr0.1977.41.2.661

Kleinspehn-Ammerlahn, A., Kotter-Grühn, D., & Smith, J. (2008). Self-perceptions of aging: Do subjective age and satisfaction with aging change during old age? *The Journals of Gerontology. Series B, Psychological Sciences and Social Sciences, 63,* P377–P385. http://dx.doi.org/10.1093/geronb/63.6.P377

Kotter-Grühn, D., Kleinspehn-Ammerlahn, A., Gerstorf, D., & Smith, J. (2009). Self-perceptions of aging predict mortality and change with approaching death: 16-year longitudinal results from the Berlin Aging Study. *Psychology and Aging, 24,* 654–667. http://dx.doi.org/10.1037/a0016510

Lewis, M., & Brooks-Gunn, J. (1979). *Social cognition and the acquisition of self.* New York, NY: Plenum Press.

Logan, J. R., Ward, R., & Spitze, G. (1992). "As old as you feel": Age identity in middle and later life. *Social Forces, 71,* 451–467.

Lowe, S. R., Dillon, C. O., Rhodes, J. E., & Zwiebach, L. (2013). Defining adult experiences: Perspectives of a diverse sample of young adults. *Journal of Adolescent Research, 28,* 31–68. http://dx.doi.org/10.1177/0743558411435854

Macia, E., DuBoz, P., Montepare, J. M., & Gueye, L. (2012). Age identity, self-rated health, and life satisfaction among older adults in Dakar, Senegal. *European Journal of Ageing, 9,* 243–253. http://dx.doi.org/10.1007/s10433-012-0227-7

Markides, K. S. (1980). Ethnic differences in age identification: A study of older Mexican-Americans and Anglos. *Social Science Quarterly, 60,* 659–666.

Markides, K., & Boldt, J. (1983). Change in subjective age among the elderly: A longitudinal analysis. *The Gerontologist, 23,* 422–427. http://dx.doi.org/10.1093/geront/23.4.422

McFarland, C., Ross, M., & Giltrow, M. (1992). Biased recollections in older adults: The role of implicit theories of aging. *Journal of Personality and Social Psychology, 62,* 837–850. http://dx.doi.org/10.1037/0022-3514.62.5.837

Mock, S. E., & Eibach, R. P. (2011). Aging attitudes moderate the effect of subjective age on psychological well-being: Evidence from a 10-year longitudinal study. *Psychology and Aging, 26,* 979–986. http://dx.doi.org/10.1037/a0023877

Montepare, J. M. (1991). Characteristics and psychological correlates of young adult men's and women's subjective age. *Sex Roles, 24,* 323–333. http://dx.doi.org/10.1007/BF00288305

Montepare, J. M. (1996a). An assessment of adults' perceptions of their psychological, physical, and social ages. *Journal of Clinical Geropsychology, 2,* 117–128.

Montepare, J. M. (1996b). Variations in adults' subjective ages in relation to birthday nearness, age awareness, and attitudes toward aging. *Journal of Adult Development, 3,* 193–203. http://dx.doi.org/10.1007/BF02281963

Montepare, J. M. (1996c). Actual and subjective-related age differences in women's attitudes toward their bodies across the life span. *Journal of Adult Development, 3,* 171–182. http://dx.doi.org/10.1007/BF02285777

Montepare, J. M. (2009). Subjective age: A guiding life span framework. *International Journal of Behavioral Development, 33,* 42–46. http://dx.doi.org/10.1177/0165025408095551

Montepare, J. M., & Birchander, E. (1994, November). *Social circles and subjective age identities.* Paper presented at the meeting of the Gerontological Association of America, Atlanta, GA.

Montepare, J. M., & Clements, A. (1995, April). *"The denial of youth": Implications for age identification in young adult men and women.* Paper presented at the meeting of the Eastern Psychological Association, Boston, MA.

Montepare, J. M., & Clements, A. (2001). "Age schemas": Guides to processing information about the self. *Journal of Adult Development, 8,* 99–108. http://dx.doi.org/10.1023/A:1026493818246

Montepare, J. M., & Lachman, M. E. (1989). "You're only as old as you feel": Self-perceptions of age, fears of aging, and life satisfaction from adolescence to old age. *Psychology and Aging, 4,* 73–89. http://dx.doi.org/10.1037/0882-7974.4.1.73

Montepare, J. M., & Petrov, P. M. (2012, March). *Personal models of development: A life drawing analysis*. Paper presented at the meeting of the Eastern Psychological Association, Pittsburg, PA.

Montepare, J. M., Reirdan, J., Koff, E., & Stubbs, P. (1989, June). *The impact of biological events on females' subjective age identities*. Paper presented at the meeting of the Society for Menstrual Cycle Research, Salt Lake City, Utah.

Montepare, J. M., & Zebrowitz, L. A. (1998). "Person perception comes of age": The salience and significance of age in social judgments. In M. Zanna (Ed.), *Advances in experimental social psychology* (Vol. 30, pp. 93–161). San Diego, CA: Academic Press.

Nilsson, M., Sarvimäki, A., & Ekman, S. (2000). Feelingold: Being in a phase of transition in later life. *Nursing Inquiry, 7*, 41–49. http://dx.doi.org/10.1046/j.1440-1800.2000.00049.x

O'Brien-Suric, N. (2013). A cross-national comparison of perceptions of aging and older adults. A discussion of comparative analysis and findings of the five countries: Part 2. *Care Management Journals, 14*, 89–107. http://dx.doi.org/10.1891/1521-0987.14.2.89

Peters, G. R. (1971). Self-conceptions of the aged, age identification, and aging. *The Gerontologist, 11*, 69–73. http://dx.doi.org/10.1093/geront/11.4_Part_2.69

Pinquart, M., & Sörensen, S. (2001). Gender differences in self-concept and psychological well-being in old age: A meta-analysis. *The Journals of Gerontology. Series B, Psychological Sciences and Social Sciences, 56*, P123–P195.

Ross, M. (1989). Relation of implicit theories to the construction of personal histories. *Psychological Review, 96*, 341–357. http://dx.doi.org/10.1037/0033-295X.96.2.341

Ross, M., McFarland, C., & Fletcher, G. J. (1981). The effect of attitude on the recall of personal histories. *Journal of Personality and Social Psychology, 40*, 627–634. http://dx.doi.org/10.1037/0022-3514.40.4.627

Rubin, D. C., & Berntsen, D. (2006). People over forty feel 20% younger than their age: Subjective age across the life span. *Psychonomic Bulletin & Review, 13*, 776–780. http://dx.doi.org/10.3758/BF03193996

Sato, S., Shimonaka, Y., Nakazato, K., & Kawaai, C. (1997). A life span developmental study of age identity: Cohort and gender differences. *Japanese Journal of Developmental Psychology, 8*, 88–97.

Schafer, M. H. (2009). Parental death and subjective age: Indelible imprints from early in the life course? *Sociological Inquiry, 79*, 75–97. http://dx.doi.org/10.1111/j.1475-682X.2008.00270.x

Schafer, M. H., & Shippee, T. P. (2010). Age identity in context: Stress and the subjective side of aging. *Social Psychology Quarterly, 73*, 245–264. http://dx.doi.org/10.1177/0190272510379751

Settersten, R. A. (1999). *Lives in time and place: The problems and promises of developmental science*. Amityville, NY: Baywood.

Settersten, R. A., Jr., & Mayer, K. U. (1997). The measurement of age, age structuring, and the life course. *Annual Review of Sociology, 23*, 233–262. http://dx.doi.org/10.1146/annurev.soc.23.1.233

Sherman, S. (1994). Changes in age identity: Self perceptions in middle and later life. *Journal of Aging Studies, 8*, 397–412. http://dx.doi.org/10.1016/0890-4065(94)90011-6

Stephan, Y., Chalabaev, A., Kotter-Grühn, D., & Jaconelli, A. (2013). "Feeling younger, being stronger": An experimental study of subjective age and physical functioning among older adults. *The Journals of Gerontology. Series B, Psychological Sciences and Social Sciences, 68*, 1–7. http://dx.doi.org/10.1093/geronb/gbs037

Stephan, Y., Demulier, V., & Terracciano, A. (2012). Personality, self-rated health, and subjective age in a life span sample: The moderating role of chronological age. *Psychology and Aging, 27*, 875–880. http://dx.doi.org/10.1037/a0028301

Teuscher, U. (2007). Subjective age bias: A motivational and information processing approach. *International Journal of Behavioral Development, 33*, 18–27.

Uotinen, V. (1998). Age identification: A comparison between Finnish and North-American cultures. *International Journal of Aging and Human Development, 46*, 109–124. http://dx.doi.org/10.2190/WAVV-14YU-1UV3-0MPN

Uotinen, V., Rantanen, T., & Suutama, T. (2005). Perceived age as a predictor of old age mortality: A 13-year prospective study. *Age and Ageing, 34*, 368–372. http://dx.doi.org/10.1093/ageing/afi091

Uotinen, V., Rantanen, T., Suutama, T., & Ruoppila, I. (2006). Change in subjective age among older people over an eight-year follow-up: "Getting older and feeling younger?" *Experimental Aging Research, 32*, 381–393. http://dx.doi.org/10.1080/03610730600875759

Ward, R. (1977). The impact of subjective age and stigma on older persons. *Journal of Gerontology, 32*, 227–232. http://dx.doi.org/10.1093/geronj/32.2.227

Ward, R. A. (2013). Change in perceived age in middle and later life. *International Journal of Aging and Human Development, 76*, 281–297. http://dx.doi.org/10.2190/AG.76.3.e

Weiss, D., & Lang, F. R. (2012). "They" are old but "I" feel younger: Age-group dissociation as a self-protective strategy in old age. *Psychology and Aging, 27*, 153–163. http://dx.doi.org/10.1037/a0024887

Westerhof, G. J. (2008). Age identity. In D. Carr (Ed.), *Encyclopedia of the life course and human development* (Vol. 3, pp. 10–14). Farmington Hills, MI: Thomson/Gale.

Westerhof, G. J., & Barrett, A. E. (2005). Age identity and subjective well-being: A comparison of the United States and Germany. *The Journals of Gerontology. Series B, Psychological Sciences and Social Sciences, 60*, S129–S136.

Westerhof, G. J., Barrett, A. E., & Steverink, N. (2003). Forever young? A comparison of age identities in the United States and Germany. *Research on Aging, 25*, 366–383. http://dx.doi.org/10.1177/0164027503025004002

Westerhof, G. J., Whitbourne, S. K., & Freeman, G. P. (2012). The aging self in a cultural context: The relation of conceptions of aging to identity processes and self-esteem in the United States and the Netherlands. *The Journals of Gerontology. Series B, Psychological Sciences and Social Sciences, 67*, 52–60. http://dx.doi.org/10.1093/geronb/gbr075

Whitbourne, S. K. (1985). *The aging body: Physiological changes and psychological consequences.* New York, NY: Springer-Verlag.

CHAPTER 4

Experimental Research on Age Stereotypes

Insights for Subjective Aging

Mary Lee Hummert

ABSTRACT

The chapter begins with a discussion of experimental and quasi-experimental research on the content and dimensionality of age stereotypes with implications for the study of subjective age. It focuses next on research documenting the behavioral and psychological effects of age stereotypes on older individuals, highlighting the ways in which awareness of age-related change, age identity, and subjective age enter into that process. The chapter concludes with a discussion of future directions for the experimental investigation of the relationship between age stereotypes and subjective aging. Three areas for future research are highlighted: (a) investigation of the contextual cues and awareness of age-related change experiences that call forth positive and negative age stereotype and stereotype domains; (b) the role of age identification or dissociation in influencing subjective age, as well as the mediating role of subjective age in buffering or increasing the effects of age stereotypes on self-perceptions and behaviors of older persons, deserve study; and (c) examination of the extent to which behavioral assimilation to age stereotypes creates a feedback cycle involving awareness of aging experiences and subjective age.

INTRODUCTION

Age stereotypes lurk behind any discussion of subjective age, the focus of this volume of the *Annual Review of Gerontology and Geriatrics*. Age stereotypes, particularly negative age stereotypes, are referenced in research demonstrating that middle-aged and older persons report older subjective ages after being primed with age stereotypes (Kotter-Grühn & Hess, 2012; O'Brien & Hummert, 2006). Other research has examined the link between age stereotypes, subjective age, and self-perceptions, indicating that younger subjective ages may serve to distance older adults from negative age stereotypes and therefore contribute to their psychological well-being (Weiss & Lang, 2012). This chapter explores the relationship between age stereotypes and subjective age to highlight how age stereotype research can inform this study of subjective aging.

The chapter begins with a discussion of experimental and quasi-experimental research on the content and dimensionality of age stereotypes with implications for the study of subjective age. It focuses next on research documenting the behavioral and psychological effects of age stereotypes on older individuals, highlighting the ways in which awareness of age-related change, age identity, and subjective age enter into that process. The chapter concludes with a discussion of future directions for the experimental investigation of the relationship between age stereotypes and subjective aging.

RESEARCH ON THE CONTENT AND DIMENSIONALITY OF AGE STEREOTYPES

Age stereotypes have been variously conceptualized by psychologists historically. The research discussed here views age stereotypes from a *social cognitive framework* as psychological constructs, specifically as person perception schemas which facilitate interpretation of new information (Hummert, 1999, 2011; Operario & Fiske, 2004). As psychological constructs, age stereotypes exist within individuals. Although stereotypes encompass shared cultural perceptions about the characteristics of older people, they also include personal experiences—both of older people and of one's own progression through the lifespan. Thus, despite the commonality of perceptions that we associate with the label *stereotype*, the content of age stereotypes will vary to some extent across individuals (Hummert, Garstka, Shaner, & Strahm, 1994). Social cognitive research on the nature of age stereotypes has documented characteristics of their content and their effects which are relevant to subjective age.

Positive and Negative Age Stereotypes

Although early research on age stereotypes assumed that stereotypes were exclusively negative (Crockett & Hummert, 1987), social cognitive research on the content of age stereotypes revealed the coexistence of positive age stereotypes as well as multiple subtypes of the positive and negative stereotypes (Brewer, Dull, & Lui, 1981; Schmidt & Boland, 1986). Other research confirmed the positive and negative dimensions of age stereotypes while demonstrating that the stereotypes varied in complexity across age groups (Brewer & Lui, 1984; Chasteen, Schwarz, & Park, 2002; Hummert et al., 1994).

For example, Hummert et al. (1994) asked young, middle-aged, and older adult participants to sort 97 traits associated with the category *older adult* into groups by "putting the traits that would be found in the same elderly person into a single group or pile" (p. P242). The data were analyzed using cluster analysis. For all three age groups, the resulting tree diagrams revealed two high-level clusters of positive and negative traits, with several subcategories or multiple stereotypes within these two clusters. Table 4.1 presents the positive and negative subcategories for each age group with representative traits associated with those stereotypes, revealing that seven subcategories (three positive and four negative) were evident in some form in the stereotype subsets of all three age groups. Hummert et al. referred to these as "cultural archetypes of aging" (p. P249).

However, as Table 4.1 also reveals, the number of subcategories increased across the three age groups (from young to middle-aged to older adult), indicating greater complexity in the age stereotypes held by middle-aged than younger participants and by older than middle-aged participants. The additional stereotypes held by older and middle-aged participants were often subdivisions of broader stereotypes held by those in a younger age group. These results suggested that those in the two older groups made finer discriminations among types of older persons than did the young participants.

Another fact evident in Table 4.1 is that the age stereotypes held by the middle-aged and older participants may have been more complex than those of the young participants, but they were not more positive. For all age groups, the number of negative stereotypes exceeded the number of positive stereotypes. This result reflects a general pattern in age stereotype research: Negative age stereotypes predominate over positive stereotypes (Crockett & Hummert, 1987; Hess, 2006; Hummert, 2011; Kite & Johnson, 1988; Kite, Stockdale, Whitley, & Johnson, 2002; Kite & Wagner, 2002). Experimental research demonstrates that, in comparison to positive age stereotypes, negative age stereotypes are more accessible as indicated by response times on lexical decision tasks (Perdue & Gurtman, 1990; Wentura & Brandstädter, 2003) and hit/error rates on memory recognition tasks (Krings, 2004). These results hold for older participants as well as younger ones. In addition, Meisner's (2012) meta-analysis of the priming effects of positive and negative age stereotypes on the behavior of older persons revealed that the effects of negative stereotypes "were almost three times larger than positive effects, compared with a neutral referent" (p. 16).

TABLE 4.1

Positive and Negative Age Stereotypes and Representative Traits by Age Group:
Summary of Data Reported in Hummert et al. (1994)

Participant Age Group		
Young **(Aged 18–24 Years)**	**Middle-Aged** **(Aged 36–50 Years)**	**Older** **(Aged 62–84 Years)**
Positive stereotypes		
Golden ager: sociable, future-oriented, capable, +22 traits	*Golden ager:* sociable, future-oriented, capable, +20 traits	*Golden ager:* sociable, future-oriented, capable, +20 traits
Perfect grandparent: kind, family-oriented, generous, +10 more traits	*Perfect grandparent:* kind, family-oriented, generous, +10 traits	*Perfect grandparent:* kind, family-oriented, generous, +7 traits
John Wayne conservative: patriotic, retired, proud, +7 traits	*John Wayne conservative:* patriotic, retired, proud, +7 traits	*John Wayne conservative:* patriotic, retired, proud, +6 traits
	Liberal matriarch/patriarch: liberal, mellow, wealthy	*Activist:* political, sexual, health-conscious, liberal
		Small town neighbor: frugal, old-fashioned, tough, +2 traits
Negative stereotypes		
Shrew/curmudgeon: complaining, ill-tempered, bitter, +11 traits	*Shrew/curmudgeon:* complaining, ill-tempered, bitter, +7 traits	*Shrew/curmudgeon:* complaining, ill-tempered, bitter, +2 traits
Despondent: depressed, sad, lonely, +4 traits	*Despondent:* depressed, sad, lonely, +5 traits	*Despondent:* depressed, sad, neglected, +4 traits
Severely impaired: incoherent, slow-thinking, senile, +8 traits	*Severely impaired:* incoherent, slow-thinking, senile, +3 traits	*Severely impaired:* incoherent, slow-thinking, senile, +5 traits
Recluse: quiet, timid, naïve, +2 traits	*Recluse:* quiet, timid, naïve	*Recluse:* timid, poor, sedentary
Vulnerable: afraid, worried, victimized, +6 traits	*Mildly impaired:* slow-moving, tired, dependent, +8 traits	*Mildly impaired:* slow-moving, tired, dependent, +4 traits
	Self-centered: miserly, greedy, humorless, +2 traits	*Self-centered:* miserly, greedy, humorless, +5 traits
		Elitist: prejudiced, wary, snobbish, +2 traits

Domain Specificity: A New View of Stereotype Multidimensionality
In recent years, psychologists have proposed an alternative to the view of multiple positive and negative age stereotypes, which represent different types or subcategories of older persons. They propose instead that there are multiple positive and negative age stereotypes defined by specific domains or contexts (Casper, Rothermund, & Wentura, 2011; Kornadt & Rothermund, 2011, 2012; see Chapter 6 by Kornadt & Rothermund, this volume). Support for this alternative perspective on age stereotypes can be found in prior experimental research on the role of age stereotypes in person perception. For instance, reviews and meta-analyses of the age stereotype literature revealed that individuating information played a stronger role than a general negative age stereotype in experiments comparing judgments of old and young targets (Crockett & Hummert, 1987; Hummert, 1999; Kite & Johnson, 1988; Kite et al., 2005). In some experiments, older targets were judged no differently or even more positively on some dimensions than younger targets with the same characteristics. In other experiments, context affected behaviors toward and judgments of the same older target. For instance, Hummert, Shaner, Garstka, and Henry (1998) found that participants, especially young adult participants, adopted an age-adapted communication style when addressing a *golden ager* target (see Table 4.1) presented in a hospital setting, whereas presentation of the same target in a community context elicited standard adult communication.

Experiments designed to test the effects of age stereotypes on older persons' behavior also produced results which suggest the importance of specific domains (e.g., memory performance, interpersonal relations, physical strength) in influencing behavior. First, the personal relevance of the domain to the individual can increase the effects of negative stereotypes. For example, Hess, Auman, Colcombe, and Rahhal (2003) found that older adults for whom memory ability was important exhibited poorer memory after being primed with a negative age stereotype about memory than did those for whom memory ability was less important. Second, the match between stereotype domain and task may be a key factor in boosting performance via positive age stereotypes as indicated by results reported by Levy and Leifheit-Limson (2009). These researchers matched stereotype primes and behavioral tasks in a 2 (positive/negative) × 2 (cognitive/physical) × 2 (task domain: photo recall/balance task) with repeated measures on the last factor. Results showed better performance by participants in the positive prime conditions in comparison to those in the negative prime conditions only when the prime matched the behavioral task. That is, participants in the positive prime condition performed better on the balance task than those in the negative prime condition only when the positive primes (e.g., fit, hardy) and the negative primes (e.g., feeble, shaky) tapped into the physical domain but not when they primed the cognitive domain (e.g., sage, alert for positive primes; dementia, confused for negative primes). Similarly, participants in the positive prime condition performed better on the photo-recall task than those in the negative prime condition only when the positive and negative primes were cognitive in nature.

Casper et al. (2011) tested the context dependence of specific age stereotypes in two experiments using sentence and photo primes followed by a lexical decision task. Primes combined relevant or irrelevant category information (old or young photo) with a sentence relevant (e.g., *she is crossing the street*) to a specific age stereotype such as *slow* or irrelevant to the stereotype (e.g., *she is watering the flowers*). Participants responded more quickly on the lexical decision task when the lexical decision followed a photo of an older person and a sentence relevant to the age stereotype than when the photo and/or the sentence were irrelevant to the category. These results supported the importance of matching both the context and the age category to the target stereotype.

Kornadt and Rothermund (2011) examined the domain specificity of age stereotypes by asking participants to complete a 27-item questionnaire designed to assess eight life domains developed from interviews and the prior literature: (a) family and partnerships; (b) friends and acquaintances; (c) religion and spirituality; (d) leisure and social or civic activities; (e) personality and way of living; (f) financial situation and dealing with money-related issues; (g) work and employment; and (h) physical and mental fitness, health, and appearance. To gain insights into the similarities and differences in the domain stereotypes across age groups, they included participants from five birth cohorts: 1929–1938, 1939–1948, 1949–1958, 1959–1968, and 1969–1978. Participants rated each questionnaire item to indicate the positivity of their assessment of "old persons" on it. Results confirmed the validity of the eight domain stereotypes and identified both domain and cohort differences in the positivity of ratings. In general, older persons were rated most positively in the family, religion, and spirituality domains. They were rated most negatively in the friends and financial domains. Older cohorts provided more positive assessments across domains than younger cohorts with two exceptions: (a) Younger cohorts were more positive than older cohorts about the religious domain stereotype, and (b) younger cohorts evaluated the friends domain similarly to older cohorts.

Figure 4.1 illustrates how the positive and negative dimensions of the eight stereotype domains from Kornadt and Rothermund (2011) could relate to the seven positive and negative shared stereotypes identified in Hummert et al. (1994). Because older individuals operate in each of the eight domains, their characteristics and behaviors in one domain could suggest a negative age stereotype, whereas other characteristics and behaviors could activate a positive age

Stereotype Domains

Positive Stereotypes		Negative Stereotypes
Golden ager	+ Leisure and social/civic	_ *Shrew/curmudgeon*
Lively, sociable, future-	activities	Complaining, bitter, ill-
Oriented, fun-loving, happy,		Tempered, stubborn,
active, interesting, alert,	+ Friends and acquaintances	_ Demanding, prejudiced
Capable	+ Work and employment	_
		Despondent
Perfect grandparent	+ Family and partnerships	_ Depressed, sad, hopeless,
Kind, loving, family-oriented,	+ Personality and way of living	_ Afraid, neglected, lonely
Generous, understanding, wise		
	+ Physical/mental fitness,	_ *Severely impaired*
John Wayne conservative	health, and appearance	Incoherent, slow-thinking,
Patriotic, proud, determined,		senile, inarticulate,
Retired, religious, nostalgic,	+ Religion and spirituality	_ Incompetent, feeble,
Reminiscent	+ Financial situation	_ forgetful
		Recluse
		Quiet, timid, naive

FIGURE 4.1 Relationship between the seven positive and negative age stereotypes shared by young, middle-aged, and older adult participants in Hummert et al. (1994) and the eight age stereotype domains identified by Kornadt and Rothermund (2012).

stereotype. Thus, a person with the social skills of a golden ager who has age-related physical disabilities could be stereotyped positively or negatively depending on which domain is emphasized in the situation, as found in Hummert et al. (1998). From the domain perspective, the golden ager and perfect grandparent age stereotypes at the person level could represent positive stereotypes for friends and acquaintances or personality and way of living domains, whereas the shrew/curmudgeon and despondent age stereotypes could represent negative stereotypes for those domains.

AGE STEREOTYPE EFFECTS, AGE IDENTITY, AND SUBJECTIVE AGE

A substantial body of research has demonstrated that age stereotypes operate implicitly and explicitly to affect the psychological well-being and behaviors of older individuals (Hess, 2006; Hummert, 2011; Levy, 2003, 2009). The emphasis has been on behavioral assimilation to age stereotypes, whether positive or negative, and related effects on psychological measures such as self-esteem. Two psychological mechanisms have received the most attention in this research: self-stereotyping (Levy, 1996, 2003, 2009) and stereotype threat (Chasteen, Bhattacharyya, Horhota, Tam, & Hasher, 2005; Hess et al., 2003; Hess & Hinson, 2006).

According to Levy's (2009) *stereotype embodiment theory*, self-stereotyping results from older adults' internalizing cultural age stereotypes and incorporating them into their self-perceptions. Self-stereotyping predicts that only self-relevant stereotypes affect behavior as well as that the effects of stereotypes occur implicitly. Supporting this view, Levy (1996) found that older, but not younger participants, exposed to subliminal negative stereotype primes performed more poorly on memory measures than did the older participants exposed to positive primes. Stereotype threat also predicts behavioral assimilation to stereotypes of one's group but through awareness of the stereotype and the fear of confirming it as valid—and self-descriptive—through one's behavior (Steele, Spencer, & Aronson, 2002). Like self-stereotyping, stereotype threat is expected to occur only when the group stereotype is salient to the self. Consistent with this expectation, Hess et al. (2003) found that memory performance of older, but not younger, participants who read a news article confirming the age–memory stereotype declined from baseline, whereas the performance of those who read an article disconfirming the stereotype improved from baseline.

Although this description presents self-stereotyping and stereotype threat as distinct mechanisms, they produce similar effects in inducing assimilation to age stereotypes (Hess, Emery, & Queen, 2009; Hummert, 2011). In addition, situational factors such as context, time constraints, or the match between a task and a stereotype domain can increase the impact of age stereotypes on behavior (Auman, Bosworth, & Hess, 2005; Hess et al., 2009; Levy & Leifheit-Limson, 2009). Likewise, individual differences in age identity, subjective age, the experience of age stigma, or the personal importance of a domain can affect susceptibility to the effects of age stereotypes (Hess et al., 2003; Kang & Chasteen, 2009; O'Brien & Hummert, 2006; see Chapter 5 by Chasteen & Cary, this volume, for a discussion of age stigma). The role of age identity is of particular interest because of its connection to subjective age (Weiss & Lang, 2012). Two studies are illustrative in this regard.

O'Brien and Hummert (2006) collected implicit age identity measures from middle-aged participants before administering memory tests and collecting psychological measures, including subjective age (Montepare, 1996). To provide a test of stereotype threat and self-stereotyping theories, participants were told that their memory ability would be compared either to people younger than 25 years (stereotype threat) or to those older than 75 years (self-stereotyping), whereas a third group of middle-aged participants served as a control. Results were consistent with self-stereotyping theory in that participants in the old comparison group exhibited poorer recall and reported older subjective ages than those in the young comparison and control groups. However, age identity moderated the self-stereotyping effects: Only those in the old comparison group with a mixed (youthful/older) implicit age identity had poorer recall than those in the other two groups.

O'Brien and Hummert (2006) demonstrated that an older age identity could increase susceptibility to negative age stereotypes and lead to an older subjective age, but Weiss and Lang (2012, Study 2) looked at age dissociation (or disidentification) as a potential coping strategy to reduce the effects of exposure to negative age stereotypes on subjective age. They predicted that age identity would mediate the relationship between stereotype activation and subjective age bias (i.e., difference between felt age and chronological age). Weiss and Lang (2012) randomly assigned older adult participants to complete one of three online quizzes to activate age stereotypes: positive stereotype, negative stereotype, or neutral. Subsequently, participants completed an age group identity measure (e.g., "I identify with people my age") and indicated how old they felt in years. Results showed that participants in the negative stereotype condition identified less with their age group and reported greater subjective age bias (i.e., younger subjective ages) than did participants in the other two conditions. Furthermore, regression analysis supported the hypothesis that age group identity would mediate the relationship between negative stereotypes and subjective age.

Aging Experiences and Stereotypes: Effects on Subjective Age

The construct of subjective age in the research reviewed to this point has been conceptualized as how old a person feels in relation to his or her chronological age, either as measured in years or on a general rating scale (e.g., younger, about the same, older than current chronological age; Montepare, 1996; Westerhof & Barrett, 2005; see Chapter 3 by Barrett & Montepare, this volume). However, attention has turned to investigating and defining the individual experiences which make aging salient and which undergird the more general concept of subjective age. Together, these experiences constitute a new view of subjective aging termed by Diehl and Wahl (2010)—*awareness of age-related change* (AARC; see Chapter 1 by Diehl, Wahl, Brothers, & Miche, this volume). The validity of the AARC construct has been established in a daily diary study involving 225 participants aged 70–89 years old (Miche et al., 2014). Results verified five major domains (each of which contained several subdomains) in which participants reported subjective aging experiences: health and physical functioning, cognitive functioning, interpersonal relations, social–cognitive and social–emotional functioning, and life style and engagement. The experiences were also coded for positivity and negativity, revealing a greater proportion of positive than negative experiences in the social–cognitive/social–emotional domain, a comparable number of positive and negative experiences in the interpersonal relations domain, and a greater proportion of negative than positive experiences in the other three domains: health and physical functioning, cognitive functioning, and life style and engagement. Note that AARC experiences like age stereotypes are multidimensional and that the AARC domains correspond to the stereotype domains reported by Kornadt and Rothermund (2011).

Two experimental studies have successfully introduced manipulations which generated the aging experiences described by AARC investigators—experiences that are also consistent with positive or negative age stereotypes. In the first of these studies, Eibach, Mock, and Courtney (2010) conducted three experiments with participants aged 40 years and older in which they induced aging experiences and examined effects on subjective age, self-evaluations, and stereotype consistent judgments. The first experiment assigned participants to read a text in one of three visual fluency conditions: fluency (16 pt. regular black font), disfluency (8 pt. italicized grayscale font) explained as caused by a photo-copying problem, and disfluency with no explanation. The second experiment used a 2 stereotype prime (positive/negative) × 2 visual disfluency (explained/unexplained) design. The first two experiments thus were aimed at inducing an experience in the physical functioning domain of the AARC and the stereotype of age-related decline in visual acuity. The third experiment focused on the stereotype that learning becomes more difficult with age by creating a generation gap experience, consistent with the cognitive functioning domain of the AARC. Participants were asked to determine the meaning of symbols that were described as emoticons used by young people in the generation gap condition but as transcription techniques used by stenographers in the control condition. Participants were assigned to these conditions in a 2 stereotype (confirmation/disconfirmation) × 2 (generation gap/control) design.

Results were similar in all three experiments. Participants in the conditions designed to induce an experience of aging (i.e., unexplained visual disfluency, generation gap) reported subjective ages which were significantly closer to their chronological age (i.e., older) than did participants in the other conditions. Participants in the aging experience/negative stereotype conditions had lower self-evaluations and were more likely to endorse stereotype consistent views than those in the other three conditions. However, the potential role of subjective age as a mediator between the negative aging experiences and the other outcome measures was not explored.

In the second study examining aging experiences, age stereotypes, and subjective age, Stephan, Chalabaev, Kotter-Grühn, and Jaconelli (2013) focused on creating a positive aging experience through a social comparison manipulation in the physical functioning domain of the AARC to counter the negative age stereotype associated with that domain. Older adult participants (52–91 years of age) first completed a subjective age measure, then read a passage emphasizing the importance of grip strength as a measure of health and functioning for older individuals, followed by a test of their grip strength. Participants in the experimental group then received feedback that their grip strength exceeded that of others in their age group by 80%, whereas those in the control group received no feedback. All participants subsequently completed a questionnaire, which included a second subjective age measure and manipulation check items as well as filler questions. Last, participants completed a second grip strength test. Results indicated that the social comparison manipulation resulted not only in a younger subjective age in comparison to baseline for those in the experimental group but also an improvement in their grip strength from baseline. In contrast, control group members showed no change from baseline in either subjective age or grip strength.

Summary

Together, the experimental studies of the effects of age stereotypes illuminate three aspects of their relationship to subjective aging. First, experimental induction of negative age experiences and stereotypes can lead to older subjective ages for older individuals as well as decrements in performance. In contrast, manipulations that call forth positive experiences and stereotypes can lead to younger subjective ages and improved performance, but for these beneficial effects to occur, the positive stereotype must match the performance domain. Second, age group identity may serve to moderate the impact of negative age stereotypes on subjective age and performance so that an older age identity may increase susceptibility to negative age stereotypes, whereas a younger age identity may protect against the effect of negative age stereotypes. Third, social comparison processes that induce dissociation from the older age group can serve to buffer subjective age and performance from the effects of the negative age stereotypes that are commonly associated with this age group.

DIRECTIONS FOR FUTURE EXPERIMENTAL RESEARCH ON AGE STEREOTYPES AND SUBJECTIVE AGING

Figure 4.2 presents a model of the relationships among key constructs discussed in this chapter—multiple age stereotypes and stereotype domains, context, awareness of age-related change, and subjective age—as they influence the behaviors of older individuals.

The model shows contextual cues and AARC leading to activation of domain-specific age stereotypes which have an indirect effect on stereotype-consistent behavior mediated by subjective age. The effects of the AARC and the domain-specific stereotype on subjective age and behavior will vary with the valence of the experiences, the stereotype, and age identity processes. Prior research suggests two possible patterns in the case of negative valence. If the negative stereotype reinforces the individual's identification with the older age group, an older subjective age will result and lead to stereotype-consistent behavior (Eibach et al., 2010; O'Brien & Hummert, 2006). However, if the negative stereotype leads to dissociation from the older age group, a younger subjective age will ensue and should reduce the likelihood of behavioral assimilation to the negative stereotype or even improved performance (Stephan et al., 2013; Weiss & Lang, 2012). The possible patterns in response to positive valence are also twofold. Priming with positive stereotypes has led to performance benefits for older individuals (Levy, 1996, 2003, 2009) and so may be associated with a younger subjective age. On the other hand, activation of positive age stereotypes can lead to older subjective ages, perhaps by increasing age salience (Kotter-Grühn & Hess, 2012). Finally, the model predicts that stereotype-consistent behavior will itself constitute an AARC experience, increasing awareness of age-related change.

Additional studies are needed to clarify the relationships outlined in the model in Figure 4.2. These include studies of the contextual cues and AARC experiences that call forth the domain-specific age stereotypes, the role of age identity and dissociation processes in the emergence of alternative subjective age mediation patterns, and the effects of stereotype-consistent behavior on increasing AARC and internalization of age stereotypes.

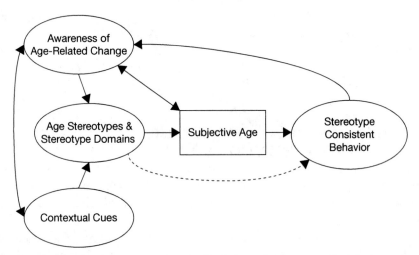

FIGURE 4.2 A mediation model with a feedback loop illustrating predicted relationships of contextual cues, AARC experiences, multiple age stereotypes, and domains to stereotype-consistent behaviors of older individuals.

AARC Experiences and Contextual Cues to Domain Stereotypes

One of the strengths of the domain-specific stereotypes proposed by Kornadt and Rothermund (2011) and the five domains that comprise the AARC construct (Diehl & Wahl, 2010; Miche et al., 2014) is their acknowledgment that stereotypes and experiences of aging can vary across contexts as well as across individuals. Earlier stereotype research has identified those cues which activate positive or negative age stereotypes in person perception studies. These include facial features indicating advanced age, contexts such as nursing homes associated with negative age stereotypes, vocal cues to age, and interpersonal communication styles associated with positive and negative age stereotypes (Hummert, Garstka, Ryan, & Bonnesen, 2004). Some prior experimental research on stereotype threat has suggested that certain contexts such as hospitals or tasks such as memory tests activate domain-specific stereotypes in older participants (Auman et al., 2005; Hess et al., 2003). However, the nature of the contextual cues and AARC experiences that activate positive or negative domain stereotypes and that affect subjective age are only beginning to be explored in experiments (Eibach et al., 2010; Stephan et al., 2013).

One area to investigate is the *role of communication* in creating AARC experiences and inducing age stereotypes. The ways in which age stereotypes are implicated in communication directed at older persons has been well-documented, with negative stereotypes associated with use of a patronizing communication style (Giles & Gasiorek, 2011; Hummert et al., 2004). This communication style may trigger negative age stereotypes in the relational and cognitive stereotype domains. Although several studies indicate that observers judge this communication style as unsatisfactory, its impact on the self-perceptions and subjective age of recipients has received limited attention.

Cues related to multiple stereotype domains varying in valence are present in natural settings, but experiments focus most often on one domain to maintain internal validity. However, just as age stereotype and contextual cues have been manipulated as separate factors in person perception studies of age stereotypes (e.g., Hummert et al., 1998), contextual cues of varying valence could be manipulated in studies of subjective aging. Such experiments would reveal the relative weight individuals put on contextual cues consistent with a positively evaluated stereotype domain such as family and partnerships in comparison to a negatively evaluated stereotype domain such as physical and cognitive functioning as well as their relationship to AARC experiences as presented in Figure 4.2. Prior experimental research suggests that perceivers place greater value on negative information as diagnostic of stable individual characteristics of targets than on positive information (Skowronski & Carlston, 1989). That is, they exhibit the *fundamental attribution error*, making internal attributions about other individuals in the face of negative information but external attributions about their own failings (Ross, 1977). Whether or not older individuals also make external attributions for negative AARC experiences or view those experiences as diagnostic of stable characteristics of the aging self is a question for investigation. The answer will carry implications for the nature of the age stereotypes activated in situations that involve both positive and negative stereotype cues.

Age Group Identification or Dissociation and Subjective Age as a Mediator

Several studies (Stephan et al., 2013; Weiss & Freund, 2012; Weiss & Lang, 2009, 2012; Weiss, Sassenberg, & Freund, 2013) have manipulated age group identification to examine its relationship to subjective age and behavioral assimilation to negative age stereotypes. Results confirm the hypothesis that dissociation from one's chronological age group is a response to negative age stereotypes, which leads to younger subjective ages and serves a protective psychological function for older persons. Stephan et al. (2013) found that dissociation contributed to improved performance on a physical task. When age identity has been assessed prior to experimental manipulations or in correlational studies, however, results suggest that dissociation is not an automatic response to negative age stereotypes so that older subjective ages and behavioral assimilation to stereotypes follow (Kotter-Grühn & Hess, 2012; O'Brien & Hummert, 2006).

As indicated in Figure 4.2, subjective age has been viewed as having a mediational role in the relationship between age stereotypes and assimilation to age stereotypes (Eibach et al., 2010; Stephan et al., 2013). However, none of the studies to date has tested this hypothesis. Future research should address this oversight to provide insight into the conditions under which subjective age mediates the relationship between age stereotypes and stereotype-consistent behaviors, as well as the conditions under which it does not.

Effects of Stereotype-Consistent Behavior on AARC and Subjective Age

The model in Figure 4.2 shows that engagement in stereotype-consistent behavior may itself contribute to AARC with a related impact on subjective age. This predicted relationship is consistent with other feedback models in the aging literature such as the communicative predicament of aging (CPA) model (Ryan, Giles, Bartolucci, & Henwood, 1986). According to the CPA model, experiencing age-adapted communication from others can reinforce age stereotypes, contribute to loss of self-esteem, and result in further age-related decline in older individuals. These predictions have received empirical support (Giles & Gasiorek, 2011; Hummert et al., 2004).

The theoretical framework for AARC and age stereotype domains presented by Diehl et al. (see Chapter 1, this volume) and correlational data on the relationships between individuals' evaluations of AARC domains, age stereotype domains, and their self-evaluations are consistent with the feedback loop proposed in Figure 4.2. Kornadt and Rothermund (2012) found a positive relationship between individuals' evaluations of age stereotype domains and their current selves, which was mediated by their future self-views, and Miche et al. (2014) found a similar positive relationship between participants' assessment of the valence of AARC domains and their subjective well-being. Experimental research is necessary to provide a full test of these relationships.

CONCLUSIONS

Experimental and quasi-experimental research has been emphasized in this chapter because the experimental method offers the best opportunity to test causal relationships in theoretical models, such as those presented in Figure 4.2 (Campbell & Stanley, 1963; Crano & Brewer, 2002). At the same time, the experimental method has limitations which create challenges for all investigators but perhaps especially for developmental psychologists. One example is the tension that exists between the control necessary to establish internal validity on the one hand and the need to create ecologically valid manipulations and dependent measures that are equivalent across age groups to establish generalizability on the other. Another example is the difficulty (if not the inability) of documenting long-term effects and individual change trajectories central to developmental theories solely through experiments (Campbell & Stanley, 1963; Cook & Campbell, 1979; Crano & Brewer, 2002). Complementing experiments with correlational studies constitutes an effective way to address some of these limitations. However, experimental researchers can increase the validity of their studies through careful designs which appropriately address the threats to internal validity, such as the absence of a control group, and develop creative experimental manipulations which closely mimic experiences and activities in natural settings (as in Stephan et al., 2013).

Prior research on the multidimensionality and dual valence of age stereotypes and stereotype domains carries implications for the study of AARC experiences and subjective age as they relate to psychological well-being of older individuals and their behavioral assimilation to age stereotypes. Although some relationships have received clear support in experimental tests, additional investigation of the contextual cues and AARC experiences that call forth positive and negative age stereotype and stereotype domains is necessary. Similarly, the role of age identification or dissociation in influencing subjective age, as well as the mediating role of subjective age in buffering or increasing the effects of age stereotypes on self-perceptions and behaviors of older persons, deserve study. Finally, examination of the extent to which behavioral assimilation to age stereotypes creates a feedback cycle which affects AARC and subjective age would advance our theoretical understanding of the power of stereotype-consistent behavior in the experience of subjective aging.

REFERENCES

Auman, C., Bosworth, H. B., & Hess, T. M. (2005). Effect of health-related stereotypes on physiological responses of hypertensive middle-aged and older men. *The Journals of Gerontology. Series B, Psychological Sciences and Social Sciences, 60,* P3–P10. http://dx.doi.org/10.1093/geronb/60.1.P3

Brewer, M., Dull, V., & Lui, L. (1981). Perceptions of the elderly: Stereotypes as prototypes. *Journal of Personality and Social Psychology, 41,* 656–670. http://dx.doi.org/10.1037/0022-3514.41.4.656

Brewer, M., & Lui, L. (1984). Categorization of the elderly by the elderly. *Personality and Social Psychology Bulletin, 10,* 585–595. http://dx.doi.org/10.1177/0146167284104012

Campbell, D. T., & Stanley, J. C. (1963). *Experimental and quasi-experimental designs for research.* Boston, MA: Houghton Mifflin.

Casper, C., Rothermund, K., & Wentura, D. (2011). The activation of specific facets of age stereotypes depends on individuating information. *Social Cognition, 29,* 393–414. http://dx.doi.org/10.1521/soco.2011.29.4.393

Chasteen, A. L., Bhattacharyya, S., Horhota, M., Tam, R., & Hasher, L. (2005). How feelings of stereotype threat influence older adults' memory performance. *Experimental Aging Research, 31,* 235–260. http://dx.doi.org/10.1080/0361073059094817

Chasteen, A. L., Schwarz, N., & Park, D. C. (2002). The activation of aging stereotypes in younger and older adults. *The Journals of Gerontology. Series B, Psychological Sciences and Social Sciences, 57,* P540–P547. http://dx.doi.org/10.1093/geronb/57.6.P540

Cook, T. D., & Campbell, D. T. (1979). *Quasi-experimentation: Design and analysis for field settings.* Boston, MA: Houghton Mifflin.

Crano, W. D., & Brewer, M. B. (2002). *Principles and methods of social research* (2nd ed.). Mahwah, NJ: Lawrence Erlbaum Associates.

Crockett, W. H., & Hummert, M. L. (1987). Perceptions of aging and the elderly. *Annual Review of Gerontology and Geriatrics, 7,* 217–241.

Diehl, M. K., & Wahl, H. W. (2010). Awareness of age-related change: Examination of (mostly) unexplored concept. *The Journals of Gerontology. Series B, Psychological and Social Sciences, 65,* 340–350. http://dx.doi.org/10.1093/geronb/gbp110

Eibach, R. P., Mock, S. E., & Courtney, E. A. (2010). Having a "senior moment": Induced aging, phenomenology, subjective age, and susceptibility to ageist stereotypes. *Journal of Experimental Social Psychology, 46,* 643–649. http://dx.doi.org/10.1016/j.jesp.2010.03.002

Giles, H., & Gasiorek, J. (2011). Intergenerational communication practices. In K. W. Schaie & S. L. Willis (Eds.), *Handbook of the psychology of aging* (7th ed., pp. 233–248). San Diego, CA: Academic Press.

Hess, T. M. (2006). Attitudes toward aging and their effects on behavior. In J. E. Birren & K. W. Schaie (Eds.), *Handbook of the psychology of aging* (6th ed., pp. 379–406). San Diego, CA: Academic Press.

Hess, T. M., Auman, C., Colcombe, S. J., & Rahhal, T. A. (2003). The impact of stereotype threat on age differences in memory performance. *The Journals of Gerontology. Series B, Psychological Sciences & Social Sciences, 58,* P3–P11. http://dx.doi.org/10.1093/geronb/58.1.P3

Hess, T. M., Emery, L., & Queen, T. L. (2009). Task demands moderate stereotype threat effects on memory performance. *The Journals of Gerontology. Series B, Psychological Sciences and Social Sciences, 64,* 482–486. http://dx.doi.org/10.1093/geronb/gbp044

Hess, T. M., & Hinson, J. T. (2006). Age-related variation in the influences of aging stereotypes on memory in adulthood. *Psychology and Aging, 21,* 621–625. http://dx.doi.org/10.1037//0882-7974.21.3.621

Hummert, M. L. (1999). A social cognitive perspective on age stereotypes. In T. M. Hess & F. Blanchard-Fields (Eds.), *Social cognition and aging* (pp. 175–195). New York, NY: Academic Press.

Hummert, M. L. (2011). Age stereotypes and aging. In K. W. Schaie & S. L. Willis (Eds.), *Handbook of the psychology of aging* (7th ed., pp. 249–262). San Diego, CA: Academic Press.

Hummert, M. L., Garstka, T. A., Ryan, E. B., & Bonnesen, J. L. (2004). The role of age stereotypes in interpersonal communication. In J. F. Nussbaum & J. Coupland (Eds.), *Handbook of communication and aging research* (2nd ed., pp. 91–115). Hillsdale, NJ: Lawrence Erlbaum Associates.

Hummert, M. L., Garstka, T. A., Shaner, J. L., & Strahm, S. (1994). Stereotypes of the elderly held by young, middle-aged, and elderly adults. *Journals of Gerontology: Psychological Sciences, 49,* P240–P249.

Hummert, M. L., Shaner, J. L., Garstka, T. A., & Henry, C. (1998). Communication with older adults: The influence of age stereotypes, context, and communicator age. *Human Communication Research, 25,* 125–152.

Kang, S. K., & Chasteen, A. L. (2009). The moderating role of age-group identification and perceived threat on stereotype threat among older adults. *International Journal of Aging and Human Development, 69,* 201–220. http://dx.doi.org/10.2190/AG.69.3.c

Kite, M. E., & Johnson, B. T. (1988). Attitudes toward older and younger adults: A meta-analysis. *Psychology and Aging, 3,* 233–244. http://dx.doi.org/10.1037//0882-7974.3.2.233

Kite, M. E., Stockdale, G. D., Whitley, B. E., Jr., & Johnson, B. T. (2005). Attitudes toward younger and older adults: An updated meta-analytic review. *Journal of Social Issues, 61,* 241–266. http://dx.doi.org/10.1111/j.1540-4560.2005.00404.x

Kite, M. E., & Wagner, L. S. (2002). Attitudes toward older adults. In T. D. Nelson (Ed.), *Stereotyping and prejudice against older persons* (pp. 129–161). Cambridge, MA: MIT Press.

Kornadt, A. E., & Rothermund, K. (2011). Contexts of aging: Assessing evaluative age stereotypes in different life domains. *The Journals of Gerontology. Series B, Psychological
Sciences and Social Sciences, 66*, 547–556. http://dx.doi.org/10.1093/geronb/gbr036

Kornadt, A. E., & Rothermund, K. (2012). Internalization of age stereotypes into the
self-concept via future self-views: A general model and domain-specific differences.
Psychology and Aging, 27, 164–172. http://dx.doi.org/10.1037/a0025110

Kotter-Grühn, D., & Hess, T. M. (2012). The impact of age stereotypes on self-perceptions
of aging across the adult lifespan. *The Journals of Gerontology. Series B, Psychological
Sciences and Social Sciences, 67*, 563–571. http://dx.doi.org/10.1093/geronb/gbr153

Krings, F. (2004). Automatic and controlled influences of association with age on memory. *Swiss Journal of Psychology, 63*, 247–259. http://dx.doi.org/10.1024/1421-0185
.63.4.247

Levy, B. (1996). Improving memory in old age through implicit self-stereotyping. *Journal
of Personality and Social Psychology, 71*, 1092–1107. http://dx.doi.org/10.1037//
0022-3514.71.6.1092

Levy, B. R. (2003). Mind matters: Cognitive and physical effects of aging self-stereotypes.
The Journals of Gerontology. Series B, Psychological Sciences and Social Sciences, 58,
P203–P211. http://dx.doi.org/10.1093/geronb/58.4.P203

Levy, B. (2009). Stereotype embodiment: A psychosocial approach to aging. *Current
Directions in Psychological Science, 18*, 332–336. http://dx.doi.org/10.111/j
.1467-8721.2009.01662.x

Levy, B. R., & Leifheit-Limson, E. (2009). The stereotype-matching effect: Greater
influence on functioning when age stereotypes correspond to outcomes. *Psychology
and Aging, 24*, 230–233. http://dx.doi.org/10.1037/a0014563

Meisner, B. A. (2012). A meta-analysis of positive and negative age stereotype priming
effects on behavior among older adults. *The Journals of Gerontology. Series B,
Psychological Sciences and Social Sciences, 67*, 13–17. http://dx.doi.org/10.1093/
geronb/gbr062

Miche, M., Wahl, H. W., Diehl, M., Oswald, F., Kaspar, R., & Kolb, M. (2014). Natural
occurrence of subjective aging experiences in community-dwelling older adults.
The Journals of Gerontology. Series B, Psychological Sciences and Social Sciences, 69,
174–187. http://dx.doi.org/10.1093/geronb/gbs164

Montepare, J. M. (1996). An assessment of adults' perceptions of their psychological,
physical, and social ages. *Journal of Clinical Geropsychology, 2*, 117–128.

O'Brien, L., & Hummert, M. L. (2006). Age self-stereotyping, stereotype threat, and
memory performance in late middle-aged adults. *Social Cognition, 24*, 338–358
. http://dx.doi.org/10.1521/soco.2006.24.3.338

Operario, D., & Fiske, S. T. (2004). Stereotypes: Content, structures, processes, and
context. In M. B. Brewer & M. Hewstone (Eds.), *Social cognition* (pp. 120–141).
Malden, MA: Blackwell.

Perdue, C. W., & Gurtman, M. B. (1990). Evidence for the automaticity of ageism. *Journal
of Experimental Social Psychology, 26*, 199–216.

Ross, L. (1977). The intuitive psychologist and his shortcomings: Distortions in the attribution process. In L. Berkowitz (Ed.), *Advances in experimental social psychology* (Vol. 10, pp. 174–221). New York, NY: Academic Press.

Ryan, E. B., Giles, H., Bartolucci, G., & Henwood, K. (1986). Psycholinguistic and social psychological components of communication by and with the elderly. *Language and Communication, 6*, 1–24.

Schmidt, D. F., & Boland, S. M. (1986). The structure of impressions of older adults: Evidence for multiple stereotypes. *Psychology and Aging, 1*, 255–260. http://dx.doi.org/10.1037/0882-7974.1.3.255

Skowronski, J. J., & Carlston, D. E. (1989). Negativity and extremity biases in person perception: A review of explanations. *Psychological Bulletin, 105*, 131–142. http://dx.doi.org/10.1037/0033-2909.105.1.131

Steele, C. M., Spencer, S. J., & Aronson, J. (2002). Contending with group image: The psychology of stereotype and social identity threat. In M. P. Zanna (Ed.), *Advances in experimental social psychology* (Vol. 34, pp. 379–440). New York, NY: Academic Press.

Stephan, Y., Chalabaev, A., Kotter-Grühn, D., & Jaconelli, A. (2013). "Feeling younger, being stronger": An experimental study of subjective age and physical function among older adults. *The Journals of Gerontology. Series B, Psychological Sciences and Social Sciences, 68*, 1–7. http://dx.doi.org/10.109/geronb/gbs037

Weiss, D., & Freund, A. M. (2012). Still young at heart: Negative age-related information motivates distancing from same-aged people. *Psychology and Aging, 27*, 173–180. http://dx.doi.org/10.1037/a0024819

Weiss, D., & Lang, F. R. (2009). Thinking about my generation: Adaptive effects of a dual age identity in later adulthood. *Psychology and Aging, 24*, 729–734. http://dx.doi.org/10.1037/a0016339

Weiss, D., & Lang, F. R. (2012). "They" are old but "I" feel younger: Age-group dissociation as a self-protective strategy in old age. *Psychology and Aging, 27*, 153–163. http://dx.doi.org/10.1037/a0024887

Weiss, D., Sassenberg, K., & Freund, A. M. (2013). When feeling different pays off: How older adults can counteract negative age-related information. *Psychology and Aging, 28*(4), 1140–1146. http://dx.doi.org/10.1037/a0033811

Wentura, D., & Brandtstädter, J. (2003). Age stereotypes in younger and older women: Analyses of accommodative shifts with a sentence-priming task. *Experimental Psychology, 50*, 16–26. http://dx.doi.org/10.1027//1618-3169.50.1.16

Westerhof, G. J., & Barrett, A. E. (2005). Age identity and subjective well-being: A comparison of the United States and Germany. *The Journals of Gerontology. Series B, Psychological Sciences and Social Sciences, 60*, S129–S136. http://dx.doi.org/10.1093/geronb/60.3.S129.

CHAPTER 5

Age Stereotypes and Age Stigma

Connections to Research on Subjective Aging

Alison L. Chasteen and Lindsey A. Cary

ABSTRACT

Older adults encounter ageism in various forms on a regular basis. Their experiences of age stigma can range from benevolent ones in which they receive unwanted help to more hostile ones in which they face rejection. In this chapter, we examine how older adults may cope with ageism and consider whether feeling subjectively younger might be one way for them to disidentify from their stigmatized age group. Before exploring this proposition, we first define age stigma and review how it is manifested in terms of age stereotypes and biases toward older adults, particularly in terms of benevolent versus hostile ageism. Next, we discuss the costs of experiencing age stigma and explore individual differences in age-based rejection sensitivity as a possible moderator of older adults' susceptibility to age stigma. Finally, we examine several coping strategies older adults may use to minimize the impact of age stigma, including feeling subjectively younger. We explore whether subjective age identification may constitute a violation of prescriptive age stereotypes concerning identity and whether such violations could result in backlash. We conclude with suggested directions for future research to better understand the complex relationship between age stigma and older adults' coping responses such as subjective age identification.

© 2015 Springer Publishing Company
http://dx.doi.org/10.1891/0198-8794.35.99

INTRODUCTION

Membership in an age group comes with a prescribed set of expectations about how one ought to behave and how one ought to look. These expectations may conflict with the expectations people have for themselves. In 2008, 88-year-old World War II veteran Peter Miller was informed that he would not be bearing the flag of Britain's Royal Army Medical Corps at the Remembrance Day ceremony for the first time in 20 years. Army officials believed he had appeared frail in the previous year's ceremony, and there were concerns that he would not be able to bear the weight of the flag for the full length of the ceremony. In response, he commented, "In my experience, it's oldies like me who can take the strain at these events" (Britten, 2008).

Peter Miller's perception of his capabilities diverged from the perceptions others had of him. It is likely that he felt younger than his chronological age—a phenomenon so common that even people older than 40 years of age report feeling 20% younger than their chronological age (Rubin & Berntsen, 2006). This discrepancy is known as the subjective age bias—the difference between one's felt, or subjective age, and one's chronological age (Barak, 2009; Montepare & Lachman, 1989). Subjective age biases have been related to several positive outcomes for older adults, such that those who feel subjectively younger experience higher life satisfaction and more positive health outcomes (Montepare, 2009; Stephan, Caudroit, & Chalabaev, 2011). However, subjective age is malleable, and being reminded of the stigma and stereotypes associated with age can cause people's subjective age to increase (Hughes, Geraci, & De Forrest, 2013; Kotter-Grühn & Hess, 2012). In this chapter, we examine the relationship between age stigma and subjective age in later life. We first define age stigma and then review how it is manifested in terms of age stereotypes and biases toward older adults, particularly in terms of benevolent versus hostile ageism. Next, we discuss the costs of experiencing age stigma and explore individual differences in age-based rejection sensitivity as a possible moderator of older adults' susceptibility to age stigma. Finally, we examine several coping strategies older adults may use to minimize the consequences of age stigma, including feeling subjectively younger.

AGE STIGMA, STEREOTYPES, AND BIASES

Goffman (1963) defined stigma as an "attribute that is deeply discrediting" (p. 3). He described three categories of stigma: abominations of the body (physical deformities), blemishes of individual character (mental disorders/dementia), and tribal stigma (group membership). Each of these categories of stigma is relevant to older adults because signs of physical aging are viewed negatively in today's youth-driven culture (Schoemann & Branscombe, 2011). Minor memory lapses in older people are viewed as diagnostic of dementia (Erber, Szuchman, & Rothberg, 1990), and prejudice against older adults as a group is common (Cuddy, Norton, & Fiske, 2005; Kite, Stockdale, Whitley, & Johnson, 2005).

As with other stigmatized groups, the prejudice that older adults face originates from the stereotypes which are applied to their group. The *Stereotype Content Model* (Fiske, Cuddy, Glick, & Xu, 2002) provides a unified view for understanding stereotypes about most, if not all, groups. Although the specific content of stereotypes toward different groups (such as older adults or Asians) may be intuitively very different, the dimensions along which these stereotypes fall are the same. The Stereotype Content Model details two key dimensions along which group stereotypes fall: warmth (e.g., good-natured, friendly) and competence (e.g., intelligent, confident). Groups can be perceived as high on both, low on both, or high on one and low on the other. Data supporting the Stereotype Content Model has shown that older adults are viewed as having little power within society and as uncompetitive with other groups for resources; as a result, they are perceived as warm but incompetent (Fiske et al., 2002).

The Behaviors from Intergroup Affect and Stereotypes map extends the Stereotype Content Model by exploring how stereotype content influences behavioral outcomes (Cuddy, Fiske, & Glick, 2007; Cuddy et al., 2005). This model predicts that warm targets, such as older adults, will experience active facilitation (i.e., help). However, because they are viewed as incompetent, older adults will also experience passive harm (i.e., exclusion). Active facilitation may seem relatively benign, if not positive, whereas passive harm is more intuitively negative. However, research suggests that both are harmful. Overaccommodating or patronizing speech can be used in an attempt to help older adults in conversations. This can include simplified speech, exaggerated pitch, a demeaning emotional tone, or low quality of content (Giles, Fox, Harwood, & Williams, 1994). Although this type of behavior may seem harmless, and at times helpful, it is associated with several negative outcomes, including lowered self-esteem and communication competence (Nussbaum, Pitts, Huber, Krieger, & Ohs, 2005; Ryan, Hamilton, & Kwong See, 1994; Ryan, Hummert, & Boich, 1995). In contrast, other research has shown that if older adults are given responsibilities, rather than being overaccommodated, they will fare much better. For example, a classic study by Langer and Rodin (1976) found that assigning responsibilities to older adults in nursing homes versus performing responsibilities for them was related to several positive outcomes, including increased activity and better health outcomes. The relationship between more perceived control and more positive health outcomes has also been consistently demonstrated in more recent research (Gerstorf, Röcke, & Lachman, 2010; Infurna, Gerstorf, & Zarit, 2011; Krause & Shaw, 2003).

In addition to active facilitation, older adults may experience exclusion and disregard in various domains (Pasupathi & Löckenhoff, 2002). In the domain of employment, research shows a link between age stereotypes and employment outcomes, specifically that the stereotype of incompetence harms employment outcomes for older adults (Krings, Sczesny, & Kluge, 2011). Older adults are often perceived as unable to perform capably, even though there is little evidence to support this idea (see Posthuma & Campion, 2009, for a review). Older adults attempting to enter a new job market or maintain their current position might think to do so by emphasizing their competency through highlighting their previous achievements and successes. Unfortunately, it is unlikely that this will positively influence their outcome. Cuddy and colleagues (2005) examined the persistence of the older adult stereotype. They found that even when presented with information indicating competency, participants did not shift their competency ratings of the older target. Rather, the older target who was described as more competent experienced penalties of warmth. That is, the more competent an older target was described to be, the less warm the target was perceived to be. In terms of ratings of competence, however, describing the older target as competent failed to have an effect, and the older target was seen as relatively incompetent across all conditions. This pattern of warmth penalties combined with continued perceptions of incompetence in response to counter-stereotypical information mimics patterns seen in perceptions of women, another group that is often stereotyped as warm but incompetent (Rudman & Phelan, 2008; Tyler & McCullough, 2009).

DESCRIPTIVE AND PRESCRIPTIVE AGE STEREOTYPES

It appears to be the case, then, that older adults are often penalized in the domain of warmth when they try to counter negative age stereotypes concerning competence (Cuddy et al., 2005). Recent work by North and Fiske (2013) provides a potential explanation for why backlash such as this might occur. Specifically, they distinguish between prescriptive versus descriptive age stereotypes. Elaborating on past work that has examined the unique influence of prescriptive versus descriptive stereotypes on person perception (e.g., Rudman & Glick, 2001), North and Fiske (2013) define descriptive stereotypes as those that describe beliefs about a social group, for example, what older adults are typically like. The bulk of research on age stereotypes has focused on describing the content of those stereotypes (e.g., Hummert, Garstka, Shaner, & Strahm, 1994) as well as the activation of age stereotypes (e.g., Chasteen, Schwarz, & Park, 2002). As noted earlier, perceptions of warmth and incompetence are common components of those stereotypes (Fiske et al., 2002) and countering those stereotypes does not necessarily improve perceptions of older adults' competence (Cuddy et al., 2005). As a result, paternalistic prejudice toward older adults is likely to persist, unless those competence perceptions are improved.

Although contradicting descriptive age stereotypes may not necessarily affect the paternalistic prejudice which is expressed toward older people, contradicting prescriptive age stereotypes might produce an even more negative outcome in the form of hostile prejudice. In contrast to descriptive stereotypes, prescriptive stereotypes focus on expected or normative behaviors by group members, for example, how older adults should behave (Gill, 2004; see Rudman & Phelan, 2008, for more resources). Much of the past research on prescriptive stereotypes has examined the consequences of violating these stereotypes for perceptions of women and shows that a backlash effect occurs (Rudman & Phelan, 2008; Tyler & McCullough, 2009). For example, Tyler and McCullough (2009) found that women who present themselves as more agentic (vs. communal) in their resumes (violating prescriptive gender stereotypes) are perceived as being less likeable, competent, socially skilled, and likely to be interviewed than male agentic applicants. When women's resumes indicated more communal values (not violating prescriptive gender stereotypes), there were no differences in how the male and female resumes were evaluated.

North and Fiske (2013) presented some of the first research to examine the consequences of violating prescriptive age stereotypes for older adults. They suggest there are three domains in which prescriptive stereotypes might inform reactions to older adults: succession, consumption, and identity. Succession and consumption expectations for older adults relate to their use of shared resources. Specifically, succession is related to the transition of desirable resources (e.g., money) and positions (e.g., employment), and consumption is related to the depletion of shared resources (e.g., government spending). Prescriptive stereotypes dictate that older adults should relinquish their hold on desirable resources. In contrast, identity expectations for older adults pertain to beliefs about age-appropriate behavior. Prescriptive stereotypes in this case suggest that older adults need to "act their age."

In their examination of prescriptive age stereotype violation, North and Fiske (2013) tested whether older adults face a backlash effect, similar to women, when they violate prescriptive norms in the domains of succession, consumption, or identity. In the domain of identity, the authors conducted two studies in which young, middle-aged, and older adults read about a 74-, 44-, or 24-year-old man who enjoyed either oldies music (e.g., Frank Sinatra, Bing Crosby) or pop music (e.g., Lady Gaga, Justin Timberlake) and played it loudly on his headphones. After reading the vignette, participants rated the target on how capable and warm he seemed (both studies) as well as how much they would like to interact with him (second study). In both studies, older participants were more positive toward the older target who violated prescriptive age stereotypes by preferring pop music than were younger participants. Moreover, young adults showed the greatest discrepancy in their ratings of the older targets and evaluated the stereotype-adhering target who liked oldies music as more capable and warm and were more interested in interacting with him than the stereotype-violating target. Greater negativity among young adults toward stereotype-violating older adults also occurred in other studies which examined the domains of succession and consumption (North & Fiske, 2013). Taken together, these findings show that older adults may face hostile prejudice when they violate prescriptive age stereotypes.

HOSTILE AND BENEVOLENT AGEISM

It appears, then, that older adults may face age stigma in the form of either benevolent or hostile ageism. North and Fiske (2013) suggest that benevolent ageism arises out of descriptive age stereotypes, which depict older people as warm but incompetent. In contrast, hostile ageism arises from prescriptive age stereotypes, such that those seniors who violate stereotypes about how they should behave face repercussions in the form of backlash. It is possible that the extent to which people respond with hostile ageism to prescriptive stereotype violations may be related to the extent to which they endorse benevolent and hostile ageist beliefs. We recently explored this possibility by examining whether individual differences in hostile and benevolent ageism predicted responses to age discrimination within a hiring context (Chasteen, Cary, & Remedios, 2014). Prior to coming to the lab, young adult participants completed the Ambivalent Ageism Scale (AAS; Cary, Chasteen, & Remedios, 2014). In the lab, participants read a vignette that described a job opening for which a 60-year-old man had applied. The job was described as a managerial position in a health care organization. The man was shortlisted for the position, but ultimately, the 40-year-old interviewer decided not to hire him and gave either a neutral (other applicants were better qualified), benevolent ageist (he did not want to burden the older applicant), or hostile ageist (older people are stubborn and unmotivated) rationale for his decision.

Later on, participants read the applicant's attribution for the hiring decision, in which he indicated that he believed he was not hired either because of his interview skills or because of age discrimination. They then rated the interviewer on fairness and the candidate on competence and how much of a troublemaker he was. Surprisingly, neither the interviewer's rationale for rejecting the applicant nor the applicant's attribution (to age discrimination or interview skills) influenced perceptions of the applicant. Candidate attribution influenced

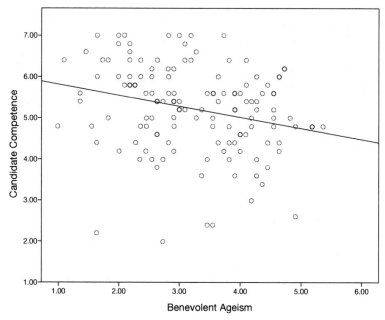

FIGURE 5.1 The relationship between benevolent ageism and candidate competence.

the extent to which participants viewed the interviewer as fair. However, the extent to which participants endorsed ageist beliefs independently predicted fairness evaluations, beyond the attribution effect. Specifically, benevolent ageism was positively associated with perceptions of the interviewer's fairness, such that regardless of rationale and attribution, the interviewer was perceived as more fair by participants high in benevolent ageism. Similarly, participants high in benevolent ageism were also more likely to view the older candidate as incompetent across conditions (Figure 5.1).

Hostile ageism was predictive of how much of a troublemaker and how nice the candidate was perceived to be. The more participants endorsed hostile ageist statements, the more they regarded him as a troublemaker (Figure 5.2) regardless of hiring rationale or attribution. These findings demonstrate that both benevolent and hostile ageism predict people's reactions to older individuals and to ageism situations.

The results of Chasteen et al. (2014) also provide further evidence for the costs of violating prescriptive age stereotypes, particularly the norm of succession. It is probable that an older adult seeking employment in a high-status position (managerial level) violates the norm of succession whereby older adults should be leaving the workforce later in life. That hostile ageism predicted how

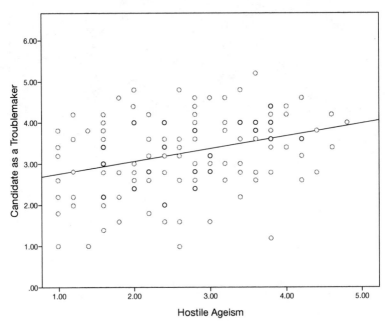

FIGURE 5.2 The relationship between hostile ageism and perceptions of the candidate as a troublemaker.

much the applicant was viewed as a troublemaker, regardless of whether he made an attribution to age discrimination, suggests that young adults did not like the idea of a 60-year-old taking an available job. This supports the idea that the young participants in this study viewed the older applicant as violating succession norms, consistent with North and Fiske's (2013) proposition that hostile ageism is related to prescriptive age stereotype violations.

EFFECTS OF AGE STIGMA ON OLDER ADULTS

Given the different types of age stereotypes (descriptive and prescriptive) and prejudices (benevolent and hostile) that older adults face, it is not surprising that age-based stigma can negatively affect them. Indeed, it is likely that older adults are not only aware of age stereotypes, having been exposed to them from a young age, but have also internalized these stereotypes, believing them to be true (Levy, 2003). A relatively large body of research has shown that older adults' capability worsens when they are directly exposed to negative age stereotypes (e.g., Levy, 1996; Meisner, 2012; for a review, see Chasteen, Kang, & Remedios, 2011). As well, other work has shown that older adults like other stigmatized groups are vulnerable to the effects of stereotype threat. Stereotype threat refers to a phenomenon in which members of a negatively stereotyped group experience concerns about confirming a negative group stereotype during a stereotype-relevant situation. These concerns can hamper their performance and, ironically, lead to stereotype confirmation (Steele & Aronson, 1995).

The influence of stereotype threat on older adults' performance has been examined in several domains, with a focus on their performance on memory tasks (for a review, see Chasteen et al., 2011). For example, Rahhal, Hasher, and Colcombe (2001) found that older adults' memory performance was poorer when the task was described as a memory task compared to a test of learning. Similarly, Hess, Hinson, and Hodges (2009) found that older adults performed worse on a memory task when they were first told the goal of the study was to see why there were performance differences between older and younger adults compared to performance similarities. Research from our lab suggests that the degree to which older adults perceive and experience stereotype threat helps account for performance differences between young and older adults on some memory tasks (Chasteen, Bhattacharyya, Horhota, Tam, & Hasher, 2005) and that the degree to which older adults perceive stereotype threat can moderate the degree to which their memory performance suffers under threat conditions (Kang & Chasteen, 2009a). Overall, a robust literature has developed showing that older adults' function can be negatively impacted by the age stigma they face.

INDIVIDUAL DIFFERENCES IN VULNERABILITY TO AGE STIGMA

Although a large body of research has demonstrated the negative impact of age stereotypes on older adults' cognitive function, there may be individual differences in the extent to which older adults are influenced by age stigma. As noted earlier, it has been suggested that older adults may have internalized negative aging stereotypes because of their exposure to those negative images throughout their lives (Levy, 2003). However, it is likely that older people vary in the degree to which they have internalized those stereotypes. As well, there are likely individual differences in the degree to which older adults are concerned about being stigmatized because of their age and having negative age stereotypes applied to them. Work with other stigmatized groups has shown that members differ in the extent to which they perceive and experience stigma. For example, Mendoza-Denton, Downey, Purdie, Davies, and Pietrzak (2002) showed that individual differences in people's sensitivity to rejection based on their race were an important moderator of their perceptions of and reactions to prejudice.

In our lab, we extended the rejection-sensitivity conceptualization to the case of age and developed the Age-Based Rejection-Sensitivity Questionnaire

(RSQ-Age; Kang & Chasteen, 2009b). Respondents were asked to imagine 15 different scenarios in which they might be stigmatized because of their age. An example of one item is "Imagine that you are involved in a minor accident while driving. It is unclear who is at fault." After imagining each scenario, respondents are asked to rate how concerned/anxious they would be that the blame for the accident might be placed on them because of their age. They were also asked to rate the extent to which they expect that the blame for the accident might be placed on them because of their age. Recent work with some of our collaborators has shown that age-based stigma-sensitivity is an important predictor of self-perceptions and function in older adults. Chasteen, Pichora-Fuller, Dupuis, Singh, and Smith (2014) found that older adults' sensitivity to age-based stigma, in combination with their fear of aging, predicted their self-views of both cognitive and perceptual abilities, which then predicted their actual function. This suggests that assessing older adults' concerns about age-based stigma is an important variable to consider when trying to understand what influences their function.

It remains unknown whether older adults' individual differences in age-based rejection sensitivity moderate the extent to which they are able to feel subjectively younger than their actual age. Given that individuals high in other types of stigma sensitivity are more vulnerable to the effects of negative stereotypes about their group (Brown & Pinel, 2003), it is likely that older adults who are high in age-based rejection sensitivity are less able to disengage from that identity through subjective age identification. However, it could be argued that those older individuals who are most concerned about age stigma might be the most motivated to avoid it and thus subjectively identify with a younger age. Future work should explore whether older people's age stigma concerns moderate subjective age bias.

COPING WITH AGE STIGMA

So far, we have seen how age stigma is manifested in terms of the stereotypes and prejudices which are applied to older people. As well, we have reviewed some of the ways that older adults are negatively affected by age stigma as well as possible individual differences in those effects. An important issue to examine next is how older people deal with age stigma. Several models have been proposed about how people cope with stigma when they encounter it (e.g., Major & O'Brien, 2005; Miller & Kaiser, 2001; Trawalter, Richeson, & Shelton, 2009). A key similarity among these models is that they propose viewing stigma as a stressor and adopting a stress and coping framework, similar to one posited by Lazarus and Folkman (1984). For the purposes of this chapter, we will focus on instances in which age stigma is appraised as stressful because it might exceed an older adult's resources for coping (Miller & Kaiser, 2001). As well, we will adopt the most common categorizations of coping strategies. Specifically, we will discuss when older adults might use problem-focused or emotion-focused strategies to deal with age stigma when they encounter it.

Problem-Focused Coping

Problem-focused coping strategies refer to coping with stigmatization by trying to change the situation. An example might be an older person confronting someone for using patronizing speech. Research on confronting prejudice in terms of other types of bigotry (e.g., racism, sexism) has shown that such a problem-focused approach can be successful in reducing bias (Czopp, Monteith, & Mark, 2006; Mallett & Wagner, 2011). However, there can also be a cost because confronters are viewed more negatively than non-confronters when a bigoted remark is made (Czopp et al., 2006), particularly when the confronter belongs to the stigmatized group (Rasinski & Czopp, 2010). In terms of research on confronting ageism, we could find no studies on the consequences of confronting ageist speech, either for reducing age prejudice or for evaluations of an older adult confronter. Research by Good, Moss-Racusin, and Sanchez (2012) suggests that people are more willing to confront prejudice on behalf of themselves or others if they believe that will make a difference or if they were less concerned about being perceived negatively. In the case of ageism, it may be that older adults often worry about negative reactions if they confront ageist behavior such as patronizing speech. This could be because the benevolent form of ageism is often not recognized as prejudice by others because of the warmth which is expressed as part of that type of bias. Indeed, data from our lab has shown that people do not seem to recognize ageism as problematic compared to other types of prejudices because we found that both young and older adults view racism and sexism to be more serious and more common than ageism (Kang, Chasteen, & Tse, 2014). These findings bolster the idea that older adults might be reluctant to use a problem-focused strategy such as confronting ageist speech for fear of seeming unreasonable and overly sensitive.

Emotion-Focused Coping

Another type of strategy that older adults might use to cope with age stigma when they encounter it is emotion-focused coping. Emotion-focused coping refers to dealing with the emotional response to the stigmatizing situation rather than to trying to change the situation itself. For example, an older adult might explain the patronizing speech he or she is experiencing by viewing the speaker as ageist. By making an attribution of age prejudice, the older adult is able to protect his or her self-esteem by concluding that there is nothing about himself or herself which deserves this kind of treatment, but rather, the speaker is prejudiced toward older people. This type of self-protective attribution has been shown to be an effective buffer that has preserved self-esteem for other types of stigmatized groups, such as women (Major, Kaiser, & McCoy, 2003) and racial minorities (Crocker, Voelkl, Testa, & Major, 1991). Work from our lab, however, suggests that making attributions to ageism may not be an effective coping technique for older adults (Chasteen & Kang, 2014). In our study, older adults were asked to imagine being rejected for a volunteer position either because the manager was ageist and hired only young people, the manager hired only his friends, or the manager specifically did not like the older participant. Although the older adults in the ageism condition rated the manager as more prejudiced than did older adults in the other conditions, this prejudice attribution did not protect them from expecting to feel depressed and anxious. Indeed, only older adults' attributions to other external causes (e.g., something else about the manager besides being ageist) buffered their anticipated feelings of depression and anxiety in the face of rejection. Major and O'Brien (2005) suggest that attributions to discrimination are less likely to be effective in protecting well-being when prejudice is subtle rather than blatant. Perhaps the often benevolent nature of ageism makes that type of prejudice seem subtle to others, resulting in older adults feeling uncomfortable with making attributions to ageism. If older adults find attributions to ageism to be less effective in dealing with age prejudice, then they might turn to other emotion-focused coping strategies instead, such as regulating their emotional response to the age stigma which they are experiencing. For example, older adults might attempt to avoid feeling angry or anxious because of the bias they are experiencing. Research on aging and coping with other types of stressors suggests that emotion regulation might also be a successful strategy for older adults to use in response to age stigma. Findings from across the adult life span suggest that older adults tend to use emotion-focused coping when dealing with other kinds of stressors because that coping style is more adaptive in later life (Diehl et al., 2014; Diehl, Coyle, & Labouvie-Vief, 1996; Heckhausen, 1997).

Another coping strategy older adults might use to deal with age stigma involves disengagement. Disengagement coping refers to finding ways to avoid being the target of prejudice. An example would be if an older adult avoids a grocery store clerk who he or she has found to be condescending on past visits to the market. This example illustrates engaging in physical avoidance of age stigma, but there are other types of disengagement strategies available for older adults to use as well. For example, an older individual may disidentify with his or her age group to distance him or herself from the age stigma of being an older adult. One way for older adults to disidentify from their age group would be to view themselves as subjectively younger than their chronological age. By adopting a younger subjective age, they can believe that negative aging stereotypes and age prejudice do not apply to them. Recent work by Weiss and colleagues (Weiss &

Freund, 2012; Weiss & Lang, 2012) supports the notion that feeling subjectively younger may be a viable strategy for older adults to escape the negative implications of age stigma. Weiss and Lang (2012) had older adults complete a quiz which emphasized either positive or negative aspects of aging followed by measures of age group identification and subjective age. They found that when older adults were presented with negative aging information, they reported a younger subjective age than when they were presented with positive or neutral information. Moreover, older adults in the negative condition also identified with their chronological age group less than did those in the other two conditions. Weiss and Freund (2012) obtained converging evidence of older adults' disidentifying with their chronological age group. Using the same quiz method, they found that older adults presented with negative information about aging felt closer in age to a middle-aged target and less similar to an older adult target compared with those in the positive and neutral information conditions. Taken together, this work suggests that feeling subjectively younger than their chronological age is at least one way by which older adults can avoid negative aspects of growing old. It should be noted, however, that the negative information condition emphasized negative aspects of aging, such as the prevalence of dementia, and increased health problems. It remains unknown whether older adults would respond similarly if they were reminded of the age prejudice which faces their group.

Indeed, other research suggests that older adults might cope quite differently when led to think about the age discrimination they face. The Rejection-Identification Hypothesis proposes that members of stigmatized groups can cope with the discrimination they face by identifying with their stigmatized group (Branscombe, Schmitt, & Harvey, 1999). Branscombe and colleagues have shown that members of various stigmatized groups were able to protect their well-being through group identification, including African Americans (Branscombe et al., 1999), women (Schmitt, Branscombe, Kobrynowicz, & Owen, 2002), and older adults (Garstka, Schmitt, Branscombe, & Hummert, 2004). In the case of older adults, Garstka et al. (2004) found that older adults' perceptions of age discrimination were positively associated with identifying with their age group, which in turn was positively associated with well-being. This suggests that rather than using a disengagement strategy such as disidentification, older adults in some instances will cope with age stigma by embracing their older adult identity. The question, then, is when might older adults respond through identification versus disidentification? As noted earlier, one determining factor might be what type of negative aging information older adults are trying to deal with. When reminded of potential negative age-related events that could affect the self, such as developing dementia, older adults may be more likely to cope by avoiding their older adult identity and instead identify with a younger age (e.g., Weiss & Freund, 2012; Weiss & Lang, 2012). However, when led to consider the age discrimination they face, perhaps older adults are more likely to cope by boosting their feelings of acceptance through identifying with their same-aged peers (e.g., Garstka et al., 2004).

It may also be the case that when older adults identify with their age group, they are really identifying with their generation rather than their chronological age. Weiss and Lang (2009) differentiate between these two types of identities, arguing that chronological age identification leads older people to focus on their older adult identity and associated negative age stereotypes, whereas generation identification provides a sense of belongingness based on socially shared experiences over time. In support of their assertion, they found that older adults' identification with same-aged people was negatively associated with well-being, whereas generation identification was positively associated. Perhaps it is the case, then, that even when older adults use age group identification as a coping strategy in response to age stigma, they are in effect emphasizing their connections with other members of their generation rather than their shared chronological age. More research is needed to tease apart these different types of age-based identification, as well as to determine the efficacy of these identification and disidentification strategies for coping with age stigma.

Although maintaining a subjectively younger age may be at times a successful strategy for escaping age stigma, such a strategy may come with costs. As noted earlier in this chapter, older adults may face backlash and even hostile age prejudice if they violate prescriptive age stereotypes. North and Fiske (2013) found that older adults who violate prescriptive age stereotypes about identity face sanctions for not "acting their age," particularly from young adults. These findings suggest that there may be times when maintaining a subjectively younger age could backfire for older adults, such that they experience more hostile reactions for violating prescriptive age stereotypes about how older adults should behave.

It may be the case, however, that older adults would only face backlash for prescriptive stereotype violations in which they have cultural interests in common with young adults. If older adults were subjectively identifying as younger, but more within a middle-aged range, they may be viewed more positively. For example, if the older target in the North and Fiske (2013) studies preferred music which is associated more with middle-aged adults, such as by the Beatles or the Rolling Stones, it is possible that young adults would not evaluate him so negatively. It could be the case that older adults would only be penalized by young adults for not acting their age if that behavior overlapped with the behavior and preferences of younger people. More work is needed to establish whether backlash toward older adults who violate prescriptive age stereotypes by subjectively identifying as younger occurs because they overlap with a younger group's identity (such as sharing music tastes with young adults) or whether it is simply because they are not behaving in accordance with stereotype-driven expectations for their group. If it were the former, then young adults should not penalize older adults for enjoying younger music (such as The Beatles or The Rolling Stones), as long as it is not music young people also enjoy.

Older adults may also face backlash for trying to maintain a younger identity by engaging in age concealment. Chasteen, Bashir, Gallucci, and Visekruna (2011) found that young adults rated older individuals who engaged in age concealment more negatively than did older adults, regardless of the type of procedure that individuals used. Schoemann and Branscombe (2011) also found that young adults negatively evaluated older targets who attempted to look younger and that this was because of perceived threats to young adults' group identities. Thus, it appears that although feeling subjectively younger than their actual years may be a disengagement strategy that helps older adults escape age stigma, the manner in which they go about feeling younger could backfire and lead to negative reactions. It is likely that there are margins of acceptability in trying to look and feel younger than one's older age, and when those parameters are exceeded, there could be a social cost. One way to pinpoint those parameters would be to have young, middle-aged, and older adults evaluate young, middle-aged, and older targets who fail to act their age. Such a design would determine whether backlash occurs toward any targets who act younger than their age or whether such sanctions occur mainly for older targets. As well, the acceptability of violations of prescriptive age stereotypes could be examined further by varying the number of years which an older adult reports feeling subjectively younger. Perhaps it is the case that younger age groups are more accepting of older adults who feel 5 years younger than their chronological age but not 15 years younger. More work is needed to determine when older adults' violations of prescriptive age stereotypes are tolerated and when they are not.

CONCLUSIONS AND FUTURE DIRECTIONS

In a world where there are pervasive age stereotypes (Nelson, 2002), it is perhaps unsurprising that older adults would try to find ways to reduce the effects of age stigma. In this chapter, we sought to characterize different forms of age stigma by distinguishing between benevolent versus hostile forms of ageism and how older adults might cope with the stigma arising from each. The bulk of age stereotype research has focused on descriptive age stereotypes, investigating the content of those stereotypes and the effects of them on older adults, particularly in terms of their function. Descriptive age stereotypes that portray older people as warm but incompetent often lead to treating older adults benevolently through paternalistic prejudice (Cuddy et al., 2007; Fiske et al., 2002; Nelson, 2002). Although benevolent ageism may seem benign because it is expressed in a warm way, it can undermine older adults' feelings of autonomy by implying incompetence. Future research should investigate further when people detect expressions of benevolent ageism, both in terms of witnessing such prejudice as well as being the target of such prejudice. Because of the warmth aspect of benevolent ageism, it is likely that it may go undetected and therefore be difficult to fight against. By systematically testing both younger and older adults' reactions to different expressions of benevolent ageism (e.g., elderspeak vs. offering unwanted help) in different contexts, we would have a greater understanding of when prejudice against older people is most likely to go unnoticed. This could lead to a development of new policies and practices to decrease the number of age-stigmatizing situations older adults face.

Unlike benevolent ageism, hostile ageism is probably easier to detect, given the lack of warmth that is expressed toward older people in such circumstances. Recent research suggests that older adults are more likely to face hostile ageism when they violate prescriptive age stereotypes (North & Fiske, 2013). Although this research is promising in that it articulates when there is a greater likelihood of intergenerational conflict occurring, for example, when older adults violate age-based expectations regarding succession or consumption, more studies are needed to pinpoint when older adults will face backlash. This is particularly relevant in the case of subjective age identification because older adults have been shown to be penalized by young adults when they adopt a younger identity themselves, such as through music preferences. At present, it is unknown whether such hostile ageism would be expressed if older adults adopted a younger subjective age which was more in line with middle rather than young adulthood. Is it the case that older adults would face hostile reactions for failing to act their age, or is it the case that some forms of age identity violations are more acceptable than others?

The research we have presented in this chapter highlights the multidimensionality of age stigma. The fact that age stereotypes contain both positive (warmth) and negative (incompetence) elements means that prejudice toward older people often takes a benevolent form, making it difficult to detect and confront. This means that older adults likely have to rely on various coping strategies in response, such as subjective age identification. The complexity of these processes necessitates that similarly complex methods are needed to both understand and ultimately reduce age stigma and its impact on older adults.

ACKNOWLEDGMENTS

This research was supported by grants from the Social Sciences and Humanities Research Council of Canada awarded to the first author (ALC) and an Ontario Graduate Scholarship awarded to the second author (LAC).

REFERENCES

Barak, B. (2009). Age identity: A cross-cultural global approach. *International Journal of Behavioral Development, 29,* 2–11. http://dx.doi.org/10.1177/0165025408099485

Branscombe, N. R., Schmitt, M. T., & Harvey, R. D. (1999). Perceiving pervasive discrimination among African Americans: Implications for group identification and well-being. *Journal of Personality and Social Psychology, 77,* 135–149. http://dx.doi.org/10.1037/0022-3514.77.1.135

Britten, N. (2008, Nov 7). Army veteran told he is too old to be Remembrance Day standard bearer. *The Telegraph.* Retrieved from http://www.telegraph.co.uk/news/uknews /3397755/Army-veteran-told-he-is-too-old-to-be-Remembrance-Day-standard-bearer.html

Brown, R. P., & Pinel, E. C. (2003). Stigma on my mind: Individual differences in the experience of stereotype threat. *Journal of Experimental Social Psychology, 39,* 626–633. http://dx.doi.org/10.1016/S0022-1031(03)00039-8

Cary, L. A., Chasteen, A. L., & Remedios, J. D. (2014). *Development of the ambivalent ageism scale.* Manuscript in preparation.

Chasteen, A. L., Bashir, N., Gallucci, C., & Visekruna, A. (2011). Age and anti-aging technique influence reactions to age concealment. *The Journals of Gerontology. Series B, Psychological Sciences and Social Sciences, 66,* 719–724. http://dx.doi.org/10.1093/geronb/gbr063

Chasteen, A. L., Bhattacharyya, S., Horhota, M., Tam, R., & Hasher, L. (2005). How feelings of stereotype threat influence older adults' memory performance. *Experimental Aging Research, 31,* 235–260. http://dx.doi.org/10.1080/03610730590948177

Chasteen, A. L., Cary, L. A., & Remedios, J. D. (2014). *Benevolent and hostile ageism influence reactions to age discrimination.* Manuscript in preparation.

Chasteen, A. L., & Kang, S. K. (2014). *Do attributions to discrimination protect targets of ageism?* Manuscript submitted for publication.

Chasteen, A. L., Kang, S. K., & Remedios, J. D. (2011). Aging and stereotype threat: Development, process, and interventions. In M. Inzlicht & T. Schmader (Eds), *Stereotype threat: Theory, process, and application* (pp. 202–216). New York, NY: Oxford University Press.

Chasteen, A. L., Pichora-Fuller, K., Dupuis, K., Singh, G., & Smith, S. (2014). *How negative views of aging influence metacognitive beliefs and memory and hearing function.* Manuscript in preparation.

Chasteen, A. L., Schwarz, N., & Park, D. C. (2002). The activation of aging stereotypes in younger and older adults. *The Journals of Gerontology. Series B, Psychological Sciences and Social Sciences, 57,* P540–P547.

Crocker, J., Voelkl, K., Testa, M., & Major, B. (1991). Social stigma: The affective consequences of attributional ambiguity. *Journal of Personality and Social Personality, 60,* 218–228. http://dx.doi.org/10.1037/0022-3514.60.2.218

Cuddy, A. J., Fiske, S. T., & Glick, P. (2007). The BIAS Map: Behaviours from intergroup affect and stereotypes. *Journal of Personality and Social Psychology, 92,* 631–648. http://dx.doi.org/10.1037/0022-3514.92.4.631

Cuddy, A. J., Norton, M. I., & Fiske, S. T. (2005). This old stereotype: The pervasiveness and persistence of the elderly stereotype. *Journal of Social Issues, 61*, 267–285. http://dx.doi.org/10.1111/j.1540-4560.2005.00405.x

Czopp, A. M., Monteith, M. J., & Mark, A. Y. (2006). Standing up for a change: Reducing bias through interpersonal confrontation. *Journal of Personality and Social Psychology, 90*, 784–803. http://dx.doi.org/10.1037/0022-3514.90.5.784

Diehl, M., Chui, H., Hay, E. L., Lumley, M. A., Grühn, D., & Labouvie-Vief, G. (2014). Change in coping and defense mechanisms across adulthood: Longitudinal findings in a European American sample. *Developmental Psychology, 50*, 634–648. http://dx.doi.org/10.1037/a0033619

Diehl, M., Coyle, N., & Labouvie-Vief, G. (1996). Age and sex differences in strategies of coping and defense across the lifespan. *Psychology and Aging, 11*, 127–139. http://dx.doi.org/10.1037.0882-7974.11.1.127

Erber, J. T., Szuchman, L. T., & Rothberg, S. T. (1990). Age, gender, and individual differences in memory failure appraisal. *Psychology and Aging, 5*, 600–603. http://dx.doi.org/10.1037/0882-7974.5.4.600

Fiske, S. T., Cuddy, A. J. C., Glick, P., & Xu, J. (2002). A model of (often mixed) stereotype content: Competence and warmth respectively from perceived status and competition. *Journal of Personality and Social Psychology, 82*, 878–902. http://dx.doi.org/10.1037/0022-3514.82.6.878

Garstka, T. A., Schmitt, M. T., Branscombe, N. R., & Hummert, M. L. (2004). How young and older adults differ in their responses to perceived age discrimination. *Psychology and Aging, 19*, 326–335. http://dx.doi.org/10.1037/0882-7974.19.2.326

Gerstorf, D., Röcke, C., & Lachman, M. E. (2010). Antecedent-consequent relations of perceived control to health and social support: Longitudinal evidence for between-domain associations across adulthood. *The Journals of Gerontology. Series B, Psychological Sciences and Social Sciences, 66*, 61–71. http://dx.doi.org/10.1093/geronb/gbq077

Giles, H., Fox, S., Harwood, J., & Williams, A. (1994). Talking age and aging talk: Communicating through the life span. In M. Hummert, J. Wiemann, & J. Nussbaum (Eds.), *Interpersonal communication in older adulthood: Interdisciplinary theory and research* (pp. 130–161). New York, NY: Sage.

Gill, M. J. (2004). When information does not deter stereotyping: Prescriptive stereotyping can foster bias under conditions that deter descriptive stereotyping. *Journal of Experimental Social Psychology, 40*, 619–632. http://dx.doi.org/10.1016/j.jesp.2003.12.001

Goffman, E. (1963). *Stigma: Notes on the management of spoiled identity*. New York, NY: Simon and Schuster.

Good, J. J., Moss-Racusin, C. A., & Sanchez, D. T. (2012). When do we confront? Perceptions of costs and benefits predict confronting discrimination on behalf of the self and others. *Psychology of Women Quarterly, 36*, 210–226. http://dx.doi.org/10.1177/0361684312440958

Heckhausen, J. (1997). Developmental regulation across adulthood: Primary and secondary control of age-related changes. *Developmental Psychology, 33*, 176–187. http://dx.doi.org/10.1037/0012-1649.33.1.176

Hess, T. M., Hinson, J., & Hodges, E. (2009). Moderators of and mechanisms underlying stereotype threat effects on older adults' memory performance. *Experimental Aging Research, 3,* 153–177. http://dx.doi.org/10.1080/03610730802716413

Hughes, M. L., Geraci, L., & De Forrest, R. L. (2013). Aging 5 years in 5 minutes: The effect of taking a memory test on older adults' subjective age. *Psychological Science,* http://dx.doi.org/10.1177/0956797613494853

Hummert, M. L., Garstka, T. A., Shaner, J. L., & Strahm, S. (1994). Stereotypes of the elderly held by young, middle-aged, and elderly adults. *Journal of Gerontology, 49,* P240–P249. http://dx.doi.org/10.1093/geronj/49.5.P240

Infurna, F. J., Gerstorf, D., & Zarit, S. H. (2011). Examining dynamic links between perceived control and health: Longitudinal evidence for differential effects in midlife and old age. *Developmental Psychology, 47,* 9–18. http://dx.doi.org/10.1037/a0021022

Kang, S. K., & Chasteen, A. L. (2009a). The moderating role of age-group identification and perceived threat on stereotype threat among older adults. *International Journal of Aging and Human Development, 69,* 201–220.

Kang, S. K., & Chasteen, A. L. (2009b). The development and validation of the age-based rejection-sensitivity questionnaire (RSQ-Age). *The Gerontologist, 49,* 303–316. http://dx.doi.org/10.1093/geront/gnp035

Kang, S. K., Chasteen, A. L., & Tse, C. (2014). *Perceptions of ageism, racism, and sexism among younger and older adults.* Manuscript in preparation.

Kite, M. E., Stockdale, G. D., Whitley, B. E., & Johnson, B. T. (2005). Attitudes toward younger and older adults: An updated meta-analytic review. *Journal of Social Issues, 61,* 241–266. http://dx.doi.org/10.1111/j.1540-4560.2005.00404.x

Kotter-Grühn, D., & Hess, T. M. (2012). The impact of age stereotypes on self-perceptions of aging across the adult lifespan. *The Journals of Gerontology. Series B, Psychological Sciences and Social Sciences, 67,* 563–571. http://dx.doi.org/10.1093/geronb/gbr153

Krause, N., & Shaw, B. A. (2003). Role-specific control, personal meaning, and health in late life. *Research on Aging, 25,* 559–586. http://dx.doi.org/10.1177/0164027503256695

Krings, F., Sczesny, S., & Kluge, A. (2011). Stereotypical inferences as mediators of age discrimination: The role of competence and warmth. *British Journal of Management, 22,* 187–201. http://dx.doi.org/10.1111/j.1467-8551.2010.00721.x

Langer, E. J., & Rodin, J. (1976). The effects of choice and enhanced personal responsibility for the aged: A field experiment in an institutional setting. *Journal of Personality and Social Psychology, 34,* 191–198. http://dx.doi.org/10.1037/0022-3514.34.2.191

Lazarus, R. S., & Folkman, S. (1984). *Stress, appraisal, and coping.* New York, NY: Springer Publishing.

Levy, B. R. (1996). Improving memory in old age by implicit self-stereotyping. *Journal of Personality and Social Psychology, 71,* 1092–1107. http://dx.doi.org/10.1037/0022-3514.71.6.1092

Levy, B. R. (2003). Mind matters: Cognitive and physical effects of aging self-stereotypes. *The Journals of Gerontology. Series B, Psychological Sciences and Social Sciences, 58,* P203–P211. http://dx.doi.org/10.1093/geronb/58.4.P203

Major, B., Kaiser, C. R., & McCoy, S. K. (2003). It's not my fault: When and why attributions to prejudice protect self-esteem. *Personality and Social Psychology Bulletin, 29*, 772–781. http://dx.doi.org/10.1177/0146167203252858

Major, B., & O'Brien, L. T. (2005). The social psychology of stigma. *Annual Review of Psychology, 56*, 393–421. http://dx.doi.org/10.1146/annurev.psych.56.091103.070137

Mallett, R. K., & Wagner, D. E. (2011). The unexpectedly positive consequences of confrontation. *Journal of Experimental Social Psychology, 47*, 215–220. http://dx.doi.org/10.1016/j.jesp.2010.10.001

Meisner, B. A. (2012). A meta-analysis of positive and negative age stereotype priming effects on behavior among older adults. *The Journals of Gerontology. Series B, Psychological Sciences and Social Sciences, 67*, 13–17. http://dx.doi.org/10.1093/geronb/gbr062

Mendoza-Denton, R., Downey, G., Purdie, V., Davis, A., & Pietrzak, J. (2002). Sensitivity to status-based rejection: Implications for African American students' college experience. *Journal of Personality and Social Psychology, 83*, 896–918. http://dx.doi.org/10.1037/0022-3514.83.4.896

Miller, C. T., & Kaiser, C. R. (2001). A theoretical perspective on coping with stigma. *Journal of Social Issues, 57*, 73–92. http://dx.doi.org/10.1111/0022-4537.00202

Montepare, J. M. (2009). Subjective age: Toward a guiding lifespan framework. *International Journal of Behavioral Development, 33*, 42–46. http://dx.doi.org/10.1177/0165025408095551

Montepare, J. M., & Lachman, M. E. (1989). "You're only as old as you feel": Self-perceptions of age, fears of aging, and life satisfaction from adolescence to old age. *Psychology and Aging, 4*, 73–78. http://dx.doi.org/10.1037/0882-7974.4.1.73

Nelson, T. D. (Ed.) (2002). *Ageism: Stereotyping and prejudice against older adults.* Cambridge, MA: MIT Press.

North, M. S., & Fiske, S. T. (2013). Act your (old) age: Prescriptive, ageist biases over succession, consumption, and identity. *Personality and Social Psychology Bulletin, 39*, 720–734. http://dx.doi.org/10.1177/0146167213480043

Nussbaum, J. F., Pitts, M. J., Huber, F. N., Krieger, J. L. R., & Ohs, J. E. (2005). Ageism and ageist language across the life span: Intimate relationships and non-intimate interactions. *Journal of Social Issues, 61*, 287–305. http://dx.doi.org/10.1111/j.1540-4560.2005.00406.x

Pasupathi, M., & Löckenhoff, C. E. (2002). Ageist behavior. In T. D. Nelson (Ed.), *Ageism: Stereotyping and prejudice against older persons* (pp. 201–246). Cambridge, MA: MIT Press.

Posthuma, R. A., & Campion, M. A. (2009). Age stereotypes in the workplace: Common stereotypes, moderators, and future research directions. *Journal of Management, 35*, 158–188. http://dx.doi.org/10.1177/0149206308318617

Rahhal, T. A., Hasher, L., & Colcombe, S. J. (2001). Instructional manipulations and age differences in memory: Now you see them, now you don't. *Psychology and Aging, 16*, 697–706. http://dx.doi.org/10.1037//0882-7974.16.4.697

Rasinski, H. M., & Czopp, A. M. (2010). The effect of target status on witnesses' reactions to confrontations of bias. *Basic & Applied Social Psychology, 32*, 8–16. http://dx.doi.org/10.1080/01973530903539754

Rubin, D. C., & Berntsen, D. (2006). People over forty feel 20% younger than their age: Subjective age across the life span. *Psychonomic Bulletin & Review, 13*, 776–780. http://dx.doi.org/10.3758/BF03193996

Rudman, L. A., & Glick, P. (2001). Prescriptive gender stereotypes and backlash toward agentic women. *Journal of Social Issues, 57*, 743–762. http://dx.doi.org/10.1111/0022-4537.00239

Rudman, L. A., & Phelan, J. E. (2008). Backlash effects for disconfirming gender stereotypes in organizations. In A. P. Brief & B. M. Staw (Eds.), *Research in organizational behavior* (Vol. 4, pp. 61–79). New York, NY: Elsevier.

Ryan, E. B., Hamilton, J. M., & Kwong See, S. (1994). Patronizing the old: How do younger and older adults respond to baby talk in the nursing home? *International Journal of Aging and Human Development, 39*, 21–32. http://dx.doi.org/10.2190/M52C-M2D2-R6C2-3PBM

Ryan, E. B., Hummert, M. L., & Boich, L. H. (1995). Communication predicaments of aging: Patronizing behavior toward older adults. *Journal of Language and Social Psychology, 14*, 144–166. http://dx.doi.org/10.1177/0261927X95141008

Schmitt, M. T., Branscombe, N. R., Kobrynowicz, D., & Owen, S. (2002). Perceiving discrimination against one's gender group has different implications for well-being in women and men. *Personality and Social Psychology Bulletin, 28*, 197–210. http://dx.doi.org/10.1177/0146167202282006

Schoemann, A. M., & Branscombe, N. R. (2011). Looking young for your age: Perceptions of anti-aging actions. *European Journal of Social Psychology, 41*, 86–95. http://dx.doi.org/10.1002/ejsp.738

Steele, C. M., & Aronson, J. (1995). Stereotype threat and the intellectual test performance of African Americans. *Journal of Personality and Social Psychology, 69*, 797–811. http://dx.doi.org/10.1037/0022-3514.69.5.797

Stephan, Y., Caudroit, J., & Chalabaev, A. (2011). Subjective health and memory self-efficacy as mediators in the relation between subjective age and life satisfaction among older adults. *Aging & Mental Health, 15*, 428–436. http://dx.doi.org/10.1080/13607863.2010.536138

Trawalter, S., Richeson, J. A., & Shelton, J. N. (2009). Predicting behavior during inter-racial interactions: A stress and coping approach. *Personality and Social Psychology Review, 13*, 243–268. http://dx.doi.org/10.1177/1088868309345850

Tyler, J. M., & McCullough, J. D. (2009). Violating prescriptive stereotypes on job resumes: A self-presentational perspective. *Management Communication Quarterly, 23*, 272–287. http://dx.doi.org/10.1177/0893318903411412

Weiss, D., & Freund, A. M. (2012). Still young at heart: Negative age-related information motivates distancing from same-aged people. *Psychology and Aging, 27*, 173–180. http://dx.doi.org/10.1037/a0024819

Weiss, D., & Lang, F. R. (2009). Thinking about my generation: Adaptive effects of a dual age identity in later adulthood. *Psychology and Aging, 24*, 729–734. http://dx.doi.org/10.1037/a0016339

Weiss, D., & Lang, F. R. (2012). "They" are old but "I" feel younger: Age-group dissociation as a self-protective strategy in old age. *Psychology and Aging, 27*, 153–163. http://dx.doi.org/10.1037/a0024887

CHAPTER 6

Views on Aging

Domain-Specific Approaches and Implications for Developmental Regulation

Anna E. Kornadt and Klaus Rothermund

ABSTRACT

Views on aging affect development across the life span through different pathways: They create a developmental context for older people by influencing behavior toward them (stereotyping, ageism), and they become incorporated into the self-concept of older people (self-stereotyping, internalization), which influences their attitudes toward their own age and aging, aging-related behaviors, life satisfaction, and even mortality. In this chapter, we argue that views on aging should be conceived as a domain-specific construct. We provide theoretical arguments for such a view that stems from life span research, as well as empirical evidence from studies that investigate the content and activation of views on aging as well as their consequences for developmental outcomes. We argue that a domain-specific perspective provides a fruitful and more comprehensive framework for addressing the role of views on aging in developmental regulation across the life span.

INTRODUCTION

Views on aging reflect a set of beliefs about "the changes that occur between birth and death, and about the social roles and activities that are to occur in different periods of life" (Settersten, 2009, p. 74). By influencing judgments of as well as attitudes and behavior toward older persons, they exert a direct impact on the developmental opportunities of older persons (Bowen & Staudinger, 2013; Nelson, 2011; Rothermund & Mayer, 2009; Ryan, Hummert, & Boich, 1995). Another, more subtle way how views on aging can influence development is through processes of self-stereotyping and stereotype internalization (Levy, 2009; Rothermund, 2005; Rothermund & Brandtstädter, 2003): One character-istic that distinguishes views on aging from other perceptions of social groups and individuals is that getting older is associated with becoming a member of the former out-group. That is, as we grow older, we become older persons ourselves, and views of old age and aging increasingly tend to color the views which we hold of ourselves in the present and in the future.

For a long time, it has been assumed that views on aging are mainly nega-tive and comprise images of losses as well as an overall deterioration of function-ing and well-being (Kite, Stockdale, Whitley, & Johnson, 2005; Nelson, 2011). However, if one thinks about older persons and aging, other things might come to mind as well: gains in wisdom and tenderness, generosity, experience, fam-ily orientation, or the freedom to pursue long-cherished activities and projects without the time constraints, which are inherent to middle-age working life. Thus, there are many reasons to assume that views on aging are complex and multidimensional: They comprise gains as well as losses, and they relate to dif-ferent areas of functioning and attributes. One such case of multidimensionality is the differentiation of views on aging regarding contexts or life domains, such as health or the work context. Considering the effects that views on aging have on aging individuals themselves, this complexity and variability in content and direction should also be reflected in the developmental outcomes which are asso-ciated with views on aging.

In the literature, a multitude of concepts and constructs have been used to describe different facets of the beliefs that people hold with respect to old age and aging (for a critical overview, see Diehl et al., 2014). We chose to use "views on aging" as an umbrella term which encompasses age stereotypes (men-tal representation of the characteristics and behaviors of older persons in gen-eral), aging stereotypes (generalized beliefs about the aging process), as well as personal expectations regarding age and aging, such as self-perceptions of one's own aging and future self-views. Focusing on those constructs, in this chapter we will highlight theoretical arguments for and determinants of the domain specific-ity of views on aging. We will also review empirical evidence from research on the content and activation of views on aging that further supports this assump-tion. Subsequently, we will review research that links domain-specific views on aging to behavior toward older persons as well as variables of adjustment and developmental regulation, which are indicators of successful development across

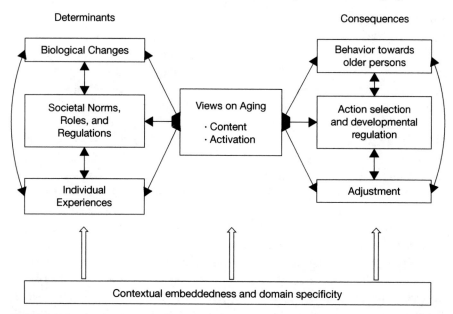

FIGURE 6.1 The domain-specific nature of views on aging, their determinants, and their consequences.

the adult life span (see Figure 6.1). We conclude by discussing open questions and challenges for future research and practice in the realm of subjective aging.

WHY CAN WE ASSUME THAT VIEWS ON AGING ARE DOMAIN SPECIFIC?

Views on aging have long been operationalized and assessed in a unidimensional way, with the implication that they have been described on a single positive–negative continuum (e.g., Kogan, 1961; Polizzi, 2003; Rothermund & Brandtstädter, 2003). Therefore, the resulting interpretation has often been that older persons and getting older are perceived to be rather negative in absolute values as well as relative to younger persons and to being younger. Such a unidimensional perspective, however, does not take the complexity and contextual embeddedness of views on aging into account. According to this latter perspective, views on aging are highly specific, varying in content and valence depending on the life domain to which they refer.

In the following text, we will review theoretical reasoning and empirical evidence for this perspective, supporting the assumption that views on aging are best conceptualized in a domain-specific way.

Life Span Theory

In Baltes' (1987) principles of life span developmental psychology, he describes multidimensionality and multidirectionality as being among the key concepts of life span development. According to these principles, actual development does not follow a unidimensional decline trajectory in older age. On the contrary, between and even within different domains of functioning, there is considerable variability in the direction and patterns of development and also in the criteria that can be applied to evaluate successful functioning and adjustment in different stages of the life span. This can be seen in domains such as cognitive functioning, personality development, and also physical characteristics (Baltes, Lindenberger, & Staudinger, 2006; Keil, 2006): Age-related changes in these different domains are to a certain degree independent and characterized by specific content. In addition, within and across domains both gains and losses can be observed throughout the entire life span.

These principles can be transferred directly to subjective conceptualizations of development, because what people think about the course of development and developmental trajectories is not independent of actual developmental mechanisms and processes (Chan et al., 2012; Löckenhoff et al., 2009; Mustafić & Freund, 2012; Schelling & Martin, 2008; Wood & Roberts, 2006). Thus, studies that investigated subjective conceptualizations of life span development consistently find that even though the proportion of losses increases with age, gains and losses in different domains are perceived to take place across the entire life span, showing a broad and multifaceted picture that cannot be forced onto a single positive–negative continuum (e.g., Grühn, Gilet, Studer, & Labouvie-Vief, 2011; Heckhausen, Dixon, & Baltes, 1989; Mustafić & Freund, 2012).

Furthermore, development is always a result of the interaction of an individual with the social and historical contexts in which he or she is situated in. This is captured by the principle of ontogenetic and historical contextualism (Baltes et al., 2006; Burke, Joseph, Pasick, & Barker, 2009). The implications of specific age-related biological or physiological changes for functioning or successful development strongly depend on the affordances and constraints that are provided by the social, physical, and historical contexts in which they occur (Diehl & Wahl, 2010; Keller, Leventhal, & Larson, 1989; Neugarten, Moore, & Lowe, 1965; Steverink, Westerhof, Bode, & Dittmann-Kohli, 2001; Waid & Frazier, 2003).

A focus on contextual influences also sensitizes developmental researchers to the fact that the life course is organized and structured by institutions, social norms, roles, and regulations that codetermine development by providing age-specific opportunities, challenges, and deadlines (Hagestad & Neugarten, 1985;

Heckhausen, Wrosch, & Fleeson, 2001; Kohli, 2007; Settersten, 2009; Wood & Roberts, 2006). Those institutionalized age norms and regulations, such as the work context, welfare and retirement practices, family systems, government-provided supportive structures, and so forth, as well as the social roles that are occupied by younger and older individuals, have a strong impact on what we expect from people of different ages in specific settings (Diehl, Hastings, & Stanton, 2001; Eagly, 1987; Eagly, Wood, & Diekman, 2000; Kite et al., 2005; Kruse & Schmitt, 2006; Wood & Roberts, 2006). For example, a mandatory retirement age (such as in Germany, age 65 years) implies that older people are expected not to work anymore after this age, which might go hand in hand with the implicit attribution of certain characteristics and skills (or lack thereof) to persons who are approaching this age (cf. Kite, Deaux, & Miele, 1991; Radl, 2012). Seen from the perspective of the aging person himself or herself, the existence of a mandatory retirement age might foster beliefs that one is not fit and flexible enough to participate in the work force, and it might reduce personal identification with the work role and instigate disengagement tendencies. Whereas the specification of a retirement age has implications for the perception and evaluation of older persons in the work domain regarding work-related attributes, other social norms affect views on aging in other domains: For example, the norm that grandparents should care for their grandchildren might impact our views on aging in the family domain, suggesting ascriptions of attributes such as affectionate, patient, and generous. It might also imply that it is often taken for granted that grandparents have plenty of free time.

In summary, institutionalized norms and regulations not only directly shape development via incentives and sanctions, but they also find their way into the views we have on aging and development in specific life domains. These internalized beliefs and expectations influence our perceptions of older people in a specific way, depending on the context in which they are encountered. In particular, deviations from age-related expectations (being "off-time" or not "acting one's age"; Neugarten et al., 1965) give rise to ascriptions of specific traits or personality characteristics—for example, someone who is still working after retirement age might be perceived as being overeager or stubborn, and refusing to take care of one's grandchildren might suggest attributes such as being selfish or cold-hearted (Kalicki, 1996).

From these theoretical arguments, it should be clear that views on aging are directly tied to and influenced by the contextual settings in which development takes place (see arrows connecting the left and middle parts of Figure 6.1). That this is not merely a theoretical assumption, but can be backed up by findings from empirical studies that investigate the content, activation, and consequences of views on aging, will be demonstrated in the following section.

Content and Activation of Domain-Specific Views on Aging

A large number of studies attest to the domain specificity of views on aging by highlighting differences in the content and valence of age-related beliefs and stereotypes. In their seminal studies, Brewer, Dull, and Lui (1981) and later Schmidt and Boland (1986), Hummert (1990), and Hummert, Garstka, Shaner, and Strahm (1994) used card-sorting tasks to determine whether prototypes of older persons could be identified. Indeed, instead of one prototypical "old person," they found several, distinct subtypes of older persons, with specifically assigned traits and descriptions, such as the "curmudgeon," the "perfect grandparent," the "severely impaired," or the "John Wayne conservative." These heterogeneous subtypes exemplify differences in aging-related developmental pathways and personality profiles, but they also refer to views of old people in different contexts (e.g., in social interactions, in political discussions, in a family setting, in a nursing home).

The most common method to assess the content of age stereotypes, however, has been to apply explicit questionnaire measures, asking participants about their beliefs about old persons and/or age-related changes. In those questionnaires, either sentences or adjectives are presented, and participants have to rate whether and to what extent the respective characteristic applies to older persons. Many scales were constructed to measure one underlying dimension: whether views on aging are either more positive or rather negative, on an absolute level, or when comparing evaluations of older and younger persons (e.g., Kogan, 1961; Polizzi, 2003). Other studies used one-dimensional subscales of questionnaires (e.g., the Attitudes Toward Own Aging subscale of the Philadelphia Geriatric Center Morale Scale; Lawton, 1975).

However, it was soon discovered that a one-dimensional structure has its shortcomings and is unable to account for the heterogeneity of aging-related beliefs and evaluations. In addition, the complexity of views on aging has been found to increase with advancing age (Heckhausen et al., 1989; Hummert, 1990). Therefore, a wide array of measures has been developed with multiple dimensions based on the assumption that the description of and attitudes toward older persons and aging are more complex than can be described with a simple dichotomy of positive and negative. Those measures range from two dimensions, assuming competence and warmth as the two underlying dimensions along which social groups are evaluated (Fiske, Cuddy, Glick, & Xu, 2002), to various attribute dimensions on semantic differential scales (Chumbler, 1994; Gluth, Ebner, & Schmiedek, 2010; Rosencranz & McNevin, 1969) and to scales which assess dimensions of everyday life and functioning associated with getting older and older persons (Kornadt & Rothermund, 2011a; Kruse & Schmitt, 2006; Sarkisian, Hays, Berry, & Mangione, 2002; Steverink et al.,

2001; Wahl, Konieczny, & Diehl, 2013). Because of differences in response for-
mat, different selections of items, and specification of different targets that have
to be rated, the proposed measures differ regarding the dimensions which are
suggested as constituting basic dimensions of aging-related beliefs and attitudes.
Still, the general conclusion that can be drawn from these studies is that apparently, separable and independent dimensions of views on old age and aging can
be identified and that a single bipolar dimension is not capable of describing the
complex system of beliefs that people hold regarding old age and aging in different contexts.

In an attempt to systematically capture the contextual embeddedness of
age-related beliefs and evaluations, Kornadt and Rothermund (2011a) developed
scales in which old persons had to be evaluated with respect to eight different life
domains (family, friends, religion, leisure, lifestyle, money, work, health). Each
life domain was represented by a set of statements specifying descriptions of
positive and negative attributes within the respective domain. Evaluations of old
people within each domain were assessed with bipolar scales, the end points of
which were anchored with opposite positive and negative stereotypic statements.
Factor analyses yielded independent factors for the eight domains. Besides the differentiation in views on aging, studies applying this questionnaire also provided
evidence for domain-specific age group differences in the evaluation of older
persons (Kornadt & Rothermund, 2011a; Kornadt, Voss, & Rothermund, 2013).
Interestingly, older people showed less negative views on aging particularly for
those domains in which strongly negative stereotypes prevail in other age groups
(health and fitness, work and employment). However, they showed less positive evaluations of old age targets for domains in which positive stereotypes are
salient for younger people (leisure activities and civic commitment, religion and
spirituality; Kornadt et al., 2013). These findings indicate that stereotypes are
more differentiated and less extreme during old age. This process might reflect an
incorporation of personal experiences into views on aging as people grow older
(Kornadt & Rothermund, 2012; Rothermund & Brandtstädter, 2003). Such age-
related changes in domain-specific evaluations might also result from accommodative shifts in views on aging that help older people to maintain a positive
outlook on their lives in those domains which are important for their well-being
(Brandtstädter & Rothermund, 2002; Rothermund, Wentura, & Brandtstädter,
1995). The complex pattern of age differences in views on aging for different
contexts and life domains provides further evidence for the necessity and useful-
ness of a domain-specific approach when investigating views on aging.

Besides investigating the content that constitutes views on aging in different life domains, which was the main focus of the questionnaire studies cited
earlier, several studies also addressed the question of when and how those beliefs

become activated. Social cognition researchers typically assume that attitudes toward and stereotypes of social groups become activated in an automatic and generalized manner, suggesting that if a person is categorized as old, all evaluations and attributes that are related to "old persons" are activated simultaneously and subsequently influence judgments of and behavior toward older people. In line with such a view, some studies investigated the activation of implicit evaluations which are related to the category "old," using the Implicit Association Test (IAT; Greenwald, McGhee, & Schwartz, 1998) or evaluative priming measures. These studies reported negative implicit attitudes toward the category old compared to the category "young" (Chasteen, Schwartz, & Park, 2002; de Paula Couto & Wentura, 2012; Hummert, Garstka, O'Brien, Greenwald, & Mellott, 2002; Nosek, Banaji, & Greenwald, 2002; Perdue & Gurtman, 1990). The methods that were used in these studies always assessed attitudes toward the category old and "old people" in a general and supposedly context-neutral way. The general negativity effects that were found with those measures, however, might emerge because they tend to activate the health context by default. This might be because of the frequent use of health-related stimuli or simply because health is the most salient context that comes to mind when thinking about older people. De Paula Couto and Wentura (2012), for example, contrasted everyday pictures of old people with decline-related stimuli, which depicted frail older people in a nursing home context. These results should thus not be taken as indicators for a general and context-neutral activation of negative evaluations with respect to the category old. It rather seems to be the case that these situations also encompass implicit context clues that lead to stereotype activation, which is specific for the respective situation.

As our own findings show, specifying contexts leads to an activation of corresponding evaluations of old age and aging, which can be negative, neutral, or positive. For example, Casper, Rothermund, and Wentura (2011) used a dual-prime technique in which category primes (i.e., pictures of old vs. young faces) and context primes (i.e., sentences describing specific situations and behavioral activities) were combined. They found that the activation of specific age-related trait attributes was dependent on the context in which the face of an older or a younger person was presented. Significant priming effects emerged only for matching combinations of age categories, contexts, and stereotypical attributes. That is, the picture of an old woman facilitated processing of the word "slow" only in combination with the sentence "she is walking across the street," but not in combination with the sentence "she is watering the flowers." These findings extend previous studies by showing that specific facets of stereotypes are activated in a highly context-specific way and that social categories alone typically do not suffice to activate stereotypic attributes on a large scale (Casper &

Rothermund, 2012; Casper et al., 2010; Mendoza-Denton, Park, & O'Conner, 2008; Müller & Rothermund, 2012; Yeh & Barsalou, 2006). Apparently, this also holds for the activation of age-related stereotypes: Age stereotypes do not form a single homogeneous cluster that is activated as a whole; instead, different facets of the age stereotype are represented as separate and independent mental schemas, each of which consists of a connection between the category information old and a specific combination of a situational context and matching trait attribute (Casper et al., 2011). In summary, studies investigating the content and activation of age stereotypes support the assumption that views on aging are domain specific. As such, they contain positive and negative elements that are activated separately and independently in different contexts and domains.

Findings emphasizing domain specificity in the content and activation of views on aging are indicated by the upward-pointing middle arrow in Figure 6.1. As we will argue in the following text, this differentiated set of aging-related beliefs and expectations is also connected to corresponding domain-specific effects regarding the developmental outcomes which are linked to views on aging (connections between middle and right part and upward-pointing arrow in Figure 6.1).

CONSEQUENCES OF DOMAIN-SPECIFIC VIEWS ON AGING FOR DEVELOPMENTAL PROCESSES AND OUTCOMES

Views on aging have consequences for development across the life span, not only influencing behavior toward older people but also affecting the aging process of older persons themselves. This has been shown in a multitude of studies, and possible mechanisms for this influence have been discussed (e.g., Hess, 2006; Kornadt & Rothermund, 2012; Levy, 2009; Rothermund, 2005; Sargent-Cox, Anstey, & Luszcz, 2014; Wurm, Tomasik, & Tesch-Römer, 2010), even though more empirical evidence for the exact mechanisms, as well as for moderators and mediators of these mechanisms, is still needed. Matching domain-specific views on aging as predictor variables to specific criteria might lead to a better and more differentiated prediction of developmental outcomes (Diehl et al., 2014). Furthermore, domains might differ regarding their importance and self-relevance depending on a person's age. For example, the work domain might be especially relevant before the retirement transition, whereas health and family might become more relevant in later life. Considering stereotype embodiment theory (Levy, 2009) and the notion that stereotypes become self-fulfilling prophecies as they become more self-relevant, they might be especially powerful predictors shortly before or around those transitions in the respective domain. There already are some studies demonstrating that views on aging in different domains might differentially influence specific outcome variables.

Influence on Ageist Behavior

Behavior toward older adults that is guided by stereotypical assumptions regarding what one can expect from and how one perceives older adults is often referred to as ageist behavior, or age discrimination (see Chapter 5 by Chasteen & Cary, this volume; Nelson, 2011). Evidence for unfair or patronizing behavior toward older people is abundant, and age discrimination has been shown to occur in various life domains such as the work place, health care settings, banking and finances (e.g., availability of mortgages, insurance terms), and jurisdiction (for a review, see Rothermund & Mayer, 2009).

Conceptualizing views on aging as domain specific might provide evidence for a refined understanding of the underlying mechanisms of ageist behavior. For example, Diekman and Hirnisey (2007) found age-related discrimination regarding hiring decisions only when the job description was advertising a modern and flexible company but not when a stable and conservative company was described. This reflects stereotypes of older people as being less flexible but highly reliable (cf. Perry & Finkelstein, 1999). In a similar vein, current conceptualizations of age-based discrimination treat ageism as a multidimensional phenomenon. North and Fiske (2013a, 2013b) categorize ageism in terms of the facets "identity," focusing on intergroup differences; "consumption," expressing the belief that shared resources should be preferentially allocated to younger people because living in old age is no longer worth living; and "succession," seeing older people as an obstacle to society as well as dispossessing old people of relevant societal roles and positions. This differentiation has implications for behavior toward older adults depending on the context in which they are encountered. Ageist beliefs focusing on a different social identity of young and old people shape behavior in contexts of intergroup interaction, favoring segregation over integration (e.g., avoiding areas where older people live). Beliefs regarding the dimension consumption might be especially relevant when predicting behavior toward older people in situations which are characterized by scarce resources (e.g., health care decisions, changes in the level of retirement pensions). Beliefs regarding succession might be more relevant when social roles have to be negotiated, such as in the work place (North & Fiske, 2013a). Again, a domain-specific perspective provides added value when predicting specific behaviors of and toward older persons.

Implications for the Self-Views and Development of Older Persons

From an action-theoretical developmental perspective (Brandtstädter, 2006), views on aging play an important role for processes of developmental regulation. Stereotypic beliefs of old age form a background for expectations regarding one's own future development and age-related changes. By comprising opportunities as well as threats, possible gains, as well as losses, they become self-fulfilling prophecies (Levy, 2009; Wurm, Warner, Ziegelmann, Wolff, & Schüz, 2013). Again, views on aging affect processes of self-development in a highly specific way: Influences are stronger in those life domains where views on aging match the content of the specific outcome. Supporting evidence comes from studies investigating the effects of views on aging on self-views, performance, attitudes toward living in old age, and preparation for old age.

Self-Stereotyping

It is assumed that during the life course, age stereotypes color the future and current self-views of older persons through processes of internalization and self-stereotyping (Levy, 2009; Rothermund, 2005; Rothermund & Brandtstädter, 2003). Evidence for the domain specificity of this process was reported in a study by Kornadt and Rothermund (2012). We found that the internalization of age stereotypes into the self-concept via future self-views was moderated by participants' expectations of age-related changes in the respective life domain. Domain-specific future expectations regarding old age thus determine whether stereotypes have a strong influence on the self-concept and thereby on the behavior of aging persons.

Stereotype Priming

Age stereotypes can also situationally affect the performance and behavior of older persons when made salient or primed implicitly. Several studies reported evidence for the content-specific nature of these behavior-priming effects. For example, Levy and Leifheit-Limson (2009) subliminally primed stereotypes in the physical versus memory domain and found that people in the former group performed worse on a balance task, whereas the latter group performed worse on a memory task. This stereotype-matching effect was further supported by Haslam et al. (2012) who showed that people who identified with old age and who were primed with either the expectation that old age is accompanied with general cognitive versus memory decline performed worse in measures of general cognitive ability versus a memory test, respectively. Thus, the influence of stereotype priming on older adults does not affect all behaviors in a global fashion but rather works in a domain-specific way.

Attitudes Towards Living in Old Age

Evidence for domain-specific relationships between age stereotypes and people's general attitudes toward life in older age has also been provided. Kornadt and Rothermund (2011b) investigated whether age stereotypes in different life domains were related to people's beliefs on whether old age should be a time of leisure and pleasure or a time of activity and commitment to others. They showed that age stereotypes in the domains of leisure, friends, and health were positively related to their participants' opinion that life in old age should be a time of activity and commitment to others. No such effect was obtained for views on aging in other life domains. Furthermore, age stereotypes were not related to the widely shared belief that old age should be a time to enjoy one's life free of any obligations.

Action Selection and Preparation for Old Age

Behavioral pathways bridging the gap between attitudes and adjustment have also been demonstrated to operate in a domain-specific way. For example, Hoppmann, Gerstorf, Smith, and Klumb (2007) found that possible future self-views of older people predicted actual engagement in daily activities in various life domains in a highly domain-specific way. Furthermore, Meisner, Weir, and Baker (2013) provided convincing evidence for the domain-specific influence of views on aging on age-related behaviors. In two studies, they demonstrated that older adults' participation in physical activities and medical examinations were related to expectations regarding aging which matched the respective functional domain (Meisner & Baker, 2013; Meisner et al., 2013). For example, older adults' participation in physical exercise was related to expectations regarding aging in the physical domain, whereas cognitive functioning and mental health expectations did not affect this type of behavior.

In a broader approach, we investigated the relationship between views on aging and preparation for anticipated age-related changes. A recent study by Kornadt and Rothermund (2014) provided evidence for the multidimensional nature of preparation behavior, showing independent factors for domain-specific aging-related planning and preparation activities. These data also attest to the relevance of views on aging for preparation: Positive age stereotypes were related to positive future self-views in the corresponding domains, which in turn predicted related domain-specific preparation activities (Kornadt & Rothermund, 2013), and ultimately life satisfaction. Conversely, negative views on aging can thus be seen as a major risk factor for a decrease in life satisfaction during old age. By highlighting negative developmental scenarios in a specific domain, negative age stereotypes and negative future self-views apparently undermine the motivation to invest into one's own future and to engage in the respective preparation behaviors.

In summary, a multitude of studies attest to the added predictive value of specific assessment of views on aging when investigating their relationship to different forms of ageism as well as to age-related regulation processes and developmental outcomes (these relations are highlighted by the arrows connecting the middle and right part and by the upward-pointing right arrow in Figure 6.1). Our own research that takes different life domains into account also provides considerable evidence for this point. Having people imagine others or oneself as an old person who is clearly situated in a particular life domain activates corresponding highly specific attributes and associations, varying in content and evaluation. Those domain-related prospects and beliefs also bear specific relationships to matching outcomes. Furthermore, the strength of those relationships depends on the relevance of the respective domain for people who are close to age- and domain-specific transitions. The reported findings highlight the differential validity and also the added value of a domain-specific approach when linking views on aging to developmental processes throughout the life span (see Figure 6.1).

FUTURE DIRECTIONS

The research presented in this chapter demonstrates that a domain-specific conceptualization of views on aging is necessary to account for the multifacetedness and complexity of the aging process and its perceptions across the life span. Various research instruments have been developed to assess views on aging in a domain-specific way: Beliefs and attitudes concerning old age and older people were measured in a specific situational context (e.g., with respect to older workers) or regarding sets of attributes which are of particular relevance within a certain life domain (e.g., family-related attributes such as lonely, generous, or caring). Studies linking these domain-specific expectations and evaluations to processes of developmental regulation show that they differentially predict behavior toward as well as attitudes, action selection, and adjustment of older persons. However, there are still several questions that have to be addressed to make more precise and informed statements about the development, activation, and influence of domain-specific views on aging across the life span.

Origins and Sources of Views on Aging

Two of the main unsolved questions are the following: Where do views of aging originate and how do they develop and change over time? And what constitutes the basis of domain specificity of views on aging? A more detailed investigation of the sources of perceived changes which are experienced by the aging person himself or herself on the one hand and changes in the contexts in which older persons develop on the other could provide further insight into possible origins of domain specificity. The former would be represented by assumptions about personality and attribute changes in old age (Chan et al., 2012), changes in mental and physical functioning (Grühn et al., 2011), and people's general awareness of age-related changes (Diehl & Wahl, 2010; Miche et al., 2014). The latter includes an assessment of expected or experienced age-related changes in situational opportunities and constraints in different contexts such as the work context or relationships within the family (Voss, 2013). This would also lead to a more theory-driven approach regarding the assumption of changes and influences of domain-specific views on aging across the life span (Diehl et al., 2014). In particular, evidence regarding the sources of views on aging could help to clarify the distinction between domain-specific (i.e., focusing on life or functional domains) and person-specific (i.e., focusing on different attribute clusters) approaches (see left part of Figure 6.1). Disentangling the person- and context-related sources of differential views on aging could lead to a refined understanding of their content and developmental regulative function and may also have applied implications regarding the design of interventions which foster successful aging and development across the life span (see Chapter 10 by Miche, Brothers, Diehl, & Wahl, this volume).

Moderators and Influences

Other person characteristics that are per se unrelated to age, but can have an indirect influence on age-related expectations and experiences, such as gender or social class, also play a major role in determining domain-specific differences in views on aging. Taking those variables into account could therefore also lead to a better understanding of why some domains are linked with a more positive view on aging, whereas others are more likely to be linked to negative views. Although there has been a vast amount of research on the differential impact that aging might have on the perceptions of men and women, a recent study by Kornadt et al. (2013) provided evidence for the benefits of a domain-specific approach in clarifying the role of gender differences in views on aging as well: Compared to older women, older men were rated more positively in the domains of finances and work; in contrast, older women were rated more positively in most activity-related and social domains such as leisure and friendship. The implications of these results need to be taken into account when investigating aging processes from a gendered perspective.

Social class also seems to be a variable that might lead to differential views on aging depending on specific life domains. To the best of our knowledge, social class differences in facets of views on aging have not yet been investigated. However, having for example financial opportunities and the means and knowledge to ameliorate age-related changes might lead to different perceptions of older persons and of one's own aging. It thus seems reasonable to assume that social class differences should also be associated with differences in views on aging. Again, effects of social class on views on aging are probably most pronounced in life domains which are closely related to education, finances, and social influence such as work, housing, or civic engagement, but are weak or negligible in more personal life domains such as close relationships, spirituality, or personality development.

When it comes to perceived or expected context changes that have an influence on how views on aging form and develop, comparisons of different cultures or countries are also necessary (Barak, 2009). If we assume that the social policy and retirement practices as well as family structures that are prevalent in different cultures have an impact on the roles and characteristics which are attributed to older persons, then this might lead to a different perception of older adults and—by implication—different developmental trajectories during the aging process. For example, in an analysis conducted with data from the European Social Survey, it was found that countries in which older adults had a higher activity level also had more positive views on aging (Bowen & Skirbekk, 2013). Pairing this with a domain-specific approach could be an interesting avenue for gaining a better understanding of cross-cultural differences in views on aging which have been reported in previous studies (e.g., Bergman, Bodner, & Cohen-Fridel, 2013; Levy & Langer, 1994; Westerhof, Whitbourne, & Freeman, 2011). In particular, cultural differences might affect different life domains—for example, collectivistic cultures might endorse more positive views on aging in the family domain, whereas individualistic cultures might provide a more positive outlook on old age and aging in terms of financial independence and provision.

Implicit Measures

Another interesting line of research concerns the relation between implicit and explicit measures of domain-specific views on aging and their differential impact on life span development (Levy & Banaji, 2002). As outlined earlier, some studies have implicitly assessed ageism and attitudes toward aging, however, in a supposedly unidimensional way (de Paula Couto & Wentura, 2012; Hummert et al., 2002; Nosek et al., 2002). That it is also fruitful to use those measures in a domain-specific way was recently demonstrated by Kornadt, Meissner, and Rothermund (2014). We could show that implicit age stereotypes in the health and family domains that were assessed with two different IATs were uncorrelated with corresponding explicit views on aging and thus have to be considered as independent constructs. We also found valence differences for the implicit stereotypes in the two domains, as well as different age trajectories. Specifically, whereas implicit age stereotypes were clearly negative for the health domain in all age groups, IAT effects indicated neutral evaluations of older people in the family domain for younger and middle-aged participants and a positive picture of old age in the family domain for the oldest subsample of our study (Kornadt et al., 2014).

Considering the pivotal role that is assigned to implicit influences of views on aging in theories such as the stereotype embodiment theory (Levy, 2009), it seems necessary to investigate the role of domain-specific implicit views on aging more closely. This should advance our understanding of internalization processes and also of the influence that views on aging have on the functioning of older adults.

Developmental Acquisition and Differentiation of Views on Aging

The images people have of older persons or their own aging are believed to form in younger years (Gilbert & Ricketts, 2008; Isaacs & Bearison, 1986; Kwong, Sheree, Rasmussen, & Pertman, 2012) and further develop and differentiate as people grow older and move through the life course (Heckhausen et al., 1989; Hummert et al., 1994; Rothermund & Brandtstädter, 2003). This process is influenced by actual encounters with older persons, culturally transmitted views on aging, norms and regulations that are based on or associated with chronological age, and personal experiences with the aging process (e.g., Blunk & Williams, 1997; Harwood, Hewstone, Paolini, & Voci, 2005; Schelling & Martin, 2008; see left part of Figure 6.1).

From the perspective of domain specificity, it would be of great interest to investigate whether specific views on aging originate from a more global attitude toward old age and aging and undergo a process of differentiation or whether views on aging are already acquired in a domain-specific way. In general, we would expect that views on aging and age stereotypes are always transmitted in a contextualized way. Children are not taught abstract statements linking old age with a set of attributes. Instead, personal experiences with older adults, such as grandparents or the portrayal of old people in the media, typically are embedded in specific contexts or domains, even if this contextual information is rarely stated in an explicit way. Clearly, however, empirical research on the development of domain-specific views on aging, comparing children at different ages, is necessary to gain more insight into the acquisition of differentiated views on aging during the early life span.

CONCLUSION

The research that has been outlined in this chapter supports the notion that views on aging are domain specific. Combined with the already existing evidence that links views on aging to a multitude of developmental outcomes, this approach might be fruitful for a more detailed and refined understanding of the aging process. Investigating views on aging and their antecedents and consequences in a domain-specific way thus helps us to provide the basis to foster successful aging and well-being of aging persons.

ACKNOWLEDGMENTS

This work was supported by two grants of the Volkswagen Stiftung (AZ II/83 142, AZ 86 758) to Klaus Rothermund.

REFERENCES

Baltes, P. B. (1987). Theoretical propositions of life-span developmental psychology: On the dynamics between growth and decline. *Developmental Psychology*, 23, 611–626. http://dx.doi.org/10.1037/0012-1649.23.5.611

Baltes, P. B., Lindenberger, U., & Staudinger, U. M. (2006). Life span theory in developmental psychology. In W. Damon (Series Ed.) & R. M. Lerner (Vol. Ed.), *Handbook of child psychology: Vol. 1. Theoretical models of human development* (6th ed., pp. 569–664). Hoboken, NJ: Wiley.

Barak, B. (2009). Age identity: A cross-cultural global approach. *International Journal of Behavioral Development*, 33, 2–11. http://dx.doi.org/10.1177/0165025408099485

Bergman, Y. S., Bodner, E., & Cohen-Fridel, S. (2013). Cross-cultural ageism: Ageism and attitudes toward aging among Jews and Arabs in Israel. *International Psychogeriatrics*, 25, 6–15. http://dx.doi.org/10.1017/s1041610212001548

Blunk, E. M., & Williams, S. W. (1997). The effects of curriculum on preschool children's perceptions of the elderly. *Educational Gerontology*, 23, 233–241. http://dx.doi.org/10.1080/0360127970230303

Bowen, C. E., & Skirbekk, V. (2013). National stereotypes of older people's competence are related to older adults' participation in paid and volunteer work. *The Journals of Gerontology. Series B. Psychological Sciences and Social Sciences*, 68, 974–983. http://dx.doi.org/10.1093/geronb/gbt101

Bowen, C. E., & Staudinger, U. M. (2013). Relationship between age and promotion orientation depends on perceived older worker stereotypes. *The Journals of Gerontology. Series B. Psychological Sciences and Social Sciences*, 68, 59–63. http://dx.doi.org/10.1093/geronb/gbs060

Brandtstädter, J. (2006). Action perspectives on human development. In W. Damon (Series Ed.) & R. M. Lerner (Vol. Ed.), *Handbook of child psychology: Theoretical models of human development* (6th ed., Vol. 1, pp. 516–568). Hoboken, NJ: Wiley.

Brandtstädter, J., & Rothermund, K. (2002). The life-course dynamics of goal pursuit and goal adjustment: A two-process framework. *Developmental Review*, 22, 117–150. http://dx.doi.org/10.1006/drev.2001.0539

Brewer, M. B., Dull, V., & Lui, L. (1981). Perceptions of the elderly: Stereotypes as prototypes. *Journal of Personality and Social Psychology*, 41, 656–670. http://dx.doi.org/10.1037/0022-3514.41.4.656

Burke, N. J., Joseph, G., Pasick, R. J., & Barker, J. C. (2009). Theorizing social context: Rethinking behavioral theory. *Health Education & Behavior*, 36, 55S–70S. http://dx.doi.org/10.1177/1090198109335338

Casper, C., & Rothermund, K. (2012). Gender self-stereotyping is context dependent for men but not for women. *Basic and Applied Social Psychology, 34*, 434–442. http://dx.doi.org/10.1080/01973533.2012.712014

Casper, C., Rothermund, K., & Wentura, D. (2010). Automatic stereotype activation is context dependent. *Social Psychology, 41*, 131–136. http://dx.doi.org/10.1027/1864-9335/a000019

Casper, C., Rothermund, K., & Wentura, D. (2011). The activation of specific facets of age stereotypes depends on individuating information. *Social Cognition, 29*, 393–414. http://dx.doi.org/10.1521/soco.2011.29.4.393

Chan, W., McCrae, R. R., de Fruyt, F., Jussim, L., Löckenhoff, C. E., de Bolle, M., . . . Terracciano, A. (2012). Stereotypes of age differences in personality traits: Universal and accurate? *Journal of Personality and Social Psychology, 103*, 1050–1066. http://dx.doi.org/10.1037/a0029712

Chasteen, A. L., Schwartz, N., & Park, D. C. (2002). The activation of aging stereotypes in younger and older adults. *The Journals of Gerontology. Series B. Psychological Sciences and Social Sciences, 57*, P540–P547. http://dx.doi.org/10.1093/geronb/57.6.P540

Chumbler, N. R. (1994). The development and reliability of a Stereotypes Toward Older People Scale. *College Student Journal, 28*, 220–229.

De Paula Couto, M. C. P., & Wentura, D. (2012). Automatically activated facets of ageism: Masked evaluative priming allows for a differentiation of age-related prejudice. *European Journal of Social Psychology, 42*, 852–863. http://dx.doi.org/10.1002/ejsp.1912

Diehl, M., Hastings, C. T., & Stanton, J. M. (2001). Self-concept differentiation across the adult life span. *Psychology and Aging, 16*, 643–654. http://dx.doi.org/10.1037/0882-7974.16.4.643

Diehl, M. K., & Wahl, H. W. (2010). Awareness of age-related change: Examination of a (mostly) unexplored concept. *The Journals of Gerontology. Series B. Psychological Sciences and Social Sciences, 65*, 340–350. http://dx.doi.org/10.1093/geronb/gbp110

Diehl, M., Wahl, H. W., Barrett, A. E., Brothers, A. F., Miche, M., Montepare, J. M., . . . Wurm, S. (2014). Awareness of aging: Theoretical considerations on an emerging concept. *Developmental Review, 34*, 93–113. http://dx.doi.org/10.1016/j.dr.2014.01.001

Diekman, A. B., & Hirnisey, L. (2007). The effect of context on the silver ceiling: A role congruity perspective on prejudiced responses. *Personality and Social Psychology Bulletin, 33*, 1353–1366. http://dx.doi.org/10.1177/0146167207303019

Eagly, A. H. (1987). *Sex differences in social behavior: A social-role interpretation*. Hillsdale, NJ: Lawrence Erlbaum Associates.

Eagly, A. H., Wood, W., & Diekman, A. B. (2000). Social role theory of sex differences and similarities: A current appraisal. In T. Eckes & H. M. Trautner (Eds.), *The developmental social psychology of gender* (pp. 123–174). Mahwah, NJ: Lawrence Erlbaum Associates.

Fiske, S. T., Cuddy, A. J., Glick, P., & Xu, J. (2002). A model of (often mixed) stereotype content: Competence and warmth respectively follow from perceived status and competition. *Journal of Personality and Social Psychology, 82*, 878–902. http://dx.doi.org/10.1037//0022-3514.82.6.878

Gilbert, C. N., & Ricketts, K. G. (2008). Children's attitudes toward older adults and aging: A synthesis of research. *Educational Gerontology, 34*, 570–586. http://dx.doi.org/10.1080/03601270801900420

Gluth, S., Ebner, N. C., & Schmiedek, F. (2010). Attitudes toward younger and older adults: The German Aging Semantic Differential. *International Journal of Behavioral Development, 34*, 147–158. http://dx.doi.org/10.1177/0165025409350947

Greenwald, A. G., McGhee, D. E., & Schwartz, J. L. K. (1998). Measuring individual differences in implicit cognition: The implicit association test. *Journal of Personality and Social Psychology, 74*, 1464–1480. http://dx.doi.org/10.1037/0022-3514.74.6.1464

Grühn, D., Gilet, A. L., Studer, J., & Labouvie-Vief, G. (2011). Age-relevance of person characteristics: Persons' beliefs about developmental change across the lifespan. *Developmental Psychology, 47*, 376–387. http://dx.doi.org/10.1037/a0021315

Hagestad, G. O., & Neugarten, B. L. (1985). Age and the life course. In R. H. Binstock & E. Shanas (Eds.), *Handbook of aging and the social sciences* (2nd ed., pp. 46–61). New York, NY: Van Nostrand Reinhold.

Harwood, J., Hewstone, M., Paolini, S., & Voci, A. (2005). Grandparent-grandchild contact and attitudes toward older adults: Moderator and mediator effects. *Personality and Social Psychology Bulletin, 31*, 393–406. http://dx.doi.org/10.1177/0146167204271577

Haslam, C., Morton, T. A., Haslam, S. A., Varnes, L., Graham, R., & Gamaz, L. (2012). "When the Age Is In, the Wit Is Out": Age-related self-categorization and deficit expectations reduce performance on clinical tests used in dementia assessment. *Psychology and Aging, 27*, 778–784. http://dx.doi.org/10.1037/a0027754

Heckhausen, J., Dixon, R. A., & Baltes, P. B. (1989). Gains and losses in development throughout adulthood as perceived by different adult age groups. *Developmental Psychology, 25*, 109–121. http://dx.doi.org/10.1037/0012-1649.25.1.109

Heckhausen, J., Wrosch, C., & Fleeson, W. (2001). Developmental regulation before and after a developmental deadline: The sample case of "biological clock" for childbearing. *Psychology and Aging, 16*, 400–413. http://dx.doi.org/10.1037/0882-7974.16.3.400

Hess, T. M. (2006). Attitudes toward aging and their effects on behavior. In J. E. Birren & K. W. Schaie (Eds.), *Handbook of the psychology of aging* (6th ed., pp. 379–406). San Diego, CA: Academic Press.

Hoppmann, C. A., Gerstorf, D., Smith, J., & Klumb, P. L. (2007). Linking possible selves and behavior: Do domain-specific hopes and fears translate into daily activities in very old age? *The Journals of Gerontology. Series B. Psychological Sciences and Social Sciences, 62*, P104–P111. http://dx.doi.org/10.1093/geronb/62.2.P104

Hummert, M. L. (1990). Multiple stereotypes of elderly and young adults: A comparison of structure and evaluations. *Psychology and Aging, 5*, 182–193. http://dx.doi.org/10.1037/0882-7974.5.2.182

Hummert, M. L., Garstka, T. A., O'Brien, L. T., Greenwald, A. G., & Mellott, D. S. (2002). Using the implicit association test to measure age differences in implicit social cognitions. *Psychology and Aging*, *17*, 482–495. http://dx.doi.org/10.1037/0882-7974.17.3.482

Hummert, M. L., Garstka, T. A., Shaner, J. L., & Strahm, S. (1994). Stereotypes of the elderly held by young, middle-aged, and elderly adults. *Journals of Gerontology*, *49*, P240–P249. http://dx.doi.org/10.1093/geronj/49.5.P240

Isaacs, L. W., & Bearison, D. J. (1986). The development of children's prejudice against the aged. *The International Journal of Aging and Human Development*, *23*, 175–194. http://dx.doi.org/10.2190/8GVR-XJQY-LFTH-E0A1

Kalicki, B. (1996). *Lebensverläufe und Selbstbilder. Die Normalbiographie als psychologisches Regulativ* [Life courses and self-views. The normal biography as a psychological regulative]. Opladen, Germany: Leske & Budrich.

Keil, F. (2006). Patterns of knowledge growth and decline. In E. Bialystok & F. I. M. Craik (Eds.), *Lifespan cognition: Mechanisms of change* (pp. 264–273). New York, NY: Oxford University Press.

Keller, M. L., Leventhal, E. A., & Larson, B. (1989). Aging: The lived experience. *The International Journal of Aging & Human Development*, *29*, 67–82. http://dx.doi.org/10.2190/DEQQ-AAUV-NBU0-3RMY

Kite, M. E., Deaux, K., & Miele, M. (1991). Stereotypes of young and old: Does age outweigh gender? *Psychology and Aging*, *6*, 19–27. http://dx.doi.org/10.1037/0882-7974.6.1.19

Kite, M. E., Stockdale, G. D., Whitley, E. B., & Johnson, B. T. (2005). Attitudes toward younger and older adults: An updated meta-analytic review. *Journal of Social Issues*, *61*, 241–266. http://dx.doi.org/10.1111/j.1540-4560.2005.00404.x

Kogan, N. (1961). Attitudes toward old people: The development of a scale and an examination of correlates. *The Journal of Abnormal and Social Psychology*, *62*, 44–54. http://dx.doi.org/10.1037/h0048053

Kohli, M. (2007). The institutionalization of the life course: Looking back to look ahead. *Research in Human Development*, *4*, 253–271. http://dx.doi.org/10.1080/15427600701663122

Kornadt, A. E., Meissner, F., & Rothermund, K. (2014). *Implicit and explicit age stereotypes for specific life-domains across the life span: Distinct patterns and age group differences.* Manuscript submitted for publication.

Kornadt, A. E., & Rothermund, K. (2011a). Contexts of aging: Assessing evaluative age stereotypes in different life domains. *The Journals of Gerontology. Series B. Psychological Sciences and Social Sciences*, *66*, 547–556. http://dx.doi.org/10.1093/geronb/gbr036

Kornadt, A. E., & Rothermund, K. (2011b). Dimensionen und Deutungsmuster des Alterns—Vorstellungen vom Altern, Altsein und der Lebensgestaltung im Alter [Dimensions and interpretative patterns of aging—Attitudes about aging, being old and ways of living in old age]. *Zeitschrift für Gerontologie und Geriatrie*, *44*, 291–298. http://dx.doi.org/10.1007/s00391-011-0192-3

Kornadt, A. E., & Rothermund, K. (2012). Internalization of age stereotypes into the self-concept via future self-views: A general model and domain-specific differences. *Psychology and Aging, 27*, 164–172. http://dx.doi.org/10.1037/a0025110

Kornadt, A. E., & Rothermund, K. (2013, November). *Hope for the best—Prepare for the worst? Views on aging and preparation for age-related changes.* Presentation at the 66th Annual Meeting of the Gerontological Society of America, New Orleans, LA.

Kornadt, A. E., & Rothermund, K. (2014). Preparation for old age in different life domains: Dimensions and age differences. *International Journal of Behavioral Development, 38*, 228–238. http://dx.doi.org/10.1177/0165025413512065

Kornadt, A., Voss, P., & Rothermund, K. (2013). Multiple standards of aging: Gender-specific age stereotypes in different life domains. *European Journal of Ageing, 10*, 335–344. http://dx.doi.org/10.1007/s10433-013-0281-9

Kruse, A., & Schmitt, E. (2006). A multidimensional scale for the measurement of agreement with age stereotypes and the salience of age in social interaction. *Ageing and Society, 26*, 393–411. http://dx.doi.org/ 10.1017/S0144686X06004703

Kwong, S., Sheree, T., Rasmussen, C., & Pertman, S. Q. (2012). Measuring children's age stereotyping using a modified Piagetian conservation task. *Educational Gerontology, 38*, 149–165. http://dx.doi.org/10.1080/03601277.2010.515891

Lawton, M. P. (1975). The Philadelphia Geriatric Center Morale Scale: A revision. *Journal of Gerontology, 30*, 85–89. http://dx.doi.org/10.1037/t07666-000

Levy, B. R. (2009). Stereotype embodiment: A psychosocial approach to aging. *Current Directions in Psychological Science, 18*, 332–336. http://dx.doi.org/10.1111/j .1467-8721.2009.01662.x

Levy, B. R., & Banaji, M. R. (2002). Implicit ageism. In T. D. Nelson (Ed.), *Ageism: Stereotyping and prejudice against older persons* (pp. 49–75). Cambridge, MA: MIT Press.

Levy, B., & Langer, E. (1994). Aging free from negative stereotypes: Successful memory in China among the American deaf. *Journal of Personality and Social Psychology, 66*, 989–997. http://dx.doi.org/10.1037/0022-3514.66.6.989

Levy, B. R., & Leifheit-Limson, E. (2009). The stereotype-matching effect: Greater influence on functioning when age stereotypes correspond to outcomes. *Psychology and Aging, 24*, 230–233. http://dx.doi.org/10.1037/a0014563

Löckenhoff, C. E., de Fruyt, F., Terracciano, A., McCrae, R. R., de Bolle, M., Costa, P. T., Jr., . . . Yik, M. (2009). Perceptions of aging across 26 cultures and their culture-level associates. *Psychology and Aging, 24*, 941–954. http://dx.doi.org/10.1037/ a0016901

Meisner, B. A., & Baker, J. (2013). An exploratory analysis of aging expectations and health care behavior among aging adults. *Psychology and Aging, 28*, 99–104. http:// dx.doi.org/10.1037/a0029295

Meisner, B. A., Weir, P. L., & Baker, J. (2013). The relationship between aging expectations and various modes of physical activity among aging adults. *Psychology of Sport and Exercise, 14*, 569–576. http://dx.doi.org/10.1016/j.psychsport.2013.02.007

Mendoza-Denton, R., Park, S. H., & O'Connor, A. (2008). Gender stereotypes as situation-behavior profiles. *Journal of Experimental Social Psychology*, 44, 971–982. http://dx.doi.org/10.1016/j.jesp.2008.02.010

Miche, M., Wahl, H. W., Diehl, M., Oswald, F., Kaspar, R., & Kolb, M. (2014). Natural occurrence of subjective aging experiences in community-dwelling older adults. *The Journals of Gerontology. Series B. Psychological Sciences and Social Sciences*, 69, 174–187. http://dx.doi.org/10.1093/geronb/gbs164

Müller, F., & Rothermund, K. (2012). Talking loudly but lazing at work—Behavioral effects of stereotypes are context dependent. *European Journal of Social Psychology*, 42, 557–563. http://dx.doi.org/10.1002/ejsp.1869

Mustafić, M., & Freund, A. M. (2012). Multidimensionality in developmental conceptions across adulthood. *GeroPsych: The Journal of Gerontopsychology and Geriatric Psychiatry*, 25, 57–72. http://dx.doi.org/10.1024/1662-9647/a000055

Nelson, T. D. (2011). Ageism: The strange case of prejudice against the older you. In R. L. Wiener & S. L. Willborn (Eds.), *Disability and aging discrimination: Perspectives in law and psychology* (pp. 37–47). New York, NY: Springer Publishing.

Neugarten, B. L., Moore, J. W., & Lowe, J. C. (1965). Age norms, age constraints, and adult socialization. *American Journal of Sociology*, 70, 710–717.

North, M. S., & Fiske, S. T. (2013a). A prescriptive intergenerational-tension ageism scale: Succession, identity, and consumption (SIC). *Psychological Assessment*, 25, 706–713. http://dx.doi.org/10.1037/a0032367

North, M. S., & Fiske, S. T. (2013b). Subtyping ageism: Policy issues in succession and consumption. *Social Issues and Policy Review*, 7, 36–57. http://dx.doi.org/10.1111/j.1751-2409.2012.01042.x

Nosek, B. A., Banaji, M., & Greenwald, A. G. (2002). Harvesting implicit group attitudes and beliefs from a demonstration web site. *Group Dynamics: Theory, Research, and Practice*, 6, 101–115. http://dx.doi.org/10.1037//1089-2699.6.1.101

Perdue, C. W., & Gurtman, M. B. (1990). Evidence for the automaticity of ageism. *Journal of Experimental Social Psychology*, 26, 199–216. http://dx.doi.org/10.1016/0022-1031(90)90035-K

Perry, E. L., & Finkelstein, L. M. (1999). Toward a broader view of age discrimination in employment-related decisions: A joint consideration of organizational factors and cognitive processes. *Human Resource Management Review*, 9, 21–49. http://dx.doi.org/10.1016/S1053-4822(99)00010-8

Polizzi, K. G. (2003). Assessing attitudes toward the elderly: Polizzi's refined version of the aging semantic differential. *Educational Gerontology*, 29, 197–216. http://dx.doi.org/10.1080/03601270390180316

Radl, J. (2012). Too old to work, or too young to retire? The pervasiveness of age norms in Western Europe. *Work, Employment and Society*, 26, 755–771. http://dx.doi.org/10.1177/0950017012451644

Rosencranz, H. A., & McNevin, T. E. (1969). A factor analysis of attitudes toward the aged. *The Gerontologist*, 9, 55–59. http://dx.doi.org/10.1093/geront/9.1.55

Rothermund, K. (2005). Effects of age stereotypes on self-views and adaptation. In W. Greve, K. Rothermund, & D. Wentura (Eds.), *The adaptive self. Personal continuity and intentional self-development* (pp. 223–242). Göttingen, Germany: Hogrefe.

Rothermund, K., & Brandtstädter, J. (2003). Age stereotypes and self-views in later life: Evaluating rival assumptions. *International Journal of Behavioral Development, 27,* 549–554. http://dx.doi.org/10.1080/01650250344000208

Rothermund, K., & Mayer, A. K. (2009). *Altersdiskriminierung. Erscheinungsformen, Erklärungen und Interventionsansätze* [Age discrimination. Manifestations, explanations, and interventions]. Stuttgart, Germany: Kohlhammer.

Rothermund, K., Wentura, D., & Brandtstädter, J. (1995). Selbstwertschützende Verschiebungen in der Semantik des Begriffs "alt" im höheren Erwachsenenalter [Protecting self-esteem by shifting the semantics of the concept "old" in old age]. *Sprache und Kognition, 14,* 52–63.

Ryan, E. B., Hummert, M. L., & Boich, L. H. (1995). Communication predicaments of aging: Patronizing behavior toward older adults. *Journal of Language and Social Psychology, 14,* 144–166. http://dx.doi.org/10.1177/0261927x95141008

Sargent-Cox, K. A., Anstey, K. J., & Luszcz, M. A. (2014). Longitudinal change of self-perceptions of aging and mortality. *The Journals of Gerontology. Series B. Psychological Sciences and Social Sciences, 69,* 168–173. http://dx.doi.org/10.1093/geronb/gbt005

Sarkisian, C. A., Hays, R. D., Berry, S., & Mangione, C. M. (2002). Development, reliability, and validity of the expectations regarding aging (ERA-38) survey. *The Gerontologist, 42,* 534–542. http://dx.doi.org/10.1037/t00930-000

Schelling, H. R., & Martin, M. (2008). Einstellung zum eigenen Alter: Eine Alters- oder eine Ressourcenfrage? [Attitudes toward one's own aging: A question of age or of resources?] *Zeitschrift für Gerontologie und Geriatrie, 41,* 38–50. http://dx.doi.org/10.1007/s00391-007-0451-5

Schmidt, D. F., & Boland, S. M. (1986). Structure of perceptions of older adults: Evidence for multiple stereotypes. *Psychology and Aging, 1,* 255–260. http://dx.doi.org/10.1037/0882-7974.1.3.255

Settersten, R. A. (2009). It takes two to tango: The (un)easy dance between life-course sociology and life-span psychology. *Advances in Life Course Research, 14,* 74–81. http://dx.doi.org/10.1016/j.alcr.2009.05.002

Steverink, N., Westerhof, G. J., Bode, C., & Dittmann-Kohli, F. (2001). The personal experience of aging, individual resources, and subjective well-being. *The Journals of Gerontology. Series B. Psychological Sciences and Social Sciences, 56,* P364–P373. http://dx.doi.org/10.1093/geronb/56.6.P364

Voss, P. (2013). *Geschlechtsunterschiede in Altersstereotypen: Die Rolle von wahrgenommenen personen- und kontextbezogenen Veränderungen* [Gender differences in age stereotypes: The role of perceived person- and context-related changes] (Unpublished master's thesis). Friedrich-Schiller-Universität Jena, Germany.

Wahl, H. W., Konieczny, C., & Diehl, M. (2013). Zum Erleben von altersbezogenen Veränderungen im Erwachsenenalter [Experiencing age-related change in adulthood: An exploratory study based on the concept of "Awareness of Age-Related Change" (AARC)]. *Zeitschrift für Entwicklungspsychologie und Pädagogische Psychologie, 45*, 66–76. http://dx.doi.org/10.1026/0049-8637/a000081

Waid, L. D., & Frazier, L. D. (2003). Cultural differences in possible selves during later life. *Journal of Aging Studies, 17*, 251–268. http://dx.doi.org/10.1016/s0890-4065(03)00031-8

Westerhof, G. J., Whitbourne, S. K., & Freeman, G. P. (2011). The aging self in a cultural context: The relation of conceptions of aging to identity processes and self-esteem in the United States and the Netherlands. *The Journals of Gerontology. Series B. Psychological Sciences and Social Sciences, 67*, 52–60. http://dx.doi.org/10.1093/geronb/gbr075

Wood, D., & Roberts, B. W. (2006). The effect of age and role information on expectations for Big Five personality traits. *Personality and Social Psychology Bulletin, 32*, 1482–1496. http://dx.doi.org/10.1177/0146167206291008

Wurm, S., Tomasik, M., & Tesch-Römer, C. (2010). On the importance of a positive view on ageing for physical exercise among middle-aged and older adults: Cross-sectional and longitudinal findings. *Psychology and Health, 25*, 25–42. http://dx.doi.org/10.1080/08870440802311314

Wurm, S., Warner, L. M., Ziegelmann, J. P., Wolff, J. K., & Schüz, B. (2013). How do negative self-perceptions of aging become a self-fulfilling prophecy? *Psychology and Aging, 28*, 1088–1097. http://dx.doi.org/10.1037/a0032845

Yeh, W., & Barsalou, L. W. (2006). The situated nature of concepts. *The American Journal of Psychology, 119*, 349–384. http://dx.doi.org/10.2307/20445349

CHAPTER 7

Longitudinal Research on Subjective Aging, Health, and Longevity

Current Evidence and New Directions for Research

Gerben J. Westerhof and Susanne Wurm

ABSTRACT

In this chapter, we carry out a narrative review of the longitudinal impact of subjective aging on health and survival. We have a specific focus on the different pathways which can explain the relation of subjective aging to health and survival. We focus on the three most common conceptualizations of subjective age: (a) age identity, (b) self-perceptions of aging, and (c) self-perceptions of age-related growth and decline. For each concept, we present the theoretical background, the empirical studies on the effects on health and survival, and conclude with the pathways which might explain these effects. The chapter ends with a heuristic model that synthesizes the theories and findings in describing how subjective aging is related to different psychological resources, which are in turn related to health and survival. Last, we provide some possible directions for further research in this area.

INTRODUCTION

Over the past several decades, life expectancy has increased substantially. Given the fact that old age is nowadays a phase in life that is attainable for most people, the concept of subjective aging, that is, the way in which individuals think about

© 2015 Springer Publishing Company
http://dx.doi.org/10.1891/0198-8794.35.145

their own aging process, may be more important than ever before. Although life expectancy has increased, people also tend to live longer with more chronic diseases. How adults perceive and experience their own aging may contribute to how individuals try to prevent and cope with illness in later life. In this chapter, we will review evidence of the longitudinal impact of subjective aging on health and longevity. Furthermore, we will develop a heuristic model that may be useful in guiding future empirical research on how subjective aging contributes to health and survival in adulthood and old age.

One of the particularities of human beings is that they are able to reflect on themselves as persons and thereby also on their own process of growing older. People attribute meaning to the intricate mix of changes and events in biological, social, and psychological functioning, which happen as they grow older. In this process, they develop cognitive representations of their own aging process. Researchers have used different concepts to describe these cognitive representations, such as subjective age, age identity, aging self, attitudes toward one's own aging, self-perceptions of aging, or satisfaction with aging (Diehl et al., 2014). In this chapter, we will use the concept of subjective aging as an overarching term that describes different aspects of these cognitive representations.

Subjective aging is related to the physical and psychological functioning of aging individuals. Numerous studies have shown that feeling younger and having more positive representations of one's own aging process are associated with better physical health and subjective well-being (Barak & Stern, 1986; Barrett, 2003; Peters, 1971; Steverink, Westerhof, Bode, & Dittmann-Kohli, 2001; Westerhof, Whitbourne, & Freeman, 2012). Because of their cross-sectional and correlational design, these studies, however, have not permitted the determination of the directionality of effects, that is, the examination of whether subjective aging affected psychophysical functioning or whether the effects were the other way around. Thus, it is possible to argue both ways. Subjective aging may be shaped by several individual and sociocultural factors. On the individual level, one might think of personality traits, personal values, individual role models of aging (e.g., one's grandparents), individual stereotypes about older persons in general, as well as personal experiences with growing older, such as a person's own declining health. On the sociocultural level, social interactions, messages in the mass media, cultural values, social policies, social structures, and societal institutions provide a framework of aging which contributes to subjective aging (see also Chapters 2 and 9 in this volume).

Although being shaped by individual and sociocultural factors, subjective aging might also contribute to further life span development and aging processes. How people understand and attribute meaning to their own aging processes might influence how they grow old(er) themselves. For example, a person who believes that symptoms of rheumatism are part of the aging process might not seek adequate help and thus contribute to a further worsening of the symptoms (Bode, Taal, Westerhof, van Gessel, & Van der Laar, 2012; Leventhal & Prohaska, 1986). Fortunately, during the last decade or so, evidence has also been accumulating from longitudinal studies which analyzed the effects of subjective aging on health and survival. In a recent meta-analysis, we found a small but significant effect of subjective aging on health and survival (Westerhof et al., in press). In this chapter, we will add to this meta-analysis by (a) synthesizing the evidence on the psychological pathways through which subjective aging might affect health and longevity and (b) developing a heuristic model based on empirical evidence and theoretical reasoning which may guide further empirical research on how subjective aging may contribute to health and survival.

In this chapter, we carry out a narrative review of longitudinal studies. We did a similar search as in the meta-analysis, using different databases (PsycInfo, Web of Science, PubMed, and Scopus) and different search terms for subjective aging ("subjective aging," "age identity," "subjective age," "felt age," "perceived age," "self-perceptions of aging," "satisfaction with aging," "view on aging," and "aging-related cognitions") and longitudinal studies ("longitudinal," "panel," "prospective"). We did not add search terms for outcomes or pathways but included all longitudinal studies which assessed the effects of subjective aging on physical and psychological functioning later in time. The present chapter thus uses more studies than the meta-analysis because that study focused on health and longevity as outcomes.

Subjective aging has been conceptualized in several different ways in longitudinal studies. As a first step in the analysis of possible pathways, we focus on the three most common conceptualizations which were used in the studies we found in our search: (a) age identity, (b) self-perceptions of aging, and (c) self-perceptions of age-related growth and decline. Age identity refers to the difference between one's subjective (i.e., felt or perceived) and one's chronological age. Self-perceptions of aging refer to general evaluations of one's own aging process and are also referred to as satisfaction with aging. Self-perceptions of age-related growth and decline refer to perceptions of gains and losses in different domains of functioning.

In the following text, we will describe how each of these concepts stems from a somewhat different theoretical background and focuses on a different facet of subjective aging. Consequently, the pathways that are proposed in explaining the effects of subjective aging on health and survival are also different for different concepts. For each concept, we will first present the theoretical background and then the empirical studies on the effects on health and survival. We conclude with discussing the pathways which might explain these effects.

AGE IDENTITY, HEALTH, AND LONGEVITY

Conceptualization

The first conceptualization of subjective aging that has been used in longitudinal studies is *age identity*. Drawing on the cultural maxim that "one is only as old as one feels," this has mainly been studied using a single item on *subjective age*: "What age do you feel?" (Barak & Stern, 1986; Peters, 1971). Age identity is then operationalized as the difference between the person's subjective and chronological age (Westerhof, Barrett, & Steverink, 2003)—a difference that is nowadays often defined in terms of the percentage which the person feels younger than his or her chronological age (Rubin & Berntsen, 2006). In terms of a variation of this approach, Uotinen, Rantanen, and Suutama (2005) asked whether older adults felt mentally and physically younger, the same, or older than their calendar age. Other operationalizations refer to age identity in terms of identifying with a specific age group, such as middle-aged or older persons, or to cognitive age (i.e., feel-age, look-age, do-age, and interest-age; Kastenbaum, Derbin, Sabatini, & Artt, 1972). However, these operationalizations have not been used in longitudinal studies.

Subjective age was first conceived as an indicator of age that might be related stronger to a person's level of functioning than chronological age (Havighurst & Albrecht, 1953). Nowadays, theories about age identity have anchored the concept more strongly in theories about self and identity (Westerhof et al., 2012). Building on the classical work of William James (1890/1981) and Erik Erikson (1997), these theories describe different motivated processes of the self, including the need for self-consistency and self-enhancement, which underlie a person's age identity. Self-consistency refers to the motive of remaining the same stable person over time and is advocated most strongly in self-verification theory (Swann, Rentfrow, & Guinn, 2003). Self-enhancement refers to maintaining or promoting a positive self-image and mainly draws on research on self-esteem as a positive illusion (Taylor & Brown, 1988). Both processes of self-consistency and self-enhancement may be at work in shaping age identities (Keyes & Westerhof, 2012; Westerhof et al., 2012). Individuals are able to maintain consistency by assimilating new experiences into their existing self-concepts and thereby identifying with the younger age they used to be. In a culture that devalues old age, identifying with younger ages and age groups allows older adults to also enhance their self-esteem and well-being (Weiss & Lang, 2009, 2012).

Empirical Evidence

Several studies found that age identity is related to health and survival. Most of these studies controlled for sociodemographic indicators, such as age, gender, and education, as well as psychological factors such as control beliefs or loneliness, which are known causes of health and longevity. Studying middle-aged and older adults, Spuling, Miche, Wurm, and Wahl (2013) found evidence of 6-year prospective relations of younger age identities with better subjective health and less physical illnesses in the German Aging Survey. In a study on cancer patients in Germany, Boehmer (2006, 2007) asked for subjective age one month and six months after surgery for malignant tumors. She found that feeling younger and remaining to feel younger across time were related to more positive self-reported health outcomes, such as health-related quality of life, perceived disability, and recovery satisfaction. Other studies examined survival in older adults. An American study on adults aged 60 years and older found a significant association between a younger age identity and a higher chance of survival over a 4-year period (Markides & Pappas, 1982). The Finnish Evergreen Project found a significant effect on longevity of a younger physical but not a younger mental age identity in 65- to 84-year-olds (Uotinen et al., 2005). The Berlin Aging Study did find support for the relation between a younger age identity and survival in adults aged 70 years and older (Kotter-Grühn, Kleinspehn-Ammerlahn, Gerstorf, & Smith, 2009). However, Lim et al. (2013) did not find evidence that age identities were related to survival in cancer patients who were treated with chemotherapy. The authors acknowledged that their study might have been somewhat underpowered, but the study also differed from previous studies in that it focused on a patient population which was somewhat younger than previous population studies.

Pathways

To our knowledge, there have been no longitudinal studies that directly addressed the pathways through which age identities might be related to health and survival over time. Given that the motives of self-consistency and self-enhancement operate in maintaining younger age identities, a major pathway may operate through the accumulation of subjective well-being, which would result from these motives (Westerhof & Barrett, 2005; Westerhof et al., 2012). Subjective well-being has been defined as the presence of positive affect, the absence of negative affect, and satisfaction with life in general (Diener, Suh, Lucas, & Smith, 1999). Although evidence exists that health is a predictor of subjective well-being, more recent meta-analyses have shown that subjective well-being is related to physical functioning and survival in the general population as well as in patient populations, in particular in older adults (Chida & Steptoe, 2008; Lamers, Bolier, Westerhof, Smit, & Bohlmeijer, 2012; Pressman & Cohen, 2005; Veenhoven, 2008). Subjective well-being might thus be a mediator in the association of age identity with health and survival.

At least indirect support for this assumption comes from two studies which have indeed found that age identity is longitudinally related to indicators of subjective well-being. Spuling et al. (2013) found younger age identities to be associated with lower depressive symptoms over a 6-year period in participants in the German Aging Survey, whereas depressive symptoms and other health indicators did not predict subjective age over time. Similarly, Mock and Eibach (2011) found associations of younger age identities with better subjective well-being over a period of 10 years in the Midlife Development in the United States (MIDUS) study (participants' age ranged from 25 to 74 years at the first time of assessment).

Based on these findings, we can conclude that there is rather consistent empirical evidence that younger age identities are related to better health and a longer life. Furthermore, some empirical evidence suggests that maintaining younger age identities may contribute to feeling well across time, which, in turn, might result in better health and longevity. However, this pathway has not been examined explicitly in empirical studies.

GENERAL SELF-PERCEPTIONS OF AGING, HEALTH, AND LONGEVITY

Conceptualization

Self-perceptions of aging are a second conceptualization of subjective aging that has been used in longitudinal studies. The concept originated from work by Lawton (1975), who saw attitudes toward own aging as a component of morale or subjective well-being. The Attitudes Toward Own Aging Scale is part of his Philadelphia Geriatric Center Morale Scale (Lawton, 1975; Liang & Bollen, 1983) and includes items such as "Things keep getting worse as I get older," "As you get older, you are less useful," or "I am as happy now as I was when I was younger." Some authors who used this scale as an indicator of subjective aging also refer to it as measuring satisfaction with aging (e.g., Maier & Smith, 1999) or self-perceptions of aging (Levy, Slade, & Kasl, 2002). Following Levy, Slade, and Kasl (2002), we will use it as a measure of self-perceptions of aging.

Theoretically, self-perceptions of aging play an important role in Levy's (2009) *stereotype embodiment theory*. Levy mainly drew on the symbolic interactionist theories of Mead (1934) who argued that societal beliefs are internalized in the self-concept and the work of Goffman (1963) who focused on the personal consequences of social stigma. She combined this symbolic interactionist approach with the functionalist perspective of Merton (1957), who coined the concept of self-fulfilling prophecy. The stereotype embodiment theory holds that individuals internalize negative stereotypical beliefs about older persons from a very young age on. When they grow old, individuals start to apply these negative stereotypes to their own person. They thereby construe negative self-perceptions of their own aging process, which contribute to a self-fulfilling prophecy of age-related decline.

Empirical Evidence

Several studies have addressed the impact of self-perceptions of aging on health and survival, again controlling for sociodemographic and psychological factors which are known causes of health and longevity. The first study on functional health was based on the Ohio Longitudinal Study of Aging and Retirement (OLSAR), focusing on adults aged 50 years and older and using a measure of the ability to perform activities of daily life. Based on this study, Levy, Slade, and Kasl (2002) showed that individuals with more positive self-perceptions of aging were better able to maintain better functional health over a period of 20 years. In the Australian Longitudinal Study of Aging (ALSA; adults aged 65 years and older), Sargent-Cox, Anstey, and Luszcz (2014) used objective physical performance tests on balance, gait, and rising from a chair. They found evidence that more positive self-perceptions of aging had an effect on these measures of physical functioning over a period of 16 years. Moser, Spagnoli, and Santos-Eggimann (2011) used data collected in the Swiss Lausanne Cohort study (adults in the age range of 65–70 years) and found evidence of preventive effects of positive self-perceptions of aging on basic and instrumental activities of daily living, falls, and hospitalizations across a period of 1–3 years. Whereas these studies focused on the general population, Cheng, Yip, Jim, and Hui (2012) focused on a specific group of institutionalized middle-aged and older persons with schizophrenia. They found that more positive self-perceptions of aging were related to less medical events 3 months later.

All studies on survival reported positive effects of more positive self-perceptions of aging on longevity. The included studies which addressed all-cause mortality based on the OLSAR over a period of 23 years (Levy, Slade, Kunkel, & Kasl, 2002), the ALSA over a period of 15 years (Sargent-Cox et al., 2014) and the Berlin Aging Study (Kotter-Grühn et al., 2009, with a follow-up of 16 years; Maier & Smith, 1999, with a follow-up of 4.5 years). Levy and Myers (2005) also used the OLSAR study with a follow-up of 23 years but focused on survival from a specific class of diseases, namely respiratory diseases.

Pathways

The stereotype embodiment theory proposes three types of pathways from stereo-types through self-perceptions of aging to functioning in later life: psychological, behavioral, and physiological pathways (Levy, 2009). One of the psychological pathways refers to the self-fulfilling prophecy in which self-perceptions of aging act as expectations about the aging process. The behavioral pathway is mainly illustrated by engagement in health practices, with adults with more positive self-perceptions engaging in more constructive health practices. One possible physiological pathway has been illustrated in experiments, for example, on the influence of subliminal priming with stereotypes of older persons on cardiovascular functioning (Levy, Hausdorff, Hencke, & Wei, 2000). Only psychological and behavioral pathways have been examined in longitudinal studies.

Different psychological and behavioral pathways have been proposed that might explain the effects of self-perceptions of aging on health and survival. The basic idea is that more positive self-perceptions of aging help to accumulate psychological resources and guide behavioral regulation which supports health and longevity. Regarding psychological pathways, Levy, Slade and Kasl (2002) studied whether or not *personal control beliefs* mediate the association between self-perceptions of aging and functional health. Individuals who have more positive self-perceptions of aging may also believe that they have more choice among responses that are effective in achieving desired outcomes, which, in turn, may contribute to physical functioning. This mediating pathway could explain part of the longitudinal relation between self-perceptions and functional health. Another psychological pathway proposed by Levy, Slade, Kunkel and Kasl (2002) involves *will to live* in relation to survival. In particular, will to live partially mediated the relation between self-perceptions of aging and survival. In another article on the OLSAR study, Levy and Myers (2004) proposed a behavioral pathway and analyzed the effects of self-perceptions of aging on preventive health behaviors, including attending a physical examination, taking medications, dieting, exercising, as well as consuming alcohol and smoking tobacco. Although more positive self-perceptions of aging were indeed associated with these health behaviors, the study did not address their mediating role regarding physical functioning or survival.

To conclude, the effects of self-perceptions of aging on health and survival have been consistently documented with samples of adults in different Western countries, using self-reports of activities of daily living as well as objective measures of physical functioning and survival. Possible pathways include the accumulation of psychological and behavioral resources which may prevent negative self-perceptions of aging from becoming a self-fulfilling prophecy.

SELF-PERCEPTIONS OF AGE-RELATED GROWTH AND DECLINE, HEALTH, AND LONGEVITY

Conceptualization

The first longitudinal findings on the impact of self-perceptions of aging on health and longevity by Levy and colleagues (Levy, Slade, & Kasl, 2002; Levy,

Slade, Kunkel, et al., 2002b) encouraged several additional studies on this topic. As we have seen, some of these studies were also based on the previously described unidimensional scale on self-perceptions of aging. In this section, we will describe studies which have used multidimensional, domain-specific scales to assess adults' perceptions of their own aging. The multidimensional perspective on subjective aging derives from theories on life span development that emphasize the multidimensionality and multidirectionality of adult development and aging. In particular, life span developmental theorizing emphasizes that human development can be characterized by a life-long pattern of both gains and losses, even though the ratio between gains and losses becomes more negative with age (e.g., Baltes, 1987; Heckhausen, Dixon, & Baltes, 1989). Midlife marks the shift from the predominance of growth and gains to an increasing risk of age-related losses. Also, changes related to restricted time perspective and declining physical functioning tend to start in midlife and continue into old age (Heckhausen, 2001).

Building on these basic tenets of life span developmental theory about the multidimensional and multidirectional nature of aging, some researchers have studied self-perceptions of aging as a multifaceted phenomenon to understand the differential impact of various views on aging. This approach did not only draw from a theoretical perspective but was also grounded in qualitative studies on self-perceptions of aging showing that older adults often view aging as both accompanied by losses—mainly in the physical and social domain—and gains, such as more freedom and time for new interests (Connidis, 1989; Dittmann-Kohli, 1995; Keller, Leventhal, & Larson, 1989). Based on these theoretical and empirical insights, Steverink et al. (2001) developed a multidimensional scale measuring cognitions about aging as physical decline, social loss, and ongoing development. This scale has been used both in several cross-sectional studies (e.g., Steverink et al., 2001; Westerhof, 2003; Westerhof et al., 2012) as well as longitudinal studies (e.g., Wurm, Tesch-Römer, & Tomasik, 2007; Wurm, Tomasik, & Tesch-Römer, 2010). All items of this multidimensional scale begin with the stem "Aging means to me . . ." followed by domain-specific endings. Exemplary items for the view that aging is accompanied by physical losses are "Aging means to me that I am less healthy" or "Aging means to me that I am less energetic and fit," whereas the items "Aging means to me that I continue to make plans" or "Aging means to me that my capabilities are increasing" are two examples for the view of aging as ongoing development.

Empirical Evidence

The German Aging Survey is a longitudinal study on healthy aging that is based on a nationally representative sample of individuals in their second half of life (40–85 years). The longitudinal studies on subjective aging used the scales of aging as physical losses and aging as ongoing development. These two domain-specific self-perceptions of aging were significant predictors for health and subjective well-being over and above major sociodemographic and socioeconomic indicators (e.g., age, gender, education) and beyond psychological factors such as control beliefs (Wurm et al., 2007; Wurm, Tomasik, & Tesch-Römer, 2008). Moreover, both the loss-oriented self-perception of aging as physical decline and the gain-oriented view of ongoing development have been shown to be better predictors of physical health than the other way around (Wurm et al., 2007). This finding is in line with previously described studies showing a higher impact of general self-perceptions of aging on functional health than vice versa (Levy, Slade & Kasl, 2002; Sargent-Cox, Anstey, & Luszcz, 2012). In addition, a recent study on domain-specific self-perceptions of aging and longevity showed that the perception of aging as ongoing development was predictive of survival, even after controlling for sociodemographic and health indicators (i.e., self-rated health, chronic conditions, and functional limitations). The same, however, was not the case for the self-perception of aging as physical loss (Wiest & Wurm, 2012).

Pathways

To understand how the gain-related view on aging as ongoing development might impact health and longevity, Wurm et al. (2010) examined physical activity as one possible behavioral pathway. They showed that middle-aged and older individuals who viewed aging as ongoing development were physically more active and better able to maintain a higher level of activity over time than those with a less gain-related view on aging. Furthermore, the authors were interested in the question of whether the positive effect of a gain-related view on aging might come to its limits when a serious health event occurs (Wurm et al., 2008). Because serious falls and illnesses can considerably hamper the striving for ongoing development, individuals with gain-related views on aging might have more difficulties to adapt to such an event. However, this assumption was not supported by the data. Individuals with a more gain-related view were able to maintain better self-rated health and life satisfaction even after a serious health event.

Furthermore, a recent study examined the question of how domain-specific self-perceptions of aging as physical losses might impede health and well-being over a 6-month period (Wurm, Warner, Ziegelmann, Wolff, & Schüz, 2013). In this study, the occurrence of a serious health event predicted the increased use of strategies of developmental regulation: Selection, Optimization, and Compensation (SOC; Baltes & Baltes, 1990). These, in turn, predicted higher self-rated health and life satisfaction. However, this effect was moderated by the domain-specific self-perception of aging as physical losses; that is, in the case of a serious health event, a self-perception of aging as physical losses was associated with a lower use of SOC strategies. These findings point to a possible psychological pathway of how a loss-related view on aging can turn into a self-fulfilling prophecy through less effective developmental regulation strategies and, hence, can contribute to poorer health and lower life satisfaction (Wurm et al., 2013).

Taken together, domain-specific self-perceptions of aging reflect the current view on life-span development as both growth and decline and shed more light on possible mechanisms, explaining the link between self-perceptions of aging, health, and longevity. Although perceiving aging as associated with further goals and plans seems to be beneficial, the contrary was found for the self-perception of aging as physical losses.

A HEURISTIC MODEL

As mentioned earlier, we have reviewed the conceptualizations, empirical evidence, and possible pathways through which subjective aging might affect health and longevity over time. As this review shows, there is substantial evidence that subjective aging is related to health and survival in a way that more youthful age identities, more positive general self-perceptions of aging, as well as more positive perceptions of age-related decline and growth serve to protect health and contribute to longevity (Westerhof et al., in press). We have discussed several pathways which may account for the effects of subjective aging on health and longevity. We have seen that there is some, but only limited, empirical evidence for these pathways. To synthesize the reviewed studies and to guide further research, we have synthesized the theoretical pathways in a heuristic model (Figure 7.1).

The left box of Figure 7.1 shows the three different conceptualizations of subjective aging which were addressed in this chapter: age identity, general self-perceptions of aging, and self-perceptions of aging as growth and decline. The second box groups the different psychological resources which were discussed in this chapter: subjective well-being, control beliefs, will to live, developmental regulation (SOC), and health behaviors. The third box concerns different indicators of health, and the last box concerns survival. All four boxes are placed in a larger box, referring to the context in which these processes operate. The basic idea of the pathways indicated by the arrows is that subjective aging contributes to the accumulation of psychological resources that help to maintain a good health which, in turn, contribute to survival. The processes take place in a context that is indicated by the larger box. A final characteristic of the model is that we also included feedback loops. That is, the loss of psychological resources or health may affect subjective aging in a negative way.

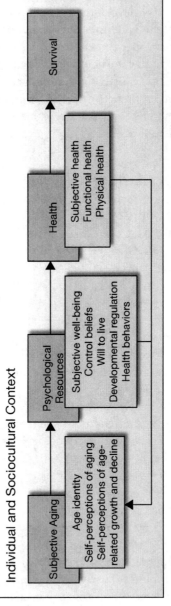

FIGURE 7.1 A heuristic model of pathways linking subjective aging to psychological resources, health, and survival.

The heuristic model can be of help in guiding further research. The first direction concerns variables which were put together in one box but might have differential contributions to different pathways. We will focus on the different aspects of subjective aging distinguished in this chapter. The second direction focuses on the role of health as a separate box between subjective aging and survival. The third direction addresses the role of the individual and sociocultural context.

Differential Contributions of Different Aspects of Subjective Aging

The impact of different aspects of subjective aging has rarely been studied together in one study. This is why the question is still open how the relations between the different indicators of subjective aging should be conceptualized; that is, how are they connected with each other and how do they differentially impact health and longevity. Little is known about the interrelations among age identities, self-perceptions of aging, and self-perceptions of age-related growth and decline. It can therefore not be ruled out that effects on health and survival do not exist independently because the different measures, as would be expected, do have some conceptual and empirical overlap (Diehl et al., 2014). Furthermore, new concepts have been proposed, such as awareness of age-related change and preparation for aging, which also need to be incorporated when further longitudinal evidence is collected (Diehl & Wahl, 2010).

Different aspects of subjective aging may have different consequences for the accumulation of psychological resources. In methodological terms, they may show differential validity. For example, the main pathway of age identity to health and survival that was addressed in this chapter was through subjective well-being. The pathways of self-perceptions of aging and age-related growth and decline were through processes such as will to live, control beliefs, health behaviors, or processes of developmental regulation. It thus remains a task for future research to further study which pathways are most important for which indicators of subjective aging and which developmental outcomes.

The Role of Health

In most studies, health is seen as an endpoint in itself. We have placed it in between psychological resources and survival because one might argue that declining health itself plays an important role in survival. We believe that it is hard to imagine a pathway from subjective aging to survival without considering the mediating role of health. However, the effects of subjective aging on survival through health have not been studied extensively yet. Rather, studies addressing the impact of subjective aging on longevity have controlled for health indicators as possible confounders. Although this is justified in establishing evidence on the unique relations of subjective aging to survival, this might also have led to an underestimation of the relation because indirect effects through health were not considered. We therefore propose to study the indirect effects of subjective aging on survival through health more intensively and in particular in a prospective longitudinal way.

The role of health might indeed be even more complex. Findings from longitudinal studies (e.g., Kleinspehn-Ammerlahn, Kotter-Grühn, & Smith, 2008; Sargent-Cox et al., 2012; Schafer & Shippee, 2010b; Uotinen, Rantanen, Suutama, & Ruoppila, 2006; Wurm et al., 2013) suggest that physical health and changes in physical health play an important role in developing older age identities and more negative self-perceptions of aging. When people experience health problems, they may attribute their health problems to age (rather than, for example, to lifestyle) and, hence, may start to feel older. This, in turn, may lead to the reinforcement of already existing negative age stereotypes and the development of more negative self-perceptions of aging. Furthermore, negative self-perceptions of aging may in turn diminish psychological resources such as subjective well-being, control beliefs, will to live, developmental regulation strategies, and health behaviors and thereby contribute to an even worse health. This would again lead to older and more negative perceptions of aging and so on. In this way, a vicious cycle of breakdown in later life could occur (Kuypers & Bengtson, 1973).

Individual and Sociocultural Context

The third focus for future research involves the inclusion of the individual and sociocultural context. Individual characteristics, such as personality traits or personal values, may affect subjective aging in fundamental ways. For example, neuroticism has been related to lower levels of subjective well-being as well as worse physical functioning and survival (e.g., Friedman & Kern, 2014; Wilson, de Leon, Bienias, Evans, & Bennett, 2004). Kotter-Grühn et al. (2009) considered neuroticism as a covariate in their analyses on subjective aging and found that the effect of subjective aging remained independently significant after emotional instability had been accounted for. Further research could clarify whether it is indeed subjective aging that results in the proposed pathways or whether other characteristics of the individual and sociocultural context can explain part of these relations. Similarly, the sociocultural context, such as social relations, media portrayals, social policies, health care systems, or institutional arrangements may influence the proposed pathways as well. For example, although social policies regarding aging have changed over the past decades, few studies have addressed how these changing social policies might have had an impact on subjective aging. It would therefore be prudent to take these individual and sociocultural contexts into account when studying the impact of subjective aging on health and longevity.

Another approach would be to assess whether individual and sociocultural contexts are conditional to the proposed pathways. For example, Schafer and Shippee (2010a) found a relationship in the MIDUS study between age identity and expectations concerning cognitive aging for women but not for men. Furthermore, findings from the German Aging Survey suggested that middle-aged individuals with more positive self-perceptions of age-related growth and decline not only engaged in sports more frequently but even increased the activity over time, provided that they were healthy enough to do so (Wurm et al., 2010). Older individuals with more positive self-perceptions of aging, however, mainly walked more regularly and increased walking over time, which is positive because walking is often the only physical activity that is even recommended in the presence of health problems (Wurm et al., 2010).

Besides individual characteristics, the sociocultural context may also play a moderating role. In our meta-analysis, we found that effects of subjective aging on health and survival were stronger in the United States than in Western Europe (Westerhof et al., in press). This finding may be related to differences in welfare state regimes (Bambra, 2007; Esping-Andersen, 1990). In the United States, which has a so-called liberal welfare regime, there is a strong need for individuals to take responsibility for their own aging process and for their financial security in old age because the social security provisions from the states and/or the federal government are very limited. In European countries, the so-called conservative welfare states, such as the German one, more state provisions and social security policies, including policies for late life, are in place. Aging individuals may thus feel less responsible for their own aging process because they feel that economic security and health care are generally provided by society. Also, in European countries, eligibilities and entitlements are still more often tied to chronological age (e.g., obligatory retirement at age 65 years), and this may make chronological age more salient for the individual. Further research could therefore assess whether individual and sociocultural contexts play a moderating role in the association between subjective aging and health and survival.

CONCLUSION

The goal of this chapter was to synthesize existing evidence from longitudinal studies and to develop a heuristic model which may guide future empirical research on how subjective aging may contribute to health and survival. We found evidence in support of the predictive value of subjective aging for health and survival and proposed three further directions for research. These directions focus on the differential contributions of different dimensions of subjective aging, the role of health, and the role of the individual and sociocultural context. It is our hope that pursuing these new directions will contribute to further evidence and insights into the processes involved in subjective aging. Specifically, such research needs to focus on the further clarification of questions about the pathways from subjective aging to survival as well as the conditions under which these pathways operate. Gaining insights into the vicious cycle that might be at work between subjective aging and physical decline would also provide the needed information to intervene in this process. Given the existing evidence, public health professionals would be well-advised to start thinking about positive and constructive interpretations of the aging process which may help adults to escape the vicious breakdown cycle, but further evidence is needed on how exactly this could be possible. First steps have been made in developing interventions aiming at changing negative self-perceptions of aging to promote a healthier lifestyle (Sarkisian, Prohaska, Davis, & Weiner, 2007; Wolff, Warner, Ziegelmann, & Wurm, 2014). However, more research in this direction is needed by simultaneously considering that overly positive views on aging might also be difficult, because aging is not only associated with gains but with increasing losses as well.

REFERENCES

Baltes, P. B. (1987). Theoretical propositions of life-span developmental psychology: On the dynamics between growth and decline. *Developmental Psychology, 23,* 611–626.

Baltes, P. B., & Baltes, M. M. (1990). Psychological perspectives on successful aging: The model of selective optimization with compensation. In P. B. Baltes & M. M. Baltes (Eds.), *Successful aging: Perspectives from the behavioral sciences* (pp. 1–34). New York, NY: Cambridge University Press.

Bambra, C. (2007). Going beyond the three worlds of welfare capitalism: Regime theory and public health research. *Journal of Epidemiological Community Health, 61,* 1098–1102. http://dx.doi.org/10.1136/jech.2007.064295

Barak, B., & Stern, B. (1986). Subjective age correlates: A research note. *The Gerontologist, 26,* 571–578.

Barrett, A. E. (2003). Socioeconomic status and age identity: The role of dimensions of health in the subjective construction of age. *The Journals of Gerontology. Series B, Psychological Sciences and Social Sciences, 58,* S101–109. http://dx.doi.org/10.1093/geronb/58.2.S101

Bode, C., Taal, E., Westerhof, G. J., van Gessel, L., & van de Laar, M. V. (2012). Experience of aging in patients with rheumatic disease: A comparison with the general population. *Aging and Mental Health, 16,* 666–672. http://dx.doi.org/10.1080/13607863.2011.651438

Boehmer, S. (2006). Does felt age reflect health-related quality of life in cancer patients? *Psychooncology, 15,* 726–738. http://dx.doi.org/10.1002/pon.1011

Boehmer, S. (2007). Relationships between felt age and perceived disability, satisfaction with recovery, self-efficacy beliefs and coping strategies. *Journal of Health Psychology*, *12*, 895–906. http://dx.doi.org/10.1177/1359105307082453

Cheng, S. T., Yip, L. C., Jim, O. T., & Hui, A. N. (2012). Self-perception of aging and acute medical events in chronically institutionalized middle-aged and older persons with schizophrenia. *International Journal of Geriatric Psychiatry*, *27*, 907–913. http://dx.doi.org/10.1002/gps.2798

Chida, Y., & Steptoe, A. (2008). Positive psychological well-being and mortality: A quantitative review of prospective observational studies. *Psychosomatic Medicine*, *70*, 741–756. http://dx.doi.org/10.1097/PSY.0b013e31818105ba

Connidis, I. A. (1989). The subjective experience of aging: Correlates of divergent views. *Canadian Journal on Aging*, *8*, 7–18. http://dx.doi.org/10.1017/S0714980800011168

Diehl, M. K., & Wahl, H. W. (2010). Awareness of age-related change: Examination of a (mostly) unexplored concept. *The Journals of Gerontology. Series B, Psychological Sciences and Social Sciences*, *65*, 340–350. http://dx.doi.org/10.1093/geronb/gbp110

Diehl, M. K., Wahl, H. W., Barrett, A. E., Brothers, A. F., Miche, M., Montepare, J. M., . . . Wurm, S. (2014). Awareness of aging: Theoretical considerations on an emerging concept. *Developmental Review*, *34*, 93–113. http://dx.doi.org/10.1016/j.dr.2014.01.001

Diener, E., Suh, E. M., Lucas, R. E., & Smith, H. L. (1999). Subjective well-being: Three decades of progress. *Psychological Bulletin*, *125*, 276–302.

Dittmann-Kohli, F. (1995). Das persönliche Sinnsystem. [The personal meaning system]. Göttingen, Germany: Hogrefe-Verlag.

Esping-Andersen, G. (1990). The three worlds of welfare capitalism. Princeton: Princeton University Press.

Erikson, E. H. (1997). *The life cycle completed*. New York, NY: Norton.

Friedman, H. S., & Kern, M. L. (2014). Personality, well-being, and health. *Annual Review of Psychology*, *65*, 719–742. http://dx.doi.org/10.1146/annurev-psych-010213-115123

Goffman, E. (1963). *Stigma*. Englewood-Cliffs, NJ: Prentice Hall.

Havighurst, R. J., & Albrecht, R. (1953). *Older people*. Oxford, United Kingdom: Longmans, Green.

Heckhausen, J. (2001). Adaptation and resilience in midlife. In M. E. Lachman (Ed.), *Handbook of midlife development* (pp. 345–391). Hoboken, NJ: Wiley.

Heckhausen, J., Dixon, R. A., & Baltes, P. B. (1989). Gains and losses in development throughout adulthood as perceived by different adult age groups. *Developmental Psychology*, *25*, 109–121. http://dx.doi.org/10.1037/0012-1649.25.1.109

James, W. (1981). *The principles of psychology*. Cambridge, MA: Harvard University Press. (Original work published 1890)

Kastenbaum, R., Derbin, V., Sabatini, P., & Artt, S. (1972). "The ages of me": Toward personal and interpersonal definitions of functional aging. *Aging and Human Development*, *3*, 197–211. http://dx.doi.org/10.2190/TUJR-WTXK-866Q-8QU7

Keller, M. L., Leventhal, E. A., & Larson, B. (1989). Aging: The lived experience. *The International Journal of Aging & Human Development*, *29*, 67–82. http://dx.doi.org/10.2190/DEQQ-AAUV-NBU0-3RMY

Keyes, C. L. M., & Westerhof, G. J. (2012). Chronological and subjective age differences in flourishing mental health and major depressive episode. *Aging and Mental Health, 16*, 67–74. http://dx.doi.org/10.1080/13607863.2011.596811

Kleinspehn-Ammerlahn, A., Kotter-Grühn, D., & Smith, J. (2008). Self-perceptions of aging: Do subjective age and satisfaction with aging change during old age? *The Journals of Gerontology. Series B, Psychological Sciences and Social Sciences, 63*, P377–P385. http://dx.doi.org/10.1093/geronb/63.6.P377

Kotter-Grühn, D., Kleinspehn-Ammerlahn, A., Gerstorf, D., & Smith, J. (2009). Self-perceptions of aging predict mortality and change with approaching death: 16-year longitudinal results from the Berlin Aging Study. *Psychology and Aging, 24*, 654–667. http://dx.doi.org/10.1037/a0016510

Kuypers, J. A., & Bengtson, V. L. (1973). Social breakdown and competence: A model of normal aging. *Human Development, 16*, 181–201.

Lamers, S. A., Bolier, L., Westerhof, G. J., Smit, F., & Bohlmeijer, E. T. (2012). The impact of emotional well-being on long-term recovery and survival in physical illness: A meta-analysis. *Journal of Behavioral Medicine, 35*, 538–547. http://dx.doi.org/10.1007/s10865-011-9379-8

Lawton, M. P. (1975). The Philadelphia Geriatric Center Morale Scale: A revision. *Journal of Gerontology, 30*, 85–89. http://dx.doi.org/10.1093/geronj/30.1.85

Leventhal, E. A., & Prohaska, T. R. (1986). Age, symptom interpretation, and health behavior. *Journal of the American Geriatrics Society, 34*, 185–191.

Levy, B. (2009). Stereotype embodiment: A psychosocial approach to aging. *Current Directions in Psychological Science, 18*, 332–336. http://dx.doi.org/10.1111/j.1467-8721.2009.01662.x

Levy, B. R., Hausdorff, J. M., Hencke, R., & Wei, J. Y. (2000). Reducing cardiovascular stress with positive self-stereotypes of aging. *The Journals of Gerontology. Series B, Psychological Sciences and Social Sciences, 55*, P205–P213. http://dx.doi.org/10.1093/geronb/55.4.P205

Levy, B. R., & Myers, L. M. (2004). Preventive health behaviors influenced by self-perceptions of aging. *Preventive Medicine, 39*, 625–629. http://dx.doi.org/10.1016/j.ypmed.2004.02.029

Levy, B. R., & Myers, L. M. (2005). Relationship between respiratory mortality and self-perceptions of aging. *Psychology & Health, 20*, 553–564. http://dx.doi.org/10.1080/14768320500066381

Levy, B. R., Slade, M. D., & Kasl, S. V. (2002). Longitudinal benefit of positive self-perceptions of aging on functional health. *The Journals of Gerontology. Series B, Psychological Sciences and Social Sciences, 57*, 409–417. http://dx.doi.org/10.1093/geronb/57.5.P409

Levy, B. R., Slade, M. D., Kunkel, S. R., & Kasl, S. V. (2002). Longevity increased by positive self-perceptions of aging. *Journal of Personality and Social Psychology, 83*, 261–270. http://dx.doi.org/ 10.1037//0022-3514.83.2.261

Liang, J., & Bollen, K. A. (1983). The structure of the Philadelphia Geriatric Center Morale Scale: A reinterpretation. *Journal of Gerontology, 38*, 181–189. http://dx.doi.org/10.1093/geronj/38.2.181

Lim, M. Y., Stephens, E. K., Novotny, P., Price, K., Salayi, M., Roeker, L., . . . Jatoi, A. (2013). Self-perceptions of age among 292 chemotherapy-treated cancer patients: Exploring associations with symptoms and survival. *Journal of Geriatric Oncology*, *4*, 249–253. http://dx.doi.org/10.1016/j.jgo.2013.02.001

Maier, H., & Smith, J. (1999). Psychological predictors of mortality in old age. *The Journals of Gerontology. Series B, Psychological Sciences and Social Sciences*, *54*, 44–54.

Markides, K. S., & Pappas, C. (1982). Subjective age, health, and survivorship in old age. *Research on Aging*, *4*, 87–96. http://dx.doi.org/10.1177/016402758241004

Mead, G. H. (1934). *Mind, self, and society*. Chicago, IL: University of Chicago Press.

Merton, R. K. (1957). *Social theory and social structure*. Glencoe, IL: Free Press.

Mock, S. E., & Eibach, R. P. (2011). Aging attitudes moderate the effect of subjective age on psychological well-being: Evidence from a 10-year longitudinal study. *Psychology and Aging*, *26*, 979–986. http://dx.doi.org/10.1037/a0023877

Moser, C., Spagnoli, J., & Santos-Eggimann, B. (2011). Self-perception of aging and vulnerability to adverse outcomes at the age of 65-70 years. *The Journals of Gerontology. Series B, Psychological Sciences and Social Sciences*, *66*, 675–680. http://dx.doi.org/10.1093/geronb/gbr052

Peters, G. R. (1971). Self-conceptions of the aged, age identification, and aging. *The Gerontologist*, *11*, 69–73. http://dx.doi.org/10.1093/geront/11.4_Part_2.69

Pressman, S. D., & Cohen, S. (2005). Does positive affect influence health? *Psychological Bulletin*, *131*, 925–971. http://dx.doi.org/10.1037/0033-2909.131.6.925

Rubin, D. C., & Berntsen, D. (2006). People over forty feel 20% younger than their age: Subjective age across the lifespan. *Psychonomic Bulletin & Review*, *13*(5), 776–780. http://dx.doi.org/10.3758/BF03193996

Sargent-Cox, K. A., Anstey, K. J., & Luszcz, M. A. (2012). The relationship between change in self-perceptions of aging and physical functioning in older adults. *Psychology and Aging*, *27*(3), 750–760. http://dx.doi.org/10.1037/a0027578

Sargent-Cox, K. A., Anstey, K. J., & Luszcz, M. A. (2014). Longitudinal change of self-perceptions of aging and mortality. *The Journals of Gerontology. Series B, Psychological Sciences and Social Sciences*, *69*, 168–173. http://dx.doi.org/10.1093/geronb/gbt005

Sarkisian, C. A., Prohaska, T. R., Davis, C., & Weiner, B. (2007). Pilot test of an attribution retraining intervention to raise walking levels in sedentary older adults. *Journal of the American Geriatrics Society*, *55*, 1842–1846. http://dx.doi.org/10.1111/j.1532-5415.2007.01427.x

Schafer, M. H., & Shippee, T. P. (2010a). Age identity, gender, and perceptions of decline: Does feeling older lead to pessimistic dispositions about cognitive aging? *The Journals of Gerontology. Series B, Psychological Sciences and Social Sciences*, *65*, 91–96. http://dx.doi.org/10.1093/geronb/gbp046

Schafer, M. H., & Shippee, T. P. (2010b). Age identity in context: Stress and the subjective side of aging. *Social Psychology Quarterly*, *73*, 245–264. http://dx.doi.org/10.1177/0190272510379751

Spuling, S. M., Miche, M., Wurm, S., & Wahl, H. (2013). Exploring the causal interplay of subjective age and health dimensions in the second half of life: A cross-lagged panel analysis. *Zeitschrift für Gesundheitspsychologie, 21*, 5–15. http://dx.doi. org/10.1026/0943-8149/a000084

Steverink, N., Westerhof, G. J., Bode, C., & Dittmann-Kohli, F. (2001). The personal experience of aging, individual resources, and subjective well-being. *The Journals of Gerontology. Series B, Psychological Sciences and Social Sciences, 56B*, P364–P373. http://dx.doi.org/10.1093/geronb/56.6.P364

Swann, W. R., Rentfrow, P. J., & Guinn, J. S. (2003). Self-verification: The search for coherence. In M. R. Leary & J. Tangney (Eds.), *Handbook of self and identity* (pp. 367–383). New York, NY: Guilford Press.

Taylor, S. E., & Brown, J. D. (1988). Illusion and well-being: A social psychological perspective on mental health. *Psychological Bulletin, 103*, 193–210. http://dx.doi .org/10.1037/0033-2909.103.2.193

Uotinen, V., Rantanen, T., & Suutama, T. (2005). Perceived age as a predictor of old age mortality: A 13-year prospective study. *Age and Ageing, 34*, 368–372. http://dx.doi .org/10.1093/ageing/afi091

Uotinen, V., Rantanen, T., Suutama, T., & Ruoppila, I. (2006). Change in subjective age among older people over an eight-year follow-up: 'Getting older and feeling younger?' *Experimental Aging Research, 32*, 381–393. http://dx.doi. org/10.1080/03610730600875759

Veenhoven, R. R. (2008). Healthy happiness: Effects of happiness on physical health and the consequences for preventive health care. *Journal Of Happiness Studies, 9*(3), 449–469. http://dx.doi.org/10.1007/s10902-006-9042-1

Weiss, D., & Lang, F. R. (2009). Thinking about my generation: Adaptive effects of a dual age identity in later adulthood. *Psychology and Aging, 24*(3), 729–734. http://dx.doi. org/10.1037/a0016339

Weiss, D., & Lang, F. R. (2012). "They" are old but "I" feel younger: Age-group dissociation as a self-protective strategy in old age. *Psychology and Aging, 27*(1), 153–163. http://dx.doi.org/10.1037/a0024887

Westerhof, G. J. (2003). De beleving van het eigen ouder worden: Multidimensionaliteit en multidirectionaliteit in relatie tot succesvol ouder worden en welbevinden [The experience of ageing: Multidimensionality and multidirectionality in relation to successful aging and well-being]. *Tijdschrift voor Gerontologie en Geriatrie, 34*, 96–103.

Westerhof, G. J., & Barrett, A. E. (2005). Age identity and subjective well-being: A comparison of the United States and Germany. *The Journals of Gerontology. Series B, Psychological Sciences and Social Sciences, 60*, S129–S136. http://dx.doi.org/10.1093/ geronb/60.3.S129

Westerhof, G. J., Barrett, A. E., & Steverink, N. (2003). Forever young? A comparison of age identities in the United States and Germany. *Research on Aging, 25*, 366–383. http://dx.doi.org/10.1177/0164027503025004002

Westerhof, G. J., Miche, M., Brothers, A. F., Barrett, A. E., Diehl, M., Montepare, J. M., . . . Wurm, S. (in press). The influence of subjective aging on psychophysical functioning and longevity: A meta-analysis of longitudinal data. *Psychology and Aging*.

Westerhof, G. J., Whitbourne, S. K., & Freeman, G. P. (2012). The aging self in a cultural context: Identity processes, perceptions of aging and self-esteem in the United States and the Netherlands. *The Journals of Gerontology. Series B, Psychological Sciences and Social Sciences*, 67, 52–60. http://dx.doi.org/10.1093/geronb/gbr075

Wiest, M., & Wurm, S. (2012, August). *Think positive about aging and you will live longer?!* Paper presented at the Conference of the European Health Psychology Society, Prague, Czech Republic.

Wilson, R. S., de Leon, C., Bienias, J. L., Evans, D. A., & Bennett, D. A. (2004). Personality and mortality in old age. *The Journals of Gerontology. Series B, Psychological Sciences and Social Sciences*, 59, P110–P116. http://dx.doi.org/10.1093/geronb/59.3.P110

Wolff, J. K., Warner, L. M., Ziegelmann, J. P., & Wurm, S. (2014). What do targeting positive views on ageing add to a physical activity intervention in older adults? Results from a randomized controlled trial. *Psychology & Health*, 29, 915–932. http://dx.doi.org/10.1080/08870446.2014.896464

Wurm, S., Tesch-Römer, C., & Tomasik, M. J. (2007). Longitudinal findings on aging-related cognitions, control beliefs, and health in later life. *The Journals of Gerontology. Series B, Psychological Sciences and Social Sciences*, 62B, 156–164. http://dx.doi.org/10.1093/geronb/62.3.P156

Wurm, S., Tomasik, M. J., & Tesch-Römer, C. (2008). Serious health events and their impact on changes in subjective health and life satisfaction: The role of age and a positive view on ageing. *European Journal of Ageing*, 5, 117–127. http://dx.doi.org/10.1007/s10433-008-0077-5

Wurm, S., Tomasik, M. J., & Tesch-Römer, C. (2010). On the importance of a positive view on ageing for physical exercise among middle-aged and older adults: Cross-sectional and longitudinal findings. *Psychology & Health*, 25, 25–42. http://dx.doi.org/10.1080/08870440802311314

Wurm, S., Warner, L. M., Ziegelmann, J. P., Wolff, J. K., & Schüz, B. (2013). How do negative self-perceptions of aging become a self-fulfilling prophecy? *Psychology and Aging*, 28, 1088–1097. http://dx.doi.org/10.1037/a0032845

CHAPTER 8

Changing Negative Views of Aging

Implications for Intervention and Translational Research

Dana Kotter-Grühn

ABSTRACT

In most Western societies, the perception of age and aging is predominantly negative, and this negativity is often integrated into older adults' self-view of age(ing). At the societal level, negative views of aging manifest themselves in the form of age stereotypes, which result in prejudice and discrimination toward older adults. At the personal level, negative views of one's own aging are related, among others, to poor health, lower well-being, and even shorter survival times. Considering these negative effects, interventions that promote positive views of aging seem warranted. This chapter discusses potential routes for changing negative (self-)views of aging and the challenges that are inherent to such efforts, such as determining and reaching the target groups for intervention programs. Strategies such as increasing the knowledge about old age, providing opportunities for children or younger adults to interact with older adults, as well as changing the portrayal of older adults in the media might be used to change societal views of aging. Because it is assumed that for some older adults age stereotypes become self-stereotypes, changing the societal view of aging might eventually also lead to a positive change in older adults' view of their own aging, and it might minimize the burden of belonging to a stigmatized group. Few strategies for changing personal views of aging (e.g., social comparison feedback) have been shown to be successful so far. Overall, more research is necessary to develop interventions which are easy to implement and universally effective.

INTRODUCTION

Negative views of aging are widespread and can have many negative consequences. Therefore, attempting to change these negative views should be on the agenda for future research. This chapter starts out at a more conceptual level by describing how perceptions of aging manifest themselves at the societal level in the form of age stereotypes and at a personal level as subjective aging experiences. This is followed by a detailed account of the consequences of negative societal and personal views of aging. Finally, the main focus of the chapter will be on theoretically (and empirically) grounded ideas for turning negative perceptions of aging into positive ones and for promoting already existing positive perceptions of aging. This part also includes a reflection on the challenges and open questions pertaining to interventions targeted at changing negative views of aging.

THE SOCIETAL PERCEPTION OF AGING

Although getting older is an integral part of life, both the aging process and the time period of old age are typically viewed in a negative light (Kite, Stockdale, Whitley, & Johnson, 2005). This negative societal perception of old age, which can be found in most cultures across the world, is mainly driven by age stereotypes—those culturally shared believes about people belonging to a certain age group (mostly referring to old age). Even though age stereotypes are multifaceted and some positive stereotypes about older adults exist (e.g., they are often seen as wise or kind), many age stereotypes are negative. Older adults are viewed, among others, as sick, dependent, weak, or lonely (Hummert, 1999). Not only are these negative attributes characterized by low controllability and low desirability (Wehr & Buchwald, 2007), but also some argue that even the positive stereotypes assigned to older adults have to be considered in a negative light because they mainly refer to characteristics which make a person rank low in competence and competitiveness (Cuddy & Fiske, 2002). According to the *stereotype content model* (Fiske, Cuddy, Glick, & Xu, 2002), older adults can be classified as high in warmth but low in competence, making them a "pitied" group. It is noteworthy that the negativity of the stereotypes assigned to older adults in their 60s and 70s even increases as they transition into their 80s and 90s (Hummert, 1994; Hummert, Garstka, & Shaner, 1997). As will be described in more detail later, these negative stereotypes about old age can have tremendous consequences for society and for individuals, which highlights the importance of trying to change negative societal perceptions of age and aging.

THE PERCEPTION OF ONE'S OWN AGING

Over the past decades, various concepts have been introduced into the literature to describe how individuals perceive not aging per se but their *own* age and aging. Among those concepts are *subjective aging*, *self-perceptions of aging*, as well as *age identity*, all of which typically refer to individuals' experiences of and beliefs about their own age and the aging process (e.g., Levy, Slade, & Kasl, 2002). Subjective aging seems to be the broadest term in that it encompasses personal experiences related to aging as well as self-perceptions of aging and age identity. The term self-perceptions of aging is mostly used to refer to a person's subjective age or his or her satisfaction with aging (Kleinspehn-Ammerlahn, Kotter-Grühn, & Smith, 2008). The term subjective age can also be subsumed under the umbrella term of age identity and refers to the age a person feels like, desires to be, or thinks he or she looks like. Throughout adulthood, most individuals are relatively satisfied with their age and aging, and they report younger subjective ages. That is, they feel younger, want to be younger, and think they look younger than they are (Kaufman & Elder, 2002; Kotter-Grühn & Hess, 2012; Montepare & Lachman, 1989; Rubin & Berntsen, 2006).

Particularly in the domain of age identity, a contrast between the predominantly negative societal view of aging and individuals' views of their own aging can be seen. If asked whether they belong to the group of middle-aged or older adults, many older individuals classify themselves as middle-aged (e.g., Logan, Ward, & Spitze, 1992), thereby potentially trying to avoid or to contrast themselves from the negativity which surrounds the old age category. Furthermore, different from what one might expect considering the negative societal view of aging, individuals' satisfaction with aging decreases only slightly with advancing age, and the discrepancy between actual and subjective age remains stable or even increases in old age (e.g., Kleinspehn-Ammerlahn et al., 2008; Kotter-Grühn, Kleinspehn-Ammerlahn, Gerstorf, & Smith, 2009). Some have argued that younger subjective ages are indicative of older adults' denial of belonging to a stigmatized age group (Bultena & Powers, 1978). If that claim was true, persons with strong fears of aging and negative views of aging—both potential precursors or indicators of a denial of aging—should report particularly young subjective ages. However, studies have found no or only weak associations between younger subjective ages and personal fears of aging or negative views of aging in older adults (e.g., Montepare & Lachman, 1989; Ward, 1977).

Other concepts dealing with individuals' perception of their own age and aging are *age awareness* as well as *awareness of age-related change* (AARC). Age awareness (also called age schematicity) refers to the personal relevance and salience of age in a person's everyday life. Strong age awareness has been shown to predict faster processing of age-related, self-relevant attributes (Montepare & Clements, 2001). The concept of AARC, on the other hand, deals with individuals' perception that changes in their physical and psychological functioning are a result of having grown older (Diehl & Wahl, 2010). Specifically, the concept looks at the positive and negative age-related changes people are aware of and tries to explain *what* makes people aware of their age and aging in several domains of life (e.g., health, lifestyle, interpersonal relationships). It is important to note that individuals are not just aware of negative age-related changes but also acknowledge positive age-related changes (Miche et al., 2014).

Taken together, a closer look at concepts that deal with individuals' perception of their own aging reveals that subjective aging, on average, is more positive than the negative societal view of aging and the negative connotation of the word *old* would suggest. Nevertheless, as will be outlined in the next section, there are interindividual differences in subjective aging experiences, and adults with more negative personal views of aging might benefit from attempts to change those negative perceptions into more positive ones. At the same time, considering that holding positive views of aging is related to more positive outcomes, it seems desirable to maintain and foster the already existing positive perceptions of age(ing).

CONSEQUENCES OF NEGATIVE VIEWS OF AGING

Before discussing the consequences of negative views of aging, it is important to recognize that most negative stereotypes about age and aging are not fully supported by empirical data. Although some information encoded in age stereotypes is typically rooted in actual experiences and observations, age stereotypes represent an overgeneralization of characteristics of older adults, and those overgeneralized features do not apply to a large proportion of older adults. In this context, it is even more surprising that not just younger adults but also older adults themselves hold negative views and stereotypes about age/aging (Hummert et al., 1994). Furthermore, in contrast to gender or racial stereotypes which apply only to a part of society, age stereotypes apply to everybody once they reach a certain age. Thus, age stereotypes will become relevant to almost everybody at one point in life, and therefore, the consequences of negative age stereotypes should be well understood.

Negative views of aging in general and negative age stereotypes in particular are omnipresent and have far-reaching consequences, such as age discrimination or prejudice toward older adults. For instance, older adults are less likely to be trained or promoted in the work place (Wood, Wilkinson, & Harcourt, 2008), they are more likely to be talked down to using patronizing speech (Hummert & Ryan, 1996), they are more likely to be treated in ways to promote dependence rather than independence (Baltes & Wahl, 1992), and physicians are sometimes more reluctant regarding the treatment of older adults' diseases (Robb, Chen, & Haley, 2002). Such forms of discrimination and prejudice are not necessarily the result of bad intentions. In fact, age stereotypes are often activated automatically simply by the exposure to age-related cues, particularly cues about old age (e.g., Perdue & Gurtman, 1990). For instance, when interacting with an older adult, one might automatically talk in a louder voice because old age stereotypes have been activated, and the information encoded in these stereotypes (e.g., older adults are hard of hearing) influences perceptions and behavior in everyday life.

As will be summarized in the following section, several experimental studies have shown that the activation of age stereotypes can affect a person's behavior, attitudes, and health even when this activation happens implicitly, that is, without the person's conscious awareness (for overviews, see Filipp & Mayer, 1999; Hess, 2006; Levy, 2003). For instance, in a study by Levy (1996), older individuals were implicitly primed with positive or negative age stereotypes. Before and after the priming, participants were given memory tests (e.g., photo recall and auditory recall). Persons who were subliminally primed with positive age stereotypes showed memory improvement. In contrast, memory decline was found in persons who were subliminally primed with negative age stereotypes. No such effects were found in younger participants. Stein, Blanchard-Fields, and Hertzog (2002) reported comparable results with the exception that in their study, older individuals' memory was not enhanced after the positive age stereotype activation. Hess and colleagues conducted a series of studies in which they investigated how the implicit and/or explicit activation of age stereotypes influences memory performance in adults. Overall, they found that memory performance was worse in older adults (but not younger adults) who were implicitly primed with negative age stereotypes as compared to those who received a positive or no age stereotype priming (Hess, Auman, Colcombe, & Rahhal, 2003; Hess, Hinson, & Statham, 2004). When older persons were aware of the manipulation (i.e., in the explicit priming conditions), their memory performance was not affected. Hess and Hinson (2006) found an interesting age-related specification of the effect of stereotype priming on memory performance. Middle-aged adults recalled more words after the negative priming than after the positive priming. Hess and Hinson (2006) interpret this as a *stereotype lift effect*; that is, as outgroup members, middle-aged adults benefitted from the negative information presented about the target group of the older adults through upward social comparisons, which, in turn, affected their performance on the memory task.

The activation of positive and/or negative age stereotypes is also related to biological parameters and behavior. Levy, Hausdorff, Hencke, and Wei (2000) demonstrated that persons who were subliminally primed with negative age stereotypes showed an increase in their autonomic responses (skin conductance, systolic blood pressure, diastolic blood pressure) from pre- to poststereotype activation, whereas no such change was found in persons who received positive age stereotype priming. Furthermore, in studies by Bargh, Chen, and Burrows (1996) and Hausdorff, Levy, and Wei (1999), the implicit activation of age stereotypes even influenced the pace with which persons walked. Note, however, that this effect could not be consistently replicated.

The societal and personal views of aging are often intertwined in that age stereotypes are likely to be integrated into the self-view of middle-aged and older adults (Rothermund & Brandtstädter, 2003). In that regard, existing age stereotypes might even be reinforced when older adults engage in self-stereotyping (cf. Levy, 2009: stereotype embodiment theory). In line with these notions, it has been shown that individuals' personal beliefs in age stereotypes and the perceptions of their own age and aging are related to several health outcomes. In a study by Levy, Slade, May, and Caracciolo (2006), older persons who had more positive age stereotypes showed better physical recovery after an acute myocardial infarction than persons who had more negative age stereotypes. This association remained significant even after controlling for factors that are typically associated with physical recovery, such as self-rated health or depressive symptoms. Similarly, older adults who became newly disabled in their activities of daily living were more likely to recover from this disability when they held positive stereotypes of aging rather than negative age stereotypes (Levy, Slade, Murphy, & Gill, 2012). In another longitudinal study, individuals between the ages of 18 and 49 years who held more negative stereotypes of aging were more likely to experience cardiovascular events such as stroke or congestive heart failure over the following 38 years of their lives compared to those who held more positive beliefs of age in young and middle adulthood (Levy, Zonderman, Slade, & Ferrucci, 2009).

An increasing number of studies has further demonstrated that negative perceptions of one's own age and aging are related to lower well-being, poorer subjective and objective health, poorer health behavior and social integration, lower self-esteem, lower optimism, and lower self-efficacy (e.g., Montepare, 2009; Steverink, Westerhof, Bode, & Dittmann-Kohli, 2001; Teuscher, 2009; Westerhof & Barrett, 2005). Perceptions of one's own aging even predict longevity. That is, those individuals who feel older and are less satisfied with their age and aging tend to die earlier than those with more positive self-perceptions of aging, even after controlling for variables which are known predictors of mortality (Kotter-Grühn, et al., 2009; Levy, Slade, Kunkel, & Kasl, 2002; Uotinen,

Rantanen, & Suutama, 2005). Taken together, there is plenty of evidence that negative views of aging at the personal and the societal level are linked to negative outcomes, and interventions that focus on changing these negative perceptions should therefore be of great interest.

CHANGING NEGATIVE VIEWS OF AGING
Should Negative Views of Aging Be Changed?

When elaborating on the question as to whether or not negative views of aging should be changed, it is important to consider the two levels at which views of aging operate: the societal and the personal level. As outlined earlier, the predominantly negative *societal* view of aging is based mostly on age stereotypes, which (a) are likely to be internalized by middle-aged and older adults, (b) lead to discrimination and prejudice, and (c) are predictive of negative outcomes for health and memory. Therefore, few people would question the importance of changing the negative societal view of aging.

The line of argumentation might be less clear when it comes to the question of whether *personal* perceptions of one's own age/aging should be changed. There are many reasons speaking in favor of changing personal views of aging. As described in more detail earlier, negative self-views of aging are related among others to poor health, low well-being, and shorter survival times. Considering these negative effects of having a negative attitude toward and perception of one's own aging, it might seem straightforward that changing personal perceptions of aging is a good idea. However, a more critical consideration might slightly dampen any initial enthusiasm. If our objective was to change personal perceptions of aging, would it not imply that something was wrong with having a negative or more realistic perception of one's age(ing)? For instance, if we wanted to change older adults' subjective ages, that is, we wanted to make them feel or look younger, the question we would have to ask is, "What is wrong about being old, feeling old, or looking old?" This would assign a negative connotation to being, feeling, or looking old, and it would in fact perpetuate the negative age stereotypes which individuals encounter in most Western youth-centered societies.

How to Change Negative Views of Aging?

If we wanted to change negative views of aging, the societal and personal level at which they operate may have to be addressed with different strategies, both of which will be discussed in the following paragraphs.

Changing the Portrayal of Older Adults in the Media

Changing societal views of aging would mean changing negative stereotypes about older adults. Thus, sources for stereotype formation need to be identified and changes would need to be implemented at that level. For instance, age ste-reotypes are reflected in the ways in which older adults are portrayed in the media. If we wanted to change the societal view of age and aging, the description and portrayal of middle-aged and older adults in the media would need to be adjusted. The group of older adults, particularly those in their 80s and 90s, is vastly underrepresented in all forms of media, including TV and print advertise-ment, TV shows, and movies (Kessler, Rakoczy, & Staudinger, 2004; Zhang et al., 2006). It has been argued that advertisers might refrain from depicting older adults with the intention to avoid connecting a specific product to the negative connotation of old age. Considering that many younger people have very little contact with older adults, increasing the frequency with which older adults are portrayed in the media would be an important step toward familiarizing people with the group of older adults and educating them about the diversity of the characteristics of older adults. Interestingly, when older characters are presented in the media, their image tends to be overly positive and depicts either posi-tive age stereotypes or a reversal of prevalent negative age stereotypes (Kessler, Schwender, & Bowen, 2010; Kessler et al., 2004). This portrayal of older adults as active, socially engaged, productive, and wise can have positive effects on viewers of all ages by taking away the societal focus on the negative aspects of aging, by providing positive role models and by highlighting the diversity of older adults' characteristics. However, the predominantly positive portrayal might also lead to overly optimistic expectations about aging, which can lead to disappointment and distancing when reality turns out to be different. Thus, with the purpose in mind to change negative societal views of aging, it seems necessary to increase the frequency of representation of older adults in the media and to offer a more realistic representation of older adults' traits and behaviors. In addition, it also seems necessary to show the vast interindividual differences among middle-aged and older adults to make the general public aware of the fact that different individuals age in very different ways.

Changing the Perception of Older Adults Through Intergenerational Contact
In social interactions, in-group versus out-group categorizations are typically made within a few minutes or even seconds based on a small number of acces-sible information, including a person's age. Thus, when younger or middle-aged adults interact with older adults, they are likely to classify the older adults as belonging to an out-group simply based on age. Although the overt behavior (e.g., verbal behavior) may not always be influenced by the in-group/out-group distinction in intergroup interactions, the nonverbal behavior often is biased (for an overview, see Richeson & Shelton, 2010). Several studies have documented an increased level of signs of anxiety and discomfort during intergroup interactions

as compared to intragroup interactions. It has been argued that differences in behavior toward in-group versus out-group members might partly be explained by a lack of familiarity with intergroup interactions. Thus, a higher level of familiarity could possibly reduce bias.

Research on intergroup interactions has shown that negative attitudes and prejudice toward members of specific groups can be changed through promoting social interactions between those who belong to the stigmatized group (out-group) and those who believe in the respective stereotypes. This so-called *contact hypothesis* has been studied extensively over the past decades and results are promising (cf. Tausch & Hewstone, 2010). It has been suggested that contact leads to a reduction in prejudice through a decrease in anxiety and an increase in empathy and knowledge regarding the out-group. Pettigrew and Tropp (2006, 2008) specify several conditions under which contact with members of stigmatized groups is most likely to result in reducing negative attitudes. For instance, contact is more effective for individuals with high levels of prejudice, for members of majority (rather than minority) groups, when individuals have no choice whether to participate in an intergroup contact situation, when members of different groups work toward or have common goals, when they are of equal social status, or when the contact receives institutional support (e.g., by law). Interestingly, contact between groups does not even have to take place in real life or in face-to-face interactions to be effective. Virtual contact through online conversations, imagined contact, as well as having an in-group friend who is friends with an out-group member (i.e., extended contact) can lead to a reduction of negative views of out-groups (e.g., Crisp & Turner, 2009).

Providing Opportunities for Intergenerational Contact

Based on the earlier described theoretical notions and empirical findings, promoting contact between older adults and younger age groups seems to be a promising avenue for changing negative societal perceptions of older adults. To be effective, opportunities for contact, specifically for positive interactions, need to be provided. Such contact opportunities could include, among others, volunteer organizations which bring younger and older people together to work on a shared task, preschool and school-aged children visiting retirement communities, or retired older adults sharing their experience with and mentoring children in schools. One program that offers such an opportunity for intergenerational contact is the Experience Corps program in which older adults volunteer in elementary schools to promote academic achievement in children (Glass et al., 2004). To my knowledge, researchers affiliated with Experience Corps have not yet investigated whether the contact between children and older adult volunteers changes the children's perception of the older adults.

Providing opportunities may be even simpler than this because studies have shown that imagined contact (i.e.,, mentally simulating interactions with out-group members) works well, too. For instance, Turner, Crisp, and Lambert (2007) showed that younger adults had more positive attitudes toward older adults after simply imagining a positive interaction with an older adult. Starting at very young ages, preschool and school curricula could include actual or imagined interactions with older adults on a regular basis. Considering that many children and young adults have very limited contact with older adults in general, providing more opportunities for contact would increase familiarity with the age group—it would increase the knowledge of children and young adults about what old age and aging looks like, provide role models, and possibly take away some of the fear related to getting old. Supporting this notion, Caspi (1984) showed that preschool children who regularly interacted with teaching aids and substitute teachers older than the age of 60 years held more positive attitudes toward them than children without such contact.

Intervention programs that follow the idea of the contact hypothesis and bring together younger and older people have become more popular, and many, although not all, programs have resulted in positive changes of attitudes toward and stereotypes about older adults (cf. Meshel & McGlynn, 2004). Moreover, intergenerational contact can benefit older adults' sense of generativity, self-esteem, or cognitive functioning (e.g., Kessler & Staudinger, 2007). The research on intergenerational interactions needs to be systematically synthesized to clearly identify those elements of intervention programs which produce positive change in the societal perception of old age. Once this is achieved, recommendations for standardized programs can be made.

Changing Self-Perceptions of Aging: General Considerations
As outlined earlier, stereotypes about old age are often integrated into the self-view of older adults. Thus, one can hope that changes in the societal views (i.e., stereotypes) of aging would eventually lead to changes in the personal view of aging. This, however, is a long-lasting process because stereotypes are learned at early ages, and current cohorts of older and even middle-aged adults would probably not change the stereotypes which are ingrained into their thinking. When thinking about ways to change older adults' self-perceptions of aging, research about correlates and antecedents of positive self-perceptions of aging might proof helpful. Unfortunately, almost all research in this area is correlational in nature and does not allow for conclusions regarding causality and directionality of effects. For instance, although higher well-being has been shown to be related to younger subjective ages, this should not lead to the conclusion that being happy makes people feel younger. The directionality of effects could

well also be the other way around. Thus, knowing about correlates of positive perceptions of aging, such as self-esteem, self-efficacy, health, or social integration, can only guide us in our conceptualization of studies which test whether some of these correlates lead to or can be manipulated so that they eventually lead to more positive self-perceptions of aging. A comprehensive approach to the study of antecedents and correlates of positive self-perceptions of aging may further identify situational variables or circumstances under which individuals feel younger and are more positive about their own aging. For example, in a daily diary study with older adults, Kotter-Grühn and Neupert (2014) showed that participants felt even younger than they normally did on days when they experienced low negative affect, low levels of pain and stress, and few physical symptoms. Although this study does not allow causal conclusions, the results suggest that age identity can change even on a day-to-day basis and that it might be worth exploring ways to explicitly create such situations in which people feel younger.

Changing Self-Perceptions of Aging: Experimental Studies
There is a limited number of experimental studies that have attempted to manipulate self-perceptions of aging. Whereas most of these studies showed that experimental manipulations could be used to make people feel older, unfortunately, so far, only a minority of studies aimed at making people feel more positive about their age and aging. In a series of investigations by Eibach, Mock, and Courtney (2010), participants were successfully induced to feel older by experiencing unexplained visual disfluency (thereby mimicking age-related vision problems) or a generation gap. This study also showed that age stereotypes had stronger effects on participants' self-evaluations after they were induced to feel older. The authors argue that individuals are more likely to apply negative age stereotypes to themselves when they feel older, and therefore, evaluations of the self and well-being are more negative. Kotter-Grühn and Hess (2012) primed younger, middle-aged, and older adults with either positive, negative, or no age stereotypes using an impression formation paradigm. Overall, after being primed with any (i.e., positive or negative) age stereotype, older adults felt older than before. Even middle-aged adults were affected by the priming in that they felt older than before after the exposure to positive age stereotypes. This study further showed that not just felt age could be manipulated but also desired age and the age a person thinks he or she looks like. After being primed with negative age stereotypes, participants throughout adulthood wanted to be younger, and participants in bad health thought they looked older than before.

As described earlier, studies have demonstrated that older adults who participate in a memory test perform worse when they receive the information that declines in memory are indicative of aging (e.g., Hess et al., 2003). Along the same lines, Hughes, Geraci, and De Forrest (2013) tested whether the participation in a memory test or the mere thought of participating in a memory test would influence older adults' subjective age. In several studies, the authors found that in fact older but not younger participants felt older after the experimental manipulation (i.e., participating in or thinking about participating in a memory study) than before.

To my knowledge, so far only a few studies attempted to change self-perceptions of aging in a positive way and not all of them were successful. As described earlier, in the Kotter-Grühn and Hess (2012) study, participants in one condition were primed with positive age stereotypes. The underlying idea was that making people aware of the positive aspects of aging would lead to more positive perceptions of one's own aging. This, however, was not the case. Participants who were primed with positive age stereotypes did not report younger subjective ages or higher aging satisfaction. On the contrary, the activation of positive age stereotypes had even negative effects on middle-aged and older adults. An experimental manipulation that led to younger subjective ages was demonstrated by Stephan, Chalabaev, Kotter-Grühn, and Jaconelli (2013). Older adults performed a task measuring handgrip strength and then received feedback about their performance. Those who were told that they had performed much better than most of their same-aged peers reported younger felt ages after the task and they even increased their performance in a second handgrip strength measure. Thus, providing favorable social comparison feedback in fact resulted in a more positive self-perception of older adults' age. Similarly, in a study by Miche and Wahl (2013), older adults performed a cognitive task after which they received social comparison feedback, which primed either positive age-related changes or negative age-related losses. In the positive priming condition, participants were told that accuracy increases with age in the task they just performed and, most importantly, that they had made less mistakes than younger adults. In the negative priming condition, participants were informed that speed decreases with age in the task they performed and that they were slower than younger adults. In comparison to a pretest, subjective age and interest age were younger after the positive priming and older after the negative priming. Thus, making people aware of positive age-related changes and providing favorable social comparison feedback was a successful strategy to change older adults' perception of their own age.

Increasing knowledge and information about successful aging may be another strategy to influence older adults' views of aging in a positive way. Wolff, Warner, Ziegelmann, and Wurm (2014) conducted a randomized controlled trial in which older adults were assigned to a physical activity intervention, an active control condition (volunteering), or a physical activity intervention which also included a "views on aging" component. In the latter condition, participants received information about positive aspects of aging, misconceptions about aging (typically negative in nature) were corrected, and positive effects of having a positive view on aging were described. Furthermore, participants were taught a technique which helps people "identify automatic, unconscious negative thoughts on ageing and, as a second step, replace them with neutral or positive ones" (Wolff et al., 2014, p. 11). Participants assigned to this condition (i.e., physical activity with views on aging) showed a positive change in their perceptions of aging, including satisfaction with aging and confidence, as compared to no change in the other experimental groups. Furthermore, a positive change in perceptions of aging was also predictive of an increase in physical activity. Thus, educating older adults about the positive aspects of aging and correcting negative misconceptions may be a good strategy to improve older adults' self-perceptions of aging.

CHALLENGES TO CHANGING NEGATIVE VIEWS OF AGING

When attempting to change negative views of aging, several challenges present themselves, most of which have already been implicitly or explicitly mentioned earlier. If we want to make people feel younger or more satisfied with their age and aging, we need to know the variables related to younger age identities. Although much research in this area exists, almost no study provides information about the direction of effects. That is, to understand the circumstances under which people are more positive about their age and aging, more longitudinal and experimental research is needed to establish cause–effect and time-ordered relationships between self-perceptions of aging and variables which might be antecedents of positive personal views of aging. This might become even more challenging when taking into account that there are most likely interindividual differences as well as intraindividual change in the factors which make people feel young and satisfied with their age and aging.

Another major challenge in changing negative views of aging pertains to finding strategies which promote positive (self-)views of aging. As described in detail earlier, although some overlap is likely, strategies that are successful in changing negative societal views of aging may differ from strategies aimed at changing negative personal views of aging. Promoting positive intergenerational interactions, educating people about age and aging, as well as changing the portrayal of older adults in the media might be successful strategies at the societal level and might consequently also change self-views of aging in future generations. At the level of personal perceptions of aging in current generations of older adults, positive social comparison feedback, making people aware of positive age-related changes, as well as providing information about positive aspects of aging have been established as successful strategies in single studies. More research is needed to replicate the findings from these studies and to document the success of such strategies.

Even when successful strategies for changing negative views of aging have been identified, questions about the stability of effects and the long-term maintenance of effects need to be considered. For instance, how long does the effect of a subjective age manipulation last? It is unlikely that a single session in which older adults receive positive social comparison feedback as in the Stephan et al.'s (2013) study will make older adults feel younger over extended periods after the experiment is over. Thus, it is a challenge to translate the one-time strategy from this specific study into a long-lasting intervention program. The specification of the group of people within the population at which interventions are aimed is another important yet potentially controversial step in planning appropriate interventions. At the societal level, *education programs* that increase knowledge about older adults would probably be most beneficial if they focused on children and young adults. In contrast, changes in the media portrayal of older adults targets society as a whole, regardless of age group. Programs fostering positive interactions between older adults and younger people may include individuals of all ages, with an emphasis on children as interaction partners given that age stereotypes are learned early in life. Programs aiming at changing negative self-views of aging should be targeted at older adults, but several questions remain open. For instance, should all older adults be targeted or only those with particularly negative self-perceptions of aging? Who would benefit most from interventions and who would in fact be willing to participate in such interventions? Selectivity effects are guaranteed if only those who are highly motivated to change their perception of aging participate in interventions.

Even if target groups can be specified, it is an open question how these target groups can be reached and convinced to participate in interventions. Should such interventions be part of a public health initiative? If so, how and by whom is the intervention delivered? Primary health care providers specializing in the field of gerontology are rare, and even if they agreed with the general goal of the program, pragmatics (e.g., time constraints) may dictate otherwise. Those who deliver the intervention also need to be trained and outcomes need to be assessed on a regular basis. Most importantly, even if all of the earlier mentioned challenges can be overcome, who pays for a program that essentially tries to make people feel better about their age and aging? Arguments about the relevance of such a public health program can be easily made even when considering the positive effects of positive self-perceptions of aging.

Taken together, when addressing the questions as to whether and how to change negative views of aging, some strategies for intervention at the personal and/or societal level can be proposed, but many challenges still remain. Particularly when aiming at changing self-views of aging, ethical concerns remain. Thus, promoting more positive self-perceptions of aging may be a viable option if we were sure that the effects are universally positive (at a societal and personal level), if we had a relatively easy strategy which works for everybody and was accessible to everybody (who is interested), and if we knew about the long-term consequences of such strategies.

REFERENCES

Baltes, M. M., & Wahl, H. W. (1992). The d-support script in institutions: Generalizations to community settings. *Psychology and Aging, 7,* 409–418. http://dx.doi.org/10.1037/0882-7974.7.3.409

Bargh, J. A., Chen, M., & Burrows, L. (1996). Automaticity of social behavior: Direct effects of trait construct and stereotype activation on action. *Journal of Personality and Social Psychology, 71,* 230–244. http://dx.doi.org/10.1037/0022-3514.71.2.230

Bultena, G. L., & Powers, E. A. (1978). Denial of aging: Age identification and reference group orientations. *Journal of Gerontology, 33,* 748–754.

Caspi, A. (1984). Contact hypothesis and inter-age attitudes: A field study of cross-age contact. *Social Psychology Quarterly, 47,* 74–80. http://dx.doi.org/10.2307/3033890

Crisp, R. J., & Turner, R. N. (2009). Can imagined interactions produce positive perceptions? Reducing prejudice through simulated social contact. *American Psychologist, 64,* 231–240. http://dx.doi.org/10.1037/a0014718

Cuddy, A. J. C., & Fiske, S. T. (2002). Doddering but dear: Process, content, and function in stereotyping of older persons. In T. D. Nelson (Ed.), *Ageism: Stereotyping and prejudice against older persons* (pp. 3–26). Cambridge, MA: MIT Press.

Diehl, M. K., & Wahl, H. W. (2010). Awareness of age-related change: Examination of a (mostly) unexplored concept. *The Journals of Gerontology. Series B, Psychological Sciences and Social Sciences, 65,* 340–350. http://dx.doi.org/10.1093/geronb/gbp110

Eibach, R. P., Mock, S. E., & Courtney, E. A. (2010). Having a "senior moment": Induced aging phenomenology, subjective age, and susceptibility to ageist stereotypes. *Journal of Experimental Social Psychology, 46,* 643–649. http://dx.doi.org/10.1016/j.jesp.2010.03.002

Filipp, S. H., & Mayer, A. K. (1999). *Bilder des Alters: Altersstereotype und die Beziehungen zwischen den Generationen* [Images of aging: Aging stereotypes and the relations between generations]. Stuttgart, Germany: Kohlhammer.

Fiske, S. T., Cuddy, A. J. C., Glick, P., & Xu, J. (2002). A model of (often mixed) stereotype content: Competence and warmth respectively follow from perceived status and competition. *Journal of Personality and Social Psychology, 82,* 878–902. http://dx.doi.org/10.1037/0022-3514.82.6.878

Glass, T. A., Freedman, M., Carlson, M. C., Hill, J., Frick, K. D., Ialongo, N., . . . Fried, L. P. (2004). Experience corps: Design of an intergenerational program to boost social capital and promote the health of an aging society. *Journal of Urban Health: Bulletin of the New York Academy of Medicine, 81,* 94–105. http://dx.doi.org/10.1093/jurban/jth096

Hausdorff, J., Levy, B., & Wei, J. (1999). The power of ageism on physical function of older persons: Reversibility of age-related gait changes. *Journal of the American Geriatrics Society, 47,* 1346–1349.

Hess, T. M. (2006). Attitudes toward aging and their effects on behavior. In J. E. Birren & K. W. Schaie (Eds.), *Handbook of the psychology of aging* (6th ed., pp. 379–406). San Diego, CA: Academic Press.

Hess, T. M., Auman, C., Colcombe, S. J., & Rahhal, T. A. (2003). The impact of stereotype threat on age differences in memory performance. *The Journals of Gerontology. Series B, Psychological Sciences and Social Sciences, 58,* P3–P11. http://dx.doi.org/10.1093/geronb/58.1.P3

Hess, T. M., & Hinson, J. T. (2006). Age-related variation in the influences of aging stereotypes on memory in adulthood. *Psychology and Aging, 21,* 621–625.

Hess, T. M., Hinson, J. T., & Statham, J. A. (2004). Explicit and implicit stereotype activation effects on memory: Do age and awareness moderate the impact of priming? *Psychology and Aging, 19,* 495–505. http://dx.doi.org/10.1037/0882-7974.19.3.495

Hughes, M. L., Geraci, L., & De Forrest, R. L. (2013). Aging 5 years in 5 minutes: The effect of taking a memory test on older adults' subjective age. *Psychological Science.* Advance online publication. http://dx.doi.org/10.1177/0956797613494853

Hummert, M. L. (1994). Physiognomic cues and the activation of stereotypes of the elderly in interaction. *International Journal of Aging & Human Development, 39,* 5–20. http://dx.doi.org/10.2190/6EF6-P8PF-YP6F-VPY4

Hummert, M. L. (1999). A social cognitive perspective on age stereotypes. In T. Hess & F. Blanchard-Fields (Eds.), *Social cognition and aging* (pp. 175–196). New York, NY: Academic Press.

Hummert, M. L., Garstka, T., & Shaner, J. (1997). Stereotyping of older adults: The role of target facial cues and perceiver characteristics. *Psychology and Aging, 12,* 107–114. http://dx.doi.org/10.1037/0882-7974.12.1.107

Hummert, M. L., Garstka, T., Shaner, J., & Strahm, S. (1994). Stereotypes of the elderly held by young, middle-aged, and elderly adults. *The Journals of Gerontology. Series B, Psychological Sciences and Social Sciences, 49,* 240–249. http://dx.doi.org/10.1093/geronj/49.5.P240

Hummert, M., & Ryan, E. B. (1996). Toward understanding variations in patronizing talk addressed to older adults: Psycholinguistic features of care and control. *International Journal of Psycholinguistics, 12,* 149–169.

Kaufman, G., & Elder, G. H., Jr. (2002). Revisiting age identity: A research note. *Journal of Aging Studies, 16,* 169–176. http://dx.doi.org/10.1016/S0890-4065(02)00042-7

Kessler, E. M., Racoczy, K., & Staudinger, U. M. (2004). The portrayal of older people in prime time television series: The mismatch with gerontological evidence. *Ageing and Society, 24,* 531–552. http://dx.doi.org/10.1017/S0144686X04002338

Kessler, E. M., Schwender, C., & Bowen, C. E. (2010). The portrayal of older people's social participation on German prime-time TV advertisements. *The Journals of*

Gerontology. Series B, Psychological Sciences and Social Sciences, 65, S97–S106. http://dx.doi.org/10.1093/geronb/gbp084

Kessler, E. M., & Staudinger, U. M. (2007). Intergenerational potential: Effects of social interaction between older adults and adolescents. *Psychology and Aging, 22*, 690–704. http://dx.doi.org/10.1037/0882-7974.22.4.690

Kite, M. E., Stockdale, G. D., Whitley, B. E., Jr., & Johnson, B. T. (2005). Attitudes toward younger and older adults: An updated meta-analytic review. *Journal of Social Issues, 61*, 241–266. http://dx.doi.org/10.1111/j.1540-4560.2005.00404.x

Kleinspehn-Ammerlahn, A., Kotter-Grühn, D., & Smith, J. (2008). Self-perceptions of aging: Do subjective age and satisfaction with aging change during old age? *The Journals of Gerontology. Series B, Psychological Sciences and Social Sciences, 63*, P377–P385. http://doi.org/10.1093/geronb/63.6.P377

Kotter-Grühn, D., & Hess, T. M. (2012). The impact of age stereotypes on self-perceptions of aging across the adult lifespan. *The Journals of Gerontology. Series B, Psychological Sciences and Social Sciences, 76*, 563–571. http://dx.doi.org/10.1037/a0023775

Kotter-Grühn, D., Kleinspehn-Ammerlahn, A., Gerstorf, D., & Smith, J. (2009). Self-perceptions of aging predict mortality and change with approaching death: 16-year longitudinal results from the Berlin Aging Study. *Psychology and Aging, 24*, 654–667. http://dx.doi/org/doi:10.1037/a0016510

Kotter-Grühn, D., & Neupert, S. D. (2014). *Feeling old today? Daily stress, affect, and health explain day-to-day changes in subjective age.* Manuscript submitted for publication.

Levy, B. R. (1996). Improving memory in old age through implicit self-stereotyping. *Journal of Personality and Social Psychology, 71*, 1092–1107. http://dx.doi.org/10.1037//0022-3514.71.6.1092

Levy, B. R. (2003). Mind matters: Cognitive and physical effects of aging self-stereotypes. *The Journal of Gerontology. Series B, Psychological Sciences and Social Sciences, 58*, P203–P211. http://dx.doi.org/10.1093/geronb/58.4.P203

Levy, B. (2009). Stereotype embodiment: A psychosocial approach to aging. *Current Directions in Psychological Science, 18*, 332–336. http://dx.doi.org/10.1111/j.1467-8721.2009.01662.x

Levy, B. R., Hausdorff, J. M., Hencke, R., & Wei, J. Y. (2000). Reducing cardiovascular stress with positive self-stereotypes of aging. *Journal of Gerontology. Series B, Psychological Sciences, 55*, P205–P213. http://dx.doi.org/10.1093/geronb/55.4.P205

Levy, B. R., Slade, M. D., & Kasl, S. V. (2002). Longitudinal benefit of positive self-perceptions of aging on functional health. *The Journals of Gerontology. Series B, Psychological Sciences and Social Sciences, 57*, P409–P417. http://dx.doi.org/10.1093/geronb/57.5.P409

Levy, B. R., Slade, M. D., Kunkel, S. R., & Kasl, S. V. Longevity increased by positive self-perceptions of aging. *Journal of Personality and Social Psychology, 83*, 261–270. http://dx.doi.org/10.1037//0022-3514.83.2.261

Levy, B. R., Slade, M., May, J., & Caracciolo, E. (2006). Physical recovery after acute myocardial infarction: Positive age self-stereotypes as a resource. *International*

Journal of Aging and Human Development, 62, 285–301. http://dx.doi.org/10.2190/EJK1-1Q0D-LHGE-7A35

Levy, B. R., Slade, M., Murphy, T. E., & Gill, T. M. (2012). Association between positive age stereotypes and recovery from disability in older persons. *Journal of the American Medical Association, 308,* 1972–1973. http://dx.doi.org/10.1001/jama.2012.14541

Levy, B. R., Zonderman, A. B., Slade, M. D., & Ferrucci, L. (2009). Age stereotypes held earlier in life predict cardiovascular events in late life. *Psychological Science, 20,* 296–298. http://dx.doi.org/10.1111/j.1467-9280.2009.02298.x

Logan, J. R., Ward, R. A., & Spitze, G. (1992). As old as you feel: Age identity in middle and later life. *Social Forces, 71,* 451–467. http://dx.doi.org/10.2307/2580019

Meshel, D. S., & McGlynn, R. P. (2004). Intergenerational contact, attitudes, and stereotypes of adolescents and older people. *Educational Gerontology, 30,* 457–479. http://dx.doi.org/10.1080/03601270490445078

Miche, M., & Wahl, H. W. (2013, November). *"It's because of my age": The influence of experimentally increased salience of age-related changes in cognitive functioning on self-perceptions of aging.* Poster presented at the 66th Annual Scientific Meeting of the Gerontological Society of America, New Orleans, LA.

Miche, M., Wahl, H. W., Diehl, M., Oswald, F., Kaspar, R., & Kolb, M. (2014). Natural occurrence of subjective aging experiences in community-dwelling older adults. *The Journals of Gerontology. Series B, Psychological Sciences and Social Sciences, 69,* 174–187. http://dx.doi.org/10.1093/geronb/gbs164

Montepare, J. M. (2009). Subjective age: Toward a guiding lifespan framework. *International Journal of Behavioral Development, 33,* 42–46. http://dx.doi.org/10.1177/0165025408095551

Montepare, J. M., & Clements, A. (2001). "Age schemas": Guides to processing information about the self. *Journal of Adult Development, 8,* 99–108. http://dx.doi.org/10.1023/a:1026493818246

Montepare, J. M., & Lachman, M. E. (1989). "You're only as old as you feel": Self-perceptions of age, fears of aging, and life satisfaction from adolescence to old age. *Psychology and Aging, 4,* 73–78. http://dx.doi.org/10.1037//0882-7974.4.1.73

Perdue, C. W., & Gurtman, M. B. (1990). Evidence for the automaticity of ageism. *Journal of Experimental Social Psychology, 26,* 199–216. http://dx.doi.org/10.1016/0022-1031(90)90035-K

Pettigrew, T. F., & Tropp, L. R. (2006). A meta-analytic test of intergroup contact theory. *Journal of Personality and Social Psychology, 90,* 751–783. http://dx.doi.org/10.1037/0022-3514.90.5.751

Pettigrew, T. F., & Tropp, L. R. (2008). How does intergroup contact reduce prejudice? Meta-analytic tests of three mediators. *European Journal of Social Psychology, 38,* 922–934. http://dx.doi.org/10.1002/ejsp.504

Richeson, J. A., & Shelton, J. N. (2010). Intergroup dyadic interactions. In J. F. Dovidio, M. Hewstone, P. Glick, & V. M. Esses (Eds.), *The Sage handbook of prejudice, stereotyping, and discrimination* (pp. 276–293). Thousand Oaks, CA: Sage.

Robb, C., Chen, H., & Haley, W. E. (2002). Ageism in mental health and health care: A critical review. *Journal of Clinical Geropsychology, 8*, 1–12. http://dx.doi.org/10.1023/A:1013013322947

Rothermund, K., & Brandtstädter, J. (2003). Age stereotypes and self-views in later life: Evaluating rival assumptions. *International Journal of Behavioral Development, 27*, 549–554. http://dx.doi.org/10.1080/01650250344000208

Rubin, D. C., & Berntsen, D. (2006). People over forty feel 20% younger than their age: Subjective age across the lifespan. *Psychonomic Bulletin & Review, 13*, 776–780. http://dx.doi.org/10.3758/BF03193996

Stein, R., Blanchard-Fields, F., & Hertzog, C. (2002). The effects of age-stereotype priming on the memory performance of older adults. *Experimental Aging Research, 28*, 169–181. http://dx.doi.org/10.1080/03610730252800184

Stephan, Y., Chalabaev, A., Kotter-Grühn, D., & Jaconelli, A. (2013). "Feeling younger, being stronger": An experimental study of subjective age and physical functioning among older adults. *The Journals of Gerontology. Series B, Psychological Sciences and Social Sciences, 68*, 1–7. http://dx.doi.org/10.1093/geronb/gbs037

Steverink, N., Westerhof, G. J., Bode, C., & Dittmann-Kohli, F. (2001). The personal experience of aging, individual resources, and subjective well-being. *The Journals of Gerontology. Series B, Psychological Sciences and Social Sciences, 56*, P364–P373. http://dx.doi.org/10.1093/geronb/56.6.P364

Tausch, N., & Hewstone, M. (2010). Intergroup contact. In J. F. Dovidio, M. Hewstone, P. Glick, & V. M. Esses (Eds.), *The Sage handbook of prejudice, stereotyping, and discrimination* (pp. 544–560). Thousand Oaks, CA: Sage.

Teuscher, U. (2009). Subjective age bias: A motivational and information processing approach. *International Journal of Behavioral Development, 33*, 22–31. http://dx.doi.org/10.1177/0165025408099487

Turner, R. N., Crisp, R. J., & Lambert, E. (2007). Imagining intergroup contact can improve intergroup attitudes. *Group Processes and Intergroup Relations, 10*, 427–441. http://dx.doi.org/10.1177/1368430207081533

Uotinen, V., Rantanen, T., & Suutama, T. (2005). Perceived age as a predictor of old age mortality: A 13-year prospective study. *Age and Ageing, 34*, 368–372. http://dx.doi.org/10.1093/ageing/afi091

Ward, R. A. (1977). The impact of subjective age and stigma on older persons. *Journal of Gerontology, 32*, 227–232.

Wehr, T., & Buchwald, F. (2007). Subjektive Vorstellungen über ältere Menschen und das Altern: Eine Untersuchung zu Typizität, Erwünschtheit, Kontrollierbarkeit und Entwicklungsperiode von 218 Personenmerkmalen [Subjective conceptions about the elderly and aging: A study of typicality, desirability, controllability, and expected onset and closing age of 218 personality traits]. *Zeitschrift für Sozialpsychologie, 38*, 163–177. http://dx.doi.org/10.1024/0044-3514.38.3.163

Westerhof, G. J., & Barrett, A. E. (2005). Age identity and subjective well-being: A comparison of the United States and Germany. *The Journals of Gerontology. Series B,*

Psychological Sciences and Social Sciences, 60, S129–S136. http://dx.doi.org/10.1093/geronb/60.3.S129

Wolff, J. K., Warner, L. M., Ziegelmann, J. P., & Wurm, S. (2014). What does targeting positive views on ageing add to a physical activity intervention in older adults? Results from a randomized controlled trial. *Psychology and Health.* Advance online publication. http://dx.doi.org/10.1080/08870446.2014.896464

Wood, G., Wilkinson, A., & Harcourt, M. (2008). Age discrimination and working life: Perspectives and contestations—A review of the contemporary literature. *International Journal of Management Reviews, 10,* 425–442. http://dx.doi.org/10.1111/j.1468-2370.2008.00236.x

Zhang, Y. B., Harwood, J., Williams, A., Ylänne-McEwen, V., Wadleigh, P. M., & Thimm, C. (2006). The portrayal of older adults in advertising. *Journal of Language and Social Psychology, 25,* 264–285. http://dx.doi.org/10.1177/0261927X06289479

CHAPTER 9

Images of Aging
Outside and Inside Perspectives

Ursula M. Staudinger

ABSTRACT

Chronological age is but one, and not the most accurate, indicator of human aging. Multiple outside (i.e., objective) and inside (i.e., subjective) perspectives on aging need to be considered to do justice to the multidimensionality of human development and aging. Outside perspectives are, for example, biological, social, and psychological ages. A chronological age of 75 years, for instance, may be linked with a different biological as well as cognitive age. Human development and aging is not only a biological process but is interactive in nature. As a result, it is characterized by impressive plasticity which entails the relativity of the meaning of chronological age. Outside perspectives are closely linked with inside perspectives on aging such as societal stereotypes, images about one's own old age and metastereotypes, that is, what we think others might think about old age. These inside perspectives, even though "invisible," are very powerful and exert effects on biological, social, and psychological ages alike and are affected by them. Future research needs to focus on furthering our understanding of the interactions taking place between biological, psychological, and sociocultural influences on the aging process and on the mechanisms linking personal, societal, and meta-images of old age.

INTRODUCTION

"What is my age and how many ages do I have?" is the first guiding question of this chapter, and it refers to the outside perspectives on aging. The second part of the chapter is concerned with the question, "What do *I think* about (my) old age and how does it influence my own aging?" and this represents the inside perspectives on aging.

The first question is meant to highlight the equivocality of the notion "age," even though we think that the answer to the question, "What is your age?" is quite straightforward. When we talk about a person's age, we usually rely on the definition of chronological age and refer to the difference between the current date and the person's birth date. The straightforward metric and the simplicity of this definition is enticing, which may be one of the reasons why, all too often, chronological age, that is, the passage of time, is bestowed with a causal power and is used to explain observed age-related changes without being aware of the actual biological, psychological, and/or social influences underlying such changes. As is often the case, it is not the most obvious and most easily available explanation that is the right one or the only one. Research in the tradition of life span psychology (Baltes, Lindenberger, & Staudinger, 2006; Baltes, Reese, & Lipsitt, 1980) as well as life course sociology (Elder, 1975; Settersten & Mayer, 1997) has shown that the meaning of age must not be reduced to that of chronological age.

Life span psychology has demonstrated that chronological age per se has no explanatory power but that it is a cover variable for the age-related processes and influences to be uncovered and understood in terms of their causal effects (Baltes et al., 2006; Baltes et al., 1980; see also Neugarten, 1977). More specifically, human development and aging—two sides of one coin—are not determined by biology, that is, in this case the genome, such that development and aging are the emergent property of elapsing time. Rather, human development and aging are the result of the continuous interaction between biological influences, sociocultural influences, and the decisions and competencies as well as beliefs and attributions of the developing individual himself or herself. Thus, age (or aging) is multidimensional. The interactive nature of aging is at the heart of its plasticity and therefore historical relativity (Staudinger, Marsiske, & Baltes, 1995). Plasticity here is defined as the modifiability of age-related change. It is a constituent characteristic of human development and aging. It is maintained throughout life unless pathological processes interfere. With increasing age, however, the degree of modifiability is reduced. Across historical time, sociocultural changes imprint themselves on the unfolding of genetic information (through epigenetic mechanisms) as well as on the age-related trajectories of psychological functioning as, for example, cognitive skills (e.g., Flynn effect), such that, the same chronological age stands for different levels of cognitive performance at different historical times and in different cultural settings. Sociocultural changes also affect images of aging and thereby also influence the inside perspectives on aging.

A comprehensive understanding of age encompasses: biological age, social age, and psychological age (e.g., Birren & Cunningham, 1985). To be clear, each of these "ages" again are multidimensional because they each encompass multiple domains and indicators. For instance, for decades, the debate about *the* indicator of biological age has been ongoing and is far from having yielded a conclusive result yet (e.g., López-Otín, Serrano, Partridge, Blasco, & Kroemer, 2013). Indicators under consideration range from muscle strength or lung capacity to telomere length. Similarly, the meaning of social and psychological age is manifold. A person's functional/performance ages within and across domains of functioning can differ and most often will diverge from the person's chronological age. Furthermore, we need to distinguish between objective and subjective indicators of domain-specific ages. The personality age of a given person (one facet of psychological age) assessed by using a test, for instance, may differ from the answer of that person when asked how old he or she feels. In this vein, I distinguish the inside from the outside perspectives on aging. Note that inside perspectives refer not only to different kinds of ages, such as felt age, but also to images of old age and aging, encompassing behaviors and characteristics that allegedly come with a person of a certain chronological age, which, in turn, influence subjective perceptions of age and subsequently expectations and behaviors.

THE POWER OF CHRONOLOGICAL AGE

Every day, we rely on the informational value of chronological age without thinking much about it. Modern societies use chronological age as an important index or marker variable to assign social roles, privileges, and responsibilities. But when is it that knowing the chronological age of a person will actually tell us something about what this person is capable of or what his or her personality and motives are like? Given the interactive nature of human development and aging that was described earlier, human beings become more different from each other as they grow older. By midlife, the informational value of chronological age has become rather limited. For instance, an 80-year-old person can function at the level of cognitive performance of an average 50-year-old and vice versa (e.g., Baltes et al., 2006). Even though the interindividual variability is reduced again at very old age, that is, around age 90 or 95 years, the conviction that old (chronological) age is in general characterized by a highly constrained cognitive capacity because it forms the core of the negative old age stereotype, which will be discussed in the second part of the chapter (e.g., Hummert, 1990), is an incorrect generalization. The performance differences between individuals during adulthood are significant and are even increasing during later life (cf. Baltes, 1987; Nelson & Dannefer, 1992). In other words, chronological age becomes less and less informative regarding the capabilities, attitudes, and typical behaviors characterizing a given older adult. Nevertheless, in many domains of life, in particular the work place, a deeply rooted belief in the unconstrained explanatory and informational value of chronological age still reigns supreme. Part of the success story of chronological age most likely lies in the ease with which it is measured. Certainly, obtaining a person's chronological age is more easily accomplished and is less intrusive than, for instance, measuring intellectual performance or telomere length. Also, it is less effortful to think in averages, for instance, the average 60-year-old, than it is to think in a differentiated way about the diversity of 60-year-olds of a given birth cohort.

BIOLOGICAL AGE: AN IMPRESSIVE EXAMPLE OF THE PLASTICITY OF HUMAN DEVELOPMENT AND AGING

As mentioned earlier, it is much more difficult to measure biological than chronological age. A rather simple approximation of biological age, however, is a person's total length of life, if we accept the disadvantage that it can only be measured after the person's death. On a population level, average life expectancy is a personally less "cruel" and more readily available measure that lends itself perfectly as a proxy to the study of historical changes in biological aging. Demographers have been doing this and have found that the human species has managed to increase its maximal average life expectancy by 40 years since 1840 (e.g., Oeppen & Vaupel, 2002). This unprecedented expansion of the life span in human history again testifies to the interactive nature of human development and aging; that is, besides biological evolution, cultural evolution plays an important role (e.g., Durham, 1990). The cultural changes discussed regarding the expansion of average life expectancy are improved hygiene and nutrition, better accident prevention (especially during the early life span), development of medical knowledge and practice, healthier work place environments, and, last but not least, increased investment in prevention as highlighted in the public health philosophy.

Besides life expectancy, however, an even more important approximation of biological aging seems to be *healthy life expectancy*, even though it is much more difficult to measure than mortality (e.g., Robine & Ritchie, 1991). Available panel studies usually are confined to indicators such as activities of daily living (ADL) or instrumental activities of daily living (IADL) as measures of functional health or self-reported number of diagnoses as an indicator of physical health. There is an ongoing debate in the fields of epidemiology and demography about whether the healthy life span has increased or not. Discrepancies in findings usually are linked with differences in the available health indicators and with actual differences between countries. It seems that within most of the industrialized world by and large, healthy life expectancy has been increasing over the last decades, such that the larger part of the added years are functionally healthy years, in the sense of active years (e.g., Christensen, Doblhammer, Rau, & Vaupel, 2009). As of recently, surprisingly the United States (and Russia) have been found to be an exception to this pattern because both average and healthy life expectancy have been declining (cf. Reither, Olshansky, & Yang, 2011). Acknowledging this exception, indeed, it seems to be the case that people not only live longer but also do so in good functional health until close to the very end of life. The health status of a 70-year-old 20 years ago is equivalent to the health status of an 80-year-old today (Vaupel, 2010).

Although the extension of healthy life expectancy is, in general, good news for aging individuals, it is also important to acknowledge that to gain more specific knowledge about the historical change in the associated biological processes, it will be necessary to conduct systematic cohort sequential comparisons on several different biological indicators. Life expectancy is only a rough proxy of biological age because it also reflects sociocultural and behavioral influences and changes. "Purer" measures of biological age, such as telomere length or average age of menarche, most likely have changed as well. No cohort comparative data on telomere length yet exist to my knowledge. But we do know that the average age of menarche has continuously decreased over the last 100 years. However, no signs have yet been observed for a postponement of the average age of onset of menopause (e.g., Te Velde & Pearson, 2002). The lack of evidence for the latter may be an indication of the limits of biological plasticity in the human species. It is also noteworthy that in contrast to the earlier onset of sexual maturity, the average age at the birth of the first child, one type of social age, has continuously increased since World War II. This phenomenon is an indication for the power of social institutions, such as educational opportunities or changed gender roles, as discussed next under the heading "Social age: A Human Necessity."

Coming full circle in terms of the focus of this section, there is more and more evidence demonstrating that the biology of the human condition is in crucial ways changed by sociocultural influences. Epigenetic research on the facilitative rather than debilitating age-related contextual influences, such as nutrition or education, may in the future help to better understand the mediating mechanisms underlying this powerful connection (Fraga & Esteller, 2007).

SOCIAL AGE: A HUMAN NECESSITY

Humans are inherently social beings. Without social support and embeddedness into relationships, a human individual could not survive. Thus, the *social age* of an individual plays a crucial role for outside and inside perspectives on aging. Within a given community, the temporal sequence of life phases is linked with a sequence of tasks and challenges as well as competences. The age-related distribution of roles serves the function to link rights as well as obligations with certain life phases which support the survival of the community. For instance, both entry into (i.e., begin of labor force participation) and exit from (i.e., retirement) adult life in the sense of being economically productive form important transitions in a person's life, which influence life planning as well as self-representations and the way a person is perceived and valued in the larger social community. However, only modern societies have assigned chronological age the importance that seems so natural nowadays (e.g., Settersten & Mayer, 1997). There are age markers and normative age expectations for entering school, entering the labor market, first marriage, birth of first child, or retirement. Despite the fact that since the 1990s the—in sociology heavily debated—*destandardization of the life course* (Kohli, 1994; Mayer & Müller, 1994) has led to a certain weakening of age norms,[1] the almost magical importance bestowed onto age markers for guiding life planning and the evaluation of one's life seems uncompromised (e.g., Heckhausen, 1989).

The sheer fact of having more years of life available without doubt contributes to the transformation of the socially defined life course structure (e.g., Wink & James, 2013). Individuals have more personal lifetime at their disposal and this, in turn, very likely results in greater interindividual variability in the ways in which developmental tasks and role expectations are encountered (e.g., Moen & Altobelli, 2006; Riley, 1986).

PSYCHOLOGICAL AGE FROM THE OUTSIDE: THE SAMPLE CASES OF COGNITION AND PERSONALITY

In the following text, the increasing discrepancy between chronological and functional age, as just discussed for biological age, will be examined for psychological dimensions of aging, such as cognitive and personality age.

Cognitive Age Deviates From Chronological Age

Several different types of evidence need to be considered here. First, the evidence on tremendous cohort improvements in cognitive functioning, for instance, from the seminal Seattle Longitudinal Study (e.g., Schaie, 1996) can be provided as evidence. Schaie (1986) showed that across 50 years of historical time (birth years 1890–1940), the level of cognitive functioning in several cognitive tests improved by 1.5 standard deviation. This indication of the impressive plasticity of cognitive performance caused by sociocultural advances, such as improved health and nutrition, more and different schooling, smaller family size, modern parenting, the rise of a visual culture, more jobs that require on-the-spot problem solving, and more leisure devoted to cognitively demanding pursuits has also been called the Flynn effect (Flynn, 1987, 2009). Evidence that seems to indicate that the Flynn effect recently may have come to a halt needs to be interpreted with care because the reference populations used to assess the effect have changed across historical time (e.g., discontinued mandatory military service or increasing migrant populations with lower language skills; Skirbekk, Stonawski, Bonsang, & Staudinger, 2013). Originally, the Flynn effect was referring to the improvement of cognitive performance levels in early adulthood, but since then, it has also been documented that it continues into middle and later adulthood (e.g., Gerstorf, Ram, Hoppmann, Willis, & Schaie, 2011; Rönnlund & Nilsson, 2008; Skirbekk et al., 2013). Moreover, we can expect the cognitive improvements across cohorts in later life to continue even after the Flynn effect in young adulthood may have stopped because the sociocultural changes linked with a "Society of Longer Lives" (Staudinger, 2012) are only starting to unfold and exert their effects on current cohorts of middle-aged and older adults. It is an interesting exercise to simulate what these cohort changes in cognitive aging might entail on a population level. When doing so, it turns out that, for instance, the United Kingdom will be cognitively younger in the year 2040 than today even though chronologically it will be older (Skirbekk et al., 2013).

Second, there is evidence from country comparisons of age-related levels of cognitive functioning. These analyses have shown that the same chronological age stands for different cognitive ages in different countries (Skirbekk, Loichinger, & Weber, 2012). Today, the average cognitive performance level of a 70-year-old in the United States is higher than the average level of a 50-year-old in India or China. This study illustrates once more how far-reaching the implications of such a perspective on chronological age are if we are to judge the productivity of an aging population.

Third and last, there is a large amount of evidence about the effects of training as well as of an active lifestyle on cognitive functioning in later adulthood (e.g., Hertzog, Kramer, Wilson, & Lindenberger, 2009). In short, this evidence is to be interpreted such that after a training intervention aiming at the improvement of cognitive functioning, be it a physical activity intervention or a cognitive training intervention, a 65-year-old can display the cognitive level of functioning that he or she has had at age 55 years. Currently, the intervention with the most generalizable effects seems to be aerobic exercise. After only 6 months of training

(3 × 45 min per week), for instance, increases in the speed of information processing have been observed and also reactivation in brain areas usually characterized by age-related decline (e.g., Voelcker-Rehage, Godde, & Staudinger, 2011; for a review of that literature, see Colcombe & Kramer, 2003). The specific contribution of the study by Voelcker-Rehage et al. (2011), for example, was to show that maintaining the physical activity regime across 12 months showed a leveling off of performance increases on the behavioral level of measurement but not on the neurophysiological level. In addition, this study highlighted the fact that different kinds of physical activity, such as aerobic exercise and coordinative training have highly differential neurophysiological effects, but after 12 months, their effects are indistinguishable in terms of performance increases.

Based on such evidence testifying to the plasticity of cognitive aging, one may ask "What are the consequences of such findings for everyday life?" Thus, it may be useful to investigate under which circumstances which kinds of working or leisure time environments are conducive to continuously challenge and support brain development across the life span. In that vein, the cumulative effect of cognitive stimulation at work and during leisure time (or the lack thereof) is currently under intensive study in different groups (e.g., Oltmanns, Godde & Staudinger, 2014; Park & Reuter-Lorenz, 2009; Stine-Morrow, Parisi, Morrow, & Park, 2008). For instance, one study currently under way examines whether many as compared to few work-task changes across a period of 16 years will make a difference to cognitive and personality outcomes. The specific strength of this study is that the number of task changes is not confounded with the level of complexity of the job or the level of qualification necessary for the position. If hypotheses are confirmed and results show that more work-task changes are related with higher levels of cognitive flexibility 16 years later, this would suggest that work biographies in a Society of Longer Lives need to provide for and incentivize regular task changes also for less complex jobs (cf. Staudinger & Kocka, 2010). Of course, the temporal pattern of work task or job changes has to match the level of complexity of a given occupation: More complex jobs may require less frequent changes than simple, physically and/or mentally exerting types of jobs.

Personality Age Is Not Set Like Plaster

Research on the plasticity of personality aging is still in its infancy compared to that on the plasticity of cognitive functioning. There seems to be less of a reason to study the plasticity of personality as rather few negative age-related changes with dysfunctional consequences for everyday life have been observed in this domain. In the realm of personality functioning, there is only one major trait that has been of concern in terms of age-related decline. In particular, data from longitudinal studies around the world (e.g., McCrae et al., 2000) have shown that after midlife, the trait of openness to new experience is on average declining (for review, see Staudinger, 2005). Because openness to new experience is a crucial personality characteristic supportive of learning as well as of staying in touch with an ever-changing world, it may be useful to find out whether the level of openness observed in a 65-year-old can be changed to reflect, for instance, this person's level of openness at age 55 years—in other words, whether it is possible to reduce a person's personality age.

And indeed, in a recently published study, it was found that exposure to preparatory training and to new activities in later life increased levels of openness to new experiences in people older than 55 years old. The study was a longitudinal field experiment that allowed the comparison of one group of volunteers, who participated in a 9-day competence training to support mastery in the volunteering context, with a group of matched volunteers on the waiting list for the training. After the three 3-day trainings, the volunteers returned to their respective volunteering settings and continued with their volunteering activities. A broad range of volunteering activities was covered in the study sample and controlling for type of volunteering activity did not compromise the finding. Across 15 months, and over and above the observed cognitive change, a significant increase in openness to new experience in the amount of about one standard deviation was found in the group of trained volunteers (Mühlig-Versen, Bowen, & Staudinger, 2012). This effect was observed in those volunteers with above median levels of internal control beliefs, suggesting that the new experiences in combination with the internal control attribution resulted in greater openness to new experience. This finding also demonstrates that the inside perspective, in this context the attributional style, played an important role regarding the efficiency of the training intervention and points to the fact that exploiting the plasticity of aging may require a personalized approach. In this particular study, the personalization concerned the attributional style. In other settings, it may be personalization according to preceding biographical experiences or to genetic polymorphisms.

As the findings from this study show, within a bit more than a year, personality age was decreased significantly if persons who believed that they can influence their life were exposed to new tasks and to task-relevant training. Personality age is indexed by the level of a given personality characteristic. Similarly as it is done when establishing the IQ, the reference for determining whether someone is younger or older in terms of personality than his or her chronological age would suggest, is the average longitudinal trajectory of the given personality dimension, in the case of the just cited study, of openness to new experiences. The average longitudinal trajectory shows the level of openness that is typical for a given chronological age at a given historical time and in a given cultural setting. Thus, when compared with this average longitudinal trajectory, a given person can be categorized as being younger or older than suggested by the average trajectory.

PSYCHOLOGICAL AGE FROM THE INSIDE: FEELING OLD MAKES OLD?

Before some of the evidence on subjective age and images of old age are discussed, it may be useful to highlight some of the sources from which these inside perspectives emerge. How do we learn about our own age-related changes? How do we learn about what it is like to be old? The following major sources need to be considered: (a) self-perceptions of physical and behavioral changes, (b) observation of and comparison with others (e.g., peers, older and younger generations), (c) feedback from and treatment by others, and (d) perception of age-related societal norms and images (e.g., media, work place). The constellations of these sources differ between people, across time and place, and depending on whether we form our own old-age image or whether we mostly adhere to a general image of old age.

Subjective Age

Subjective conceptions of age refer to the competencies, attitudes, motives, and so forth which allegedly characterize people of a given chronological age. Population-based studies can ascertain the chronological ages at which, on average, such constellations are observed at a given historical time and in a given society. A given person will be in synchrony with, exceed, or fall below these chronological age norms. A person's subjective, perceived, or felt age is among other things a reflection of this discrepancy. It is assessed using a range of different questions such as, "How old do you feel?" or "How would you describe your age when looking into the mirror?"

Research on subjective age has been conducted since the 1950s and has consistently demonstrated across many studies that adults after age 25 years subjectively feel younger than their chronological age (e.g., Westerhof & Barrett, 2005). This negative discrepancy increases until around age 40 years and subsequently stabilizes at a level of 20% underestimation (for a Danish sample, see Rubin & Berntsen, 2006). This leveling off suggests that the discrepancy is not just simply based on a denial of chronological age or elapsed time for that matter but rather than depending on chronological age as the primary informational source, the judgment of subjective age seems to incorporate information from different behavioral sources which inform the final judgment in different ways. Sociodemographic characteristics, such as gender, income, or level of education, only explain a small proportion of the variance in subjective age. An important source is a person's perception and awareness of his or her own aging process—a domain of aging research which only recently has received the systematic attention that it deserves (cf. Diehl & Wahl, 2010). In particular, the leveling off of the underestimation effect after age 40 years supports the hypothesis that subjective age judgments are grounded in individuals' real-life experiences. In this vein, it was demonstrated in a recent study that on 50% of the assessed days, the participating older adults reported experiences relevant to the perception of their own aging (Miche et al., 2014).

Interesting questions emerge in this field of study, such as how often do we update our subjective age estimate? Or what are the triggers for such updates? Or is the updating a continuous process rather than one happening in jumps? Of course, besides these processes of self-awareness, the self-enhancement effect (Sedikides & Strube, 1995) also has to be taken into consideration, which supports the underestimation of one's age as compared to the norm.

Finally, societal value orientations, such as the degree of youth centeredness of a society, most likely influence individuals' subjective age judgments. The result of a country comparison between the Unites States and Germany supports this hypothesis. The amount of underestimation observed in subjective age ratings as compared to chronological age was more pronounced in the United States than in Germany (Westerhof & Barrett, 2005). The U.S. sample also underestimated more strongly than a Finnish and a Japanese sample (Ota, Harwood, Williams, & Takai, 2000; Uotinen, 1998). Such country differences may partially also be related to differences in the political system of the respective countries, that is, the difference between a neoliberal market orientation (United States) and a social welfare state (Finland, Germany, Japan) and their related value patterns and social security policies. This interpretation is further supported by the finding that the association between subjective age and subjective health explained part of the country differences. Health is more highly valued in the United States than in Germany (Shweder, 1998). Accordingly, U.S. participants reported higher values of subjective health than participants in Germany. This finding is interesting because if objective indicators of health are used, just the opposite is the case. For example, the average life expectancy in the United States is lower than in Germany or Japan. Finally, the self-enhancement effect is also more strongly pronounced in the United States than in the other three countries and contributed to the greater difference between chronological and subjective age in the United States (Markus & Kitayama, 1991).

The subjective age judgment is most likely related to self-perceptions of physical changes. In that vein, the historical improvement in healthy life expectancy might be reflected in an increase of the underestimation of subjective as compared to chronological age. Initial evidence to support that suggestion comes from the last three waves of the German Aging Survey in 1996, 2002, and 2008. The cohort-sequential design of the study allows to tease apart age and cohort effects, and findings show that since 1996, the difference between chronological and subjective age has slightly increased in individuals age 55 years and older (Wurm & Huxhold, 2009). It remains to be seen whether this trend continues.

Images of Old Age

Images of old age refer to the expectations about the competencies, characteristics, and physical conditions of old age. Most often, the images of old age reflect prototypical societal conceptions of this last phase in life and as such are often called *old-age stereotype*. However, the image can also concern conceptions of one's own old age(ing) and should then be called *own old-age image* or *self-perceptions of old age* to avoid confusion. Finally, there are images of how we think other people might view old age. This kind of image has been called *metastereotype of old age* (cf. Bowen, Noack, & Staudinger, 2011). These three types of old-age images are closely related. Figure 9.1 presents a working model describing the interrelations between the different types of images.

Research about the old-age stereotype has shown that even though there are several positive characteristics of old age, such as agreeableness, reliability and loyalty, or experience, the negative associations, such as lack of flexibility, loss of ability to learn, dementia, sickness, or loss of autonomy, still prevail (Gordon & Arvey, 2004; Nelson, 2002). Table 9.1 lists some of the persevering stereotypes about old age and compares them against existing research evidence. Part of the perseverance of such stereotypes is grounded in the fact that they are

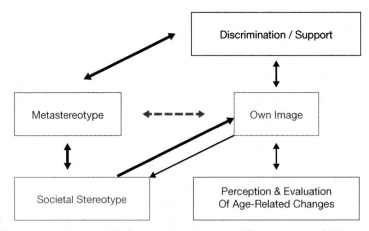

FIGURE 9.1 A working model of relationships between different images of old age.

communicated in the larger society through, for example, the mass media. For instance, a systematic study of the images of old age depicted in German TV prime time soap operas demonstrated that older adults were severely under-represented compared to other age groups and were portrayed in an one-sided fashion such that old men were either rich physicians or janitors and old women were cleaning ladies (Kessler, Rakoczy, & Staudinger, 2004).

Part of the perseverance of old-age stereotypes is also linked to the fact that we learn about old age from watching previous generations growing old. Thus, based on this source, our images of aging are doomed to lag behind one or even two generations. However, old-age stereotypes are also based on the observation of concurrent old age. This can be inferred from a finding based on data from the European Social Survey which compared data from 28 countries. Older people were indeed perceived as more competent in countries in which a greater pro-portion of older people participated in paid work or volunteer activities. This effect remained significant after controlling for country-specific life expectan-cies and educational level, as well as gender composition, and average cognitive abilities of the older population in the respective countries (Bowen & Skirbekk, 2013). Thus, even though slowly, as societal reality for old age changes, so will the old-age stereotype. In this vein, it was found in a cohort-sequential longitu-dinal study that between 1991 and 1999, the old-age stereotype became more

TABLE 9.1

*Illustration of Old-Age Stereotypes That Lag Behind the Reality of Old Age
(Based on Results of the Berlin Aging Study; Baltes et al., 1998)*

Old Age Myth	Research Evidence
Most older people feel sick.	No
Most blood parameters change with age.	No
Depression is more likely in old age.	No
Most people older than 70 years have severe cognitive constraints.	No
Older adults do have clear life goals.	Yes
Older adults primarily live in the past.	No
Most older people are not able to learn something new.	No
Most people older than 95 years live in institutions for older adults.	No

positive—in particular, when respondents older than age 70 years were considered (Rothermund & Brandtstädter, 2003).

The own old-age image seems to be more strongly influenced by the general old-age stereotype than the other way around as demonstrated in a longitudinal study (Rothermund, 2005; Rothermund & Brandtstädter, 2003; see also Figure 9.1). It is interesting to note that the own old-age image and general old-age stereotype show independent predictive relations with depressive symptoms. And there seems to be an additive effect of both images on depressive symptoms, which also implies that a rather positive general old-age image can buffer against the effect of a negative own old-age image (Rothermund, 2005).

An example for an old-age metastereotype is the old-age climate of a company; that is, how positive or negative the characteristics of older workers are perceived in a given company (cf. Noack, Bowen, & Staudinger, 2009). Of course, the older worker metastereotype is not independent of the prevailing old-age stereotype. These two concepts seem to be overlapping, but they are not synonymous (Bowen & Staudinger, 2013). Two examples may illustrate the unique qualities of the older worker metastereotype: The older worker metastereotype applies to younger age ranges than the typical old-age stereotype. Usually, employees older than 45 years are considered older workers. Second, there are major company differences implying that older worker metastereotypes are also strongly embedded in the respective company culture.

Effects of Positive and Negative Images of Old Age

Why should we even bother about images of old age? Decades of research have shown that it is more than worthwhile to reflect on one's own age. Old-age stereotypes and own old-age images strongly influence a person's self-concept as well as expectations about the person's future (e.g., Ryff, 1991; Thomae, 1970). It is this "invisible" power that makes it pivotal for "Societies of Longer Lives" (cf. Staudinger, 2012) to learn in more detail about the influences of images of old age. The more a person is convinced that aging is an inevitable process of physical decline and loss of autonomy, the less this person will believe that she or he can exert influence on his or her aging process. Convictions turn into self-fulfilling prophecies (Merton, 1948; Rosenthal & Jacobson, 1968). Thus, older adults showed less effective health behavior if they explained their physical symptoms with chronological age rather than with illness (e.g., Leventhal & Prohaska, 1986; Wurm, Warner, Ziegelmann, Wolff, & Schüz, 2013). Research on social cognition has demonstrated that the activation of negative old-age stereotypes leads to behavior matching the stereotype (assimilation affect), if the old-age category is self-relevant (e.g., Wentura & Rothermund, 2005; Wheeler & Petty, 2001). In this vein, when confronting older adults with the senility stereotype through words, such as decline, Alzheimer's disease, death, and so forth, their memory performance dropped as did their memory self-efficacy, and their attitudes toward aging became more negative (e.g., Hess, Auman, Colcombe, & Rahhal, 2003; Levy, 1996). The assimilation effect was also demonstrated regarding ideomotoric reactions (walking speed; Hausdorff, Levy, & Wei, 1999), physiological reactions (skin conductance, cardiovascular reactions to stress; see Levy, Hausdorff, Hencke, & Wei, 2000), and in terms of the will to live (Levy, 2003). These effects exist despite the fact that we feel subjectively younger than we are chronologically and despite the fact that we perceive our own aging as more positive than that of the generalized other (Heckhausen & Krueger, 1993; Montepare & Lachman, 1989; Westerhof & Barrett, 2005). Internalized negative images of old age also seem to affect performance levels and health via the stress and the anxiety they invoke (threat hypothesis; Steele & Aronson, 1995; Wurm, Tesch-Römer, & Tomasik, 2007). Stress, in turn, is linked to a worsening of the immune reaction and hence increases a person's risk for infection (Kiecolt-Glaser, McGuire, Robles, & Glaser, 2002). Most likely, it is via such mechanisms that a negative own old-age image is associated with a significant reduction in survival probability. Findings supporting this notion are maintained when controlling for socioeconomic status, objective health, and subjective well-being (Kotter-Grühn, Kleinspehn-Ammerlahn, Gerstorf, & Smith, 2009; Levy & Myers, 2004; Levy, Slade, Kunkel, & Kasl, 2002; Maier & Smith, 1999). Similarly, Wurm et al. (2007) showed that own old-age images that related aging to increased morbidity were predictive of a higher number of illnesses 6 years later. Addressing the question of the directionality of effects, findings from another study showed that the influence of old-age images on health was significantly stronger than the other way around (e.g., Spuling, Miche, Wurm, & Wahl, 2013).

The activation of a positive or negative old-age image can also play a role in the context of age-heterogeneous social interactions. When matching an older and a younger person (who do not know each other) in a situation where they are asked to discuss either a difficult life problem or a modern technology problem and to provide advice after 30 min of discussion, the activation of images of old age may play a role (Kessler & Staudinger, 2007). And indeed, it was found that the older adults who had discussed a difficult life problem with a younger person showed higher cognitive performance than the older adults who had discussed the technology problem. Consistent with the hypotheses of the study, the older persons discussing the difficult life problem felt valued by their adolescent counterpart because of their life experience which boosted their self-esteem. Accordingly, such motivational effects on cognitive age are likely to wear off after some time. It is unclear, however, whether settings that would continuously support older adults' self-esteem might yield longer lasting effects.

Aside from mortality, health, and cognitive functioning, there is also initial evidence on the effect of images of aging on job-related outcomes (Bowen et al., 2011). Through mechanisms of self-stereotyping and stereotype threat, older workers become convinced that they are less productive, more forgetful, and inflexible than they actually are. Thus, it has been demonstrated that older workers underestimate their competencies and skills. Also, older workers' self-perceptions have been found to be more similar to the negative old-age stereotype than their own actual performance (Filipp & Mayer, 1999). Furthermore, experimental evidence demonstrated that adults confronted with the fear to confirm a negative (old-age) stereotype switched from a promotion orientation, which was oriented toward success, achievement, and facilitation of performance, to an avoidance orientation, which was oriented toward avoiding failure and losses (Bowen & Staudinger, 2013; Crowe & Higgins, 1997). The regulatory focus on avoiding failure precipitates selective attention on minimizing mistakes rather than maximizing outcomes, which eventually leads to lower levels of actual performance (Hess et al., 2003; Seibt & Förster, 2004). In companies with a positive old-age climate, however, the usual age-related increase in avoidance orientation was buffered and employees reported less turnover intentions (Bowen & Staudinger, 2013).

Given what has been presented so far, the presence of a negative older worker stereotype in a company, that is, that older workers in general are less valued than younger workers, most likely has negative effects on the productivity of older workers (Bowen et al., 2011). As a result, negative relations with job satisfaction and job commitment have been ascertained (von Hippel, Kalokerinos, & Henry, 2013). Given this evidence, companies should be aware of their older worker climate.

CONCLUSION AND OUTLOOK

In summary, chronological age is often used as a convenient placeholder for many biological, psychological, and societal influences as well as their interactions which are exerted as people grow older. Chronological age has no explanatory and little informational value after young adulthood. The speed and nature of age-related processes differ greatly between people. It would therefore be much more important to know the biological, social, and psychological ages rather than the chronological age of a person. Nevertheless, modern societies heavily rely on chronological age, for instance, to determine their economic productivity in the sense of the dependency ratio. Ongoing historical changes increase the discrepancy between chronological age on the one hand and biological, cognitive, or personality age on the other hand. The same chronological age stands for better health now than 20 years ago, which entails more degrees of freedom to create new dimensions of social age yet to be implemented. These multidimensional outside perspectives on aging are complemented by a network of inside perspectives. Research has shown how powerful internalized images of old age can be. They feed back into performance and behavior which are at the basis of the outside perspectives. Future research needs to focus on furthering our understanding of the mediating mechanisms which bring about not only the historical changes of the aging process but also the mediating mechanisms linking personal, societal, and meta-images of old age.

NOTE

1. Age norms are defined as the statistical average in a given population for a certain behavior, but they can also be prescriptive in the sense that a certain behavior is expected at a given age (e.g., Hagestad, 1990).

REFERENCES

Baltes, P. B. (1987). Theoretical propositions of life-span developmental psychology: On the dynamics between growth and decline. *Developmental Psychology, 23*, 611–626. http://dx.doi.org/10.1037/0012-1649.23.5.611

Baltes, P. B., Lindenberger, U., & Staudinger, U. M. (2006). Life-span theory in developmental psychology. In W. M. Damon (Series Ed.) & R. M. Lerner (Vol. Ed.), *Handbook of child psychology: Theoretical models of development* (6th ed., Vol. 1, pp. 569–664). Hoboken, NJ: Wiley.

Baltes, P. B., Reese, H. W., & Lipsitt, L. P. (1980). Life-span developmental psychology. *Annual Review of Psychology, 31*, 65–110.

Birren, J. E., & Cunningham, W. R. (1985). Research on the psychology of aging: Principles, concepts, and theory. In J. E. Birren & K. W. Schaie (Eds.), *Handbook of the psychology of aging* (2nd ed., pp. 3–34). New York, NY: Van Nostrand Reinhold.

Bowen, C. E., Noack, C. M. G., & Staudinger, U. M. (2011). Aging in the work context. In W. Schaie & S. Willis (Eds.), *Handbook of the psychology of aging* (7th ed., pp. 263–277). San Diego, CA: Academic Press.

Bowen, C. E., & Skirbekk, V. (2013). National stereotypes of older people's competence are related to older adults' participation in paid and volunteer work. *The Journals of Gerontology. Series B, Psychological Sciences and Social Sciences, 68*, 974–983. http://dx.doi.org/10.1093/geronb/gbt101. 974983

Bowen, C. E., & Staudinger, U. M. (2013). Relationship between age and promotion orientation depends on perceived older worker stereotypes. *The Journals of Gerontology. Series B, Psychological Sciences and Social Sciences, 68*, 59–63. http://dx.doi.org/10.1093/geronb/gbs060

Christensen, K., Doblhammer, G., Rau, R., & Vaupel, J. W. (2009). Ageing populations: The challenges ahead. *Lancet, 374*, 1196–1208.

Colcombe, S., & Kramer, A. F. (2003). Fitness effects on the cognitive function of older adults: A meta-analytic study. *Psychological Science, 14*, 125–130. http://dx.doi .org/10.1111/1467-9280.t01-1-01430

Crowe, E., & Higgins, E. T. (1997). Regulatory focus and strategic inclinations: Promotion and prevention in decision-making. *Organizational Behavior and Human Decision Processes, 69*, 117–132.

Diehl, M. K., & Wahl, H. W. (2010). Awareness of age-related change: Examination of a (mostly) unexplored concept. *The Journals of Gerontology. Series B, Psychological Sciences and Social Sciences, 65*, 340–350. http://dx.doi.org/10.1093/geronb/gbp110

Durham, W. H. (1990). Advances in evolutionary culture theory. *Annual Review of Anthropology, 19*, 187–210.

Elder, G. H., Jr. (1975). Age differentiation and the life course. *Annual Review of Sociology, 1*, 165–190.

Filipp, S. H., & Mayer, A. K. (1999). *Bilder des Alters. Altersstereotype und die Beziehungen zwischen den Generationen* [Images of old age: Aging stereotypes and their connections between generations]. Stuttgart, Germany: Kohlhammer.

Flynn, J. R. (1987). Massive IQ gains in 14 nations: What IQ tests really measure. *Psychological Bulletin, 101*, 171–191. http;//dx.doi.org/10.1037/0033-2909.101.2.171

Flynn, J. (2009). Requiem for nutrition as the cause of IQ gains: Raven's gains in Britain 1938-2008. *Economics and Human Biology, 7*, 18–27. http://dx.doi.org/10.1016/ j.ehb.2009.01.009

Fraga, M. F., & Esteller, M. (2007). Epigenetics and aging: The targets and the marks. *Trends in Genetics, 23*, 413–418. http://dx.doi.org/10.1016/j.tig.2007.05.008

Gerstorf, D., Ram, N., Hoppmann, C., Willis, S. L., & Schaie, K. W. (2011). Cohort differences in cognitive aging and terminal decline in the Seattle Longitudinal Study. *Developmental Psychology, 47*, 1026–1041. http://dx.doi.org/10.1037/ a0023426

Gordon, R. A., & Arvey, R. D. (2004). Age bias in laboratory and field settings: A meta-analytic investigation. *Journal of Applied Social Psychology, 34*, 468–492. http://dx.doi.org/10.1111/j.1559-1816.2004.tb02557.x

Hausdorff, J. M., Levy, B. R., & Wei, J. Y. (1999). The power of ageism on physical function of older persons: Reversibility of age-related gait changes. *Journal of the American Geriatrics Society, 47*, 1346–1349.

Heckhausen, J. (1989). Normatives Entwicklungswissen als Bezugsrahmen zur (Re) Konstruktion der eigenen Biographie [Normative knowledge about development as frame of reference for the (re)construction of one's own biography]. In P. Alheit & E. Hoerning (Eds.), *Biographisches Wissen: Beiträge zu einer Theorie lebensgeschichtlicher Erfahrung* [Biographical knowledge: Contributions to a theory of life history experience] (pp. 202–282). Frankfurt, Germany: Campus.

Heckhausen, J., & Krueger, J. (1993). Developmental expectations for the self and most other people: Age-grading in three functions of social comparison. *Developmental Psychology, 29*, 539–548. http;//dx.doi.org/10.1037/0012-1649.29.3.539

Hertzog, C., Kramer, A. F., Wilson, R. S., & Lindenberger, U. (2009). Enrichment effects on adult cognitive development: Can the functional capacity of older adults be preserved and enhanced? *Psychological Science in the Public Interest, 9*, 1–65. http://dx.doi.org/10.1111/j.1539-6053.2009.01034.x

Hess, T. M., Auman, C., Colcombe, S., & Rahhal, T. (2003). The impact of stereotype threat on age differences in memory performance. *The Journals of Gerontology. Series B, Psychological Sciences and Social Sciences, 58*, 3–11. http://dx.doi.org/10.1093/geronb/58.1.P3

Hummert, M. L. (1990). Multiple stereotypes of elderly and young adults: A comparison of structure and evaluation. *Psychology and Aging, 5*, 182–193. http://dx.doi.org/10.1037/0882-7974.5.2.182

James, J. B., & Wink, P. (Eds.). (2006). *Annual review of gerontology and geriatrics. The crown of life: Dynamics of the early postretirement period* (Vol. 26). New York, NY: Springer Publishing.

Kessler, E. M., Rakoczy, K., & Staudinger, U. M. (2004). The portrayal of older people in prime time television series: The match with gerontological evidence. *Ageing & Society, 24*, 531–552. http://dx.doi.org/10.1017/S0144686X04002338

Kessler, E. M., & Staudinger, U. M. (2007). Intergenerational potential: Effects of social interaction between older adults and adolescents. *Psychology and Aging, 22*, 690–704. http://dx.doi.org/10.1037/0882-7974.22.4.690

Kiecolt-Glaser, J. K., McGuire, L., Robles, T. F., & Glaser, R. (2002). Emotions, morbidity, and mortality: New perspectives from psychoneuroimmunology. *Annual Review of Psychology, 53*, 83–107. http://dx.doi.org/10.1146/annurev.psych.53.100901.135217

Kohli, M. (1994). Institutionalisierung und Individualisierung der Erwerbsbiographie [Institutionalization and individualization of the professional biography]. In U. Beck & E. Beck-Gernsheim (Eds.), *Riskante Freiheiten. Individualisierung in modernen Gesellschaften* [Risky freedoms. Individualization in modern societies] (pp. 219–244). Frankfurt, Germany: Suhrkamp.

Kotter-Grühn, D., Kleinspehn-Ammerlahn, A., Gerstorf, D., & Smith, J. (2009). Self-perceptions of aging predict mortality and change with approaching death: 16-year longitudinal results from the Berlin Aging Study. *Psychology and Aging, 24*, 654–667. http://dx.doi.org/10.1037/a0016510

Leventhal, E. A., & Prohaska, T. R. (1986). Age, symptom interpretation, and health behavior. *Journal of the American Geriatrics Society, 34*, 185–191.

Levy, B. (1996). Improving memory in old age through implicit self-stereotyping. *Journal of Personality and Social Psychology, 52*, 1092–1107. http://dx.doi.org/10.1037/0022-3514.71.6.1092

Levy, B. R. (2003). Mind matters: Cognitive and physical effects of aging self-stereotypes. *The Journals of Gerontology. Series B, Psychological Sciences and Social Sciences, 58*, 203–211. http://dx.doi.org/10.1093/geronb/58.4.P203

Levy, B., Hausdorff, J., Hencke, R., & Wei, J. (2000). Reducing cardiovascular stress with positive self-stereotypes of aging. *The Journals of Gerontology. Series B,*

Psychological Sciences and Social Sciences, 55, 1–9. http://dx.doi.org/10.1093/geronb/55.4.P205

Levy, B. R., & Myers, L. M. (2004). Preventive health behaviors influenced by self-perceptions of aging. *Preventive Medicine*, 39, 625–629. http://dx.doi.org/10.1016/j.ypmed.2004.02.029

Levy, B. R., Slade, M. D., Kunkel, S. R., & Kasl, V. (2002). Longevity increased by positive self-perceptions of aging. *Journal of Personality and Social Psychology*, 83, 261–278. http://dx.doi.org/10.1037/0022-3514.83.2.261

López-Otín, C., Serrano, M., Partridge, L., Blasco, M. A., & Kroemer, G. (2013). The hallmarks of aging. *Cell*, 153, 1194–1217. http://dx.doi.org/10.1016/j.cell.2013.05.039

Maier, H., & Smith, J. (1999). Psychological predictors of mortality in old age. *The Journals of Gerontology. Series B, Psychological Sciences and Social Sciences*, 54, 44–54. http://dx.doi.org/10.1093/geronb/54B.1.P44

Markus, H., & Kitayama, S. (1991). Culture and the self: Implications for cognition, emotion, and motivation. *Psychological Review*, 98, 224–253. http://dx.doi.org/10.1037/0033-295X98.2.224

Mayer, K. U., & Müller, W. (1994). Individualisierung und Standardisierung im Strukturwandel der Moderne. Lebensverläufe im Wohlfahrtsstaat [Individualization and standardization as part of structural change during modern times. Life histories in the welfare state]. In U. Beck & E. Beck-Gernsheim (Eds.), *Riskante Freiheiten. Individualisierung in modernen Gesellschaften* [Risky freedoms: Individualization in modern societies] (pp. 265–295). Frankfurt, Germany: Suhrkamp.

McCrae, R. R., Costa, P. T., Ostendorf, F., Angleitner, A., Hrebickova, M., Avia, M. D., & Sachnez-Bernados, M. L. (2000). Nature over nurture: Temperament, personality, and life span development. *Journal of Personality and Social Psychology*, 78, 173–186. http://dx.doi.org/10.1037//O022-3514.7S.1.173

Merton, R. K. (1948). *Social theory and social structure*. New York, NY: Free Press.

Miche, M., Wahl, H. W., Diehl, M., Oswald, F., Kaspar, R., & Kolb, M. (2014). Natural occurrence of subjective aging experiences in community-dwelling older adults. *The Journals of Gerontology. Series B, Psychological Sciences and Social Sciences*, 69, 174–187. http://dx.doi.org/10.1093/geronb/gbs164

Moen, P., & Altobelli, J. (2006). Strategic selection as a retirement project: Will Americans develop hybrid arrangements? In J. B. James & P. Wink (Eds.), *Annual review of gerontology and geriatrics. The crown of life: Dynamics of the early postretirement period* (Vol. 26, pp. 61–82). New York, NY: Springer Publishing.

Montepare, J. M., & Lachman, M. E. (1989). "You're only as old as you feel": Self-perceptions of age, fears of aging, and life satisfaction from adolescence to old age. *Psychology and Aging*, 4, 73–78.

Mühlig-Versen, A., Bowen, C. E., & Staudinger, U. M. (2012). Personality plasticity in later adulthood: Contextual and personal resources are needed to increase openness to new experiences. *Psychology and Aging*, 27, 855–866. http://dx.doi.org/10.1037/a0029357

Nelson, T. D. (Ed.) (2002). Ageism. Stereotyping and prejudice against older persons. Cambridge, MA: MIT Press.

Nelson, A. E., & Dannefer, D. (1992). Aged heterogeneity: Fact or fiction? The fate of diversity in gerontological research. *The Gerontologist, 32,* 17–23. http://dx.doi .org/10.1093/geront/32.1.17

Neugarten, B. L. (1977). Personality and aging. In J. E. Birren, & K. W. Schaie (Eds.), *Handbook of the psychology of aging* (pp. 626–649). New York: Van Nostrand Reinhold.

Noack, C. M. G., Bowen, C. E., & Staudinger, U. M. (2009). *Measuring age climate in organizations (Tech. Rep.).* Bremen, Germany: Jacobs University.

Oeppen, J., & Vaupel, J. W. (2002). Broken limits to life expectancy. *Science, 296,* 1029–1031.

Oltmanns, J., Godde, B., & Staudinger, U. M. (2014). *What is the effect of work task mobility on cognitive aging?* Manuscript submitted for publication.

Ota, H., Harwood, J., Williams, A., & Takai, J. (2000). A cross-cultural analysis of age identity in Japan and the United States. *Journal of Multilingual and Multicultural Development, 21,* 33–41.

Park, D. C., & Reuter-Lorenz, P. (2009). The adaptive brain: Aging and neurocognitive scaffolding. *Annual Review of Psychology, 60,* 173–196. http://dx.doi.org/10.1146/ annurev.psych.59.103006.093656.

Reither, E. N., Olshansky, S. J., & Yang, Y. (2011). New forecasting methodology indicates more disease and earlier mortality ahead for today's younger Americans. *Health Affairs, 30,* 1562–1568. http://dx.doi.org/10.1377/hlthaff.2011.0092

Riley, M. W. (1986). Men, women, and the lengthening of the life course. In A. Rossi (Ed.), *Gender and the life course* (pp. 333–347). New York, NY: Aldine.

Robine, J. M., & Ritchie, K. (1991). Healthy life expectancy: Evaluation of global indicator of change in population health. *British Medical Journal, 302*(6774), 457–460.

Rönnlund, M., & Nilsson, L. G. (2008). The magnitude, generality, and determinants of Flynn effects on forms of declarative memory and visuospatial ability: Time-sequential analyses of data from a Swedish cohort study. *Intelligence, 36,* 192–209.

Rosenthal, R., & Jacobson, L. (1968). *Pygmalion in the classroom.* New York, NY: Holt, Rinehart & Winston.

Rothermund, K. (2005). Effects of age stereotypes on self-views and adaptation. In W. Greve, K. Rothermund, & D. Wentura (Eds.), *The adaptive self.* Göttingen, Germany: Hogrefe.

Rothermund, K., & Brandtstädter, J. (2003). Age stereotypes and self-views in later life: Evaluating rival assumptions. *International Journal of Behavioral Development, 27,* 549–554. http://dx.doi.org/10.1080/01650250344000208

Rubin, D. C., & Berntsen, D. (2006). People over forty feel 20% younger than their age: Subjective age across the life span. *Psychonomic Bulletin and Review, 13,* 776–780. http://dx.doi.org/10.3758/BF03193996

Ryff, C. D. (1991). Possible selves in adulthood and old age: A tale of shifting horizons. *Psychology and Aging, 6,* 286–295. http://dx.doi.org/10.1037/0882-7974.6.2.286

Schaie, K. W. (1996). *Adult intellectual development: The Seattle Longitudinal Study*. New York, NY: Cambridge University Press.

Sedikides, C., & Strube, M. J. (1995). "The multiply motivated self". *Personality and Social Psychology Bulletin, 21*, 1330–1335. http://dx.doi.org/10.1177/0146167295211201

Seibt, B., & Förster, J. (2004). Stereotype threat and performance: How self-stereotypes influence processing by inducing regulatory foci. *Journal of Personality and Social Psychology, 87*, 38–56.

Settersten, R. A., Jr., & Mayer, K. U. (1997). The measurement of age, age structuring, and the life course. *Annual Review of Sociology, 23*, 233–261.

Shweder, R. A. (Ed.). (1998). *Welcome to the middle age! (And other cultural fictions)*. Chicago, IL: University of Chicago Press.

Skirbekk, V., Loichinger, E., & Weber, D. (2012). Variation in cognitive functioning as a refined approach to comparing aging across countries. *Proceedings of the National Academy of Sciences, 109*(3), 770–774. http://dx.doi.org/10.1073/pnas.1112173109

Skirbekk, V., Stonawski, M., Bonsang, E., & Staudinger, U. M. (2013). The Flynn effect and population aging. *Intelligence, 41*, 169–177. http://dx.doi.org/10.1016/j.intell.2013.02.001

Spuling, S. M., Miche, M., Wurm, S., & Wahl, H. W. (2013). Exploring the causal interplay of subjective age and health dimensions in the second half of life: A cross-lagged panel analysis. *Zeitschrift für Gesundheitspsychologie, 21*, 5–15.

Staudinger, U. M. (2005). Personality and aging. In M. Johnson, V. L. Bengtson, P. G. Coleman, & T. Kirkwood (Eds.), *Cambridge handbook of age and ageing* (pp. 237–244). Cambridge, United Kingdom: Cambridge University Press.

Staudinger, U. M. (2012). Möglichkeiten und Grenzen menschlicher Entwicklungen über die Lebensspanne [Potentials and limitations of human development across the lifespan]. In J. Hacker & M. Hecker (Eds.), *Was ist Leben?* [What is life?] (Nova Acta Leopoldina, Bd. 115, Nr. 394, pp. 255–266). Stuttgart, Germany: Wissenschaftliche Verlagsgesellschaft.

Staudinger, U. M., & Kocka, J. (Eds.). (2010). *More years, more life. Recommendations of the Joint Academy Initiative on Aging (Translation of "Gewonnene Jahre"; Aging in Germany Bd. 9)*. Stuttgart, Germany: Wissenschaftliche Verlagsgesellschaft Nova Acta Leopoldina N. F. Bd. 108, Nr. 372.

Staudinger, U. M., Marsiske, M., & Baltes, P. B. (1995). Resilience and reserve capacity in later adulthood: Potentials and limits of development across the life span. In D. Cicchetti & D. Cohen (Eds.), *Developmental psychopathology: Risk, disorder, and adaptation* (Vol. 2, pp. 801–847). New York, NY: Wiley

Steele, C. M., & Aronson, J. (1995). Stereotype threat and the intellectual test performance of African Americans. *Journal of Personality and Social Psychology, 69*, 797–811. http://dx.doi.org/10.1037/0022-3514.69.5.797

Stine-Morrow, E. A. L., Parisi, J. M., Morrow, D. G., & Park, D. C. (2008). The effects of an engaged lifestyle on cognitive vitality: A field experiment. *Psychology and Aging, 23*, 778–786. http://dx.doi.org/10.1037/a0014341

Te Velde, E. R., & Pearson, P. L. (2002). The variability of female reproductive ageing. *Human Reproduction Update, 8*, 141–154.

Thomae, H. (1970). Theory of aging and cognitive theory of personality. *Human Development, 12,* 1–16.

Uotinen, V. (1998). Age identification: A comparison between Finnish and North-American cultures. *International Journal of Aging and Human Development, 46,* 109–124.

Vaupel, J. W. (2010). Biodemography of human ageing. *Nature, 464,* 536–542.

Voelcker-Rehage, C., Godde, B., & Staudinger, U. M. (2011). Cardiovascular and coordination training differentially improve cognitive performance and neural processing in older adults. *Frontiers in Human Neuroscience, 5,* 1–12. http://dx.doi .org/10.3389/fnhum.2011.00026

Von Hippel, C., Kalokerinos, E. K., & Henry, J. D. (2013). Stereotype threat among older employees: Relationship with job attitudes and turnover intentions. *Psychology and Aging, 28,* 17–27. http://dx.doi.org/10.1037/a0029825

Wentura, D., & Rothermund, K. (2005). Alterssterotype und Altersbilder [Aging stereotypes and images of aging]. In S. H. Fillip & U. M. Staudinger (Eds.), *Entwicklungspsychologie des mittleren und höheren Erwachsenenalters* [Developmental psychology of middle and late adulthood] (pp. 616–654). Göttingen, Germany: Horgrefe.

Westerhof, G. J., & Barrett, A. E. (2005). Age identity and subjective well-being: A comparison of the United States and Germany. *The Journals of Gerontology. Series B, Psychological Sciences and Social Sciences, 60,* S129–S136. http;//dx.doi.org/10.1093/geronb/60.3.S129

Wheeler, S. C., & Petty, R. E. (2001). The effects of stereotype activation on behavior: A review of possible mechanisms. *Psychological Bulletin, 127,* 797–826. http://dx.doi.org/10.1037/0033-2909.127.6.797

Wink, P., & James, J. (2013). The life course perspective on life in the post-retirement period. In M. Wang (Eds.), *The Oxford handbook of retirement* (pp. 59–72). New York: Oxford University Press.

Wurm, S., & Huxhold, O. (2009). Sozialer Wandel und individuelle Entwicklung von Altersbildern [Social change and the individual development of images of aging]. *Expertise für den 6. Altenbericht auf der Gundlage der dritten Welle des Deutschen Alterssurveys.* Berlin, Germany: Deutsches Zentrum für Altersfragen.

Wurm, S., Tesch-Römer, C., & Tomasik, M. J. (2007). Longitudinal findings on aging-related cognitions, control beliefs, and health in later life. *The Journals of Gerontology. Series B, Psychological Sciences and Social Sciences, 62,* P156–P164.

Wurm, S., Warner, L. M., Ziegelmann, J. P., Wolff, J. K., & Schüz, B. (2013). How do negative self-perceptions of aging become a self-fulfilling prophecy? *Psychology and Aging, 28,* 1088–1097. http://dx.doi.org/10.1037/a0032845

CHAPTER 10

The Role of Subjective Aging Within the Changing Ecologies of Aging

Perspectives for Research and Practice

Martina Miche, Allyson Brothers, Manfred Diehl, and Hans-Werner Wahl

ABSTRACT

The negative conceptualization of aging pervades most societies and can be seen implicitly and explicitly across many levels and contexts of society. However, there is substantial theoretical and empirical evidence to argue that a more realistic and constructive view of aging acknowledges both positive and negative changes as people grow old. In this chapter, we explore possible implications of the negative conceptualizations of aging at different bioecological levels. Then, in light of a growing body of evidence suggesting that negative views on aging have harmful effects for individuals and societies, we discuss challenges and potentials for transforming such views at the different bioecological levels to a more accurate representation of older age. Finally, we present a life-span oriented framework, which illustrates several potential avenues for research and practice at different bioecological levels, considering all points along the developmental chronosystem.

INTRODUCTION

Given the body of research on subjective aging compiled in this volume, we use this chapter to reflect on the many applications that can be made to gerontological practice and the possible implications for newly emerging views on the process of aging in the 21st century. Translating the scientific findings on subjective aging—which consistently demonstrate important influences of attitudinal variables on the aging process—is a particularly appropriate and timely task in light of the changing demographic dynamics on a regional and global level. Although the idealized dream of living forever captures our imagination in popular fiction, such a goal may not be so rosy unless we see drastic shifts in our individual and cultural treatment of older adults. As the proportion of old and very old adults rises throughout the coming decades, focused approaches to improving various aspects of the aging experience will become essential. We ask in this work what subjective aging research may have to contribute to the fundamental reasoning related to the future aging of individuals and societies. Furthermore, might the subjective aging research contribute to the emergence of a proactive culture of aging as a productive element of individual and societal development to come? The overarching term *subjective aging* will be used to refer to the ways in which aging is interpreted and constructed by society and by individuals. Constructs subsumed by the overarching term subjective aging include subjective age (how old a person feels), expectations regarding aging (ERA), age stereotypes, and self-perceptions of aging, all of which are delineated in further detail by Diehl et al. (2014).

As an organizing scheme for the chapter, we draw elements from the bioecological framework (Bronfenbrenner, 1994) because we consider this framework useful for addressing several pertinent issues. According to Bronfenbrenner (1994), ecologies are inherently biopsychosocial interactive systems and are seen as major developmental forces. Within the bioecological framework, four levels of analysis, that is, micro-, meso-, exo-, and macrosystems are differentiated. Subjective aging at the *microsystem level* is composed of an individual's interactions within an environment (e.g., the workplace, the health care system). The self-directed attitudes about aging held by an individual, including how satisfied the person is with his or her own aging process, the awareness of becoming older, and the age with which the person identifies are shaped by ongoing interactions (called proximal processes) of the aging individual with the immediate environment. Therefore, the content and structure of microsystems may foster or inhibit positive views on aging at the individual level. At the *mesosystem level*, subjective aging is negotiated through interactions between two or more microsystems. Encounters between the staff and family members of a resident at a long-term care facility, for example, might have strong influence on subjectively perceived opportunities and developmental constraints of an older person, which in turn affect his or her views of the aging process. The *exosystem* captures the indirect influence and interaction of two or more remote settings, at least one of which that does not directly involve the individual. With specific regard to subjective aging, the exosystem might refer to the influences of a physician's medical training on the individual or the influence of a family caregiver's connection (or lack of connection) to local caregiving resources and information on an aging parent. Subjective aging at the *macrosystem level* reflects those patterns made up by the micro-, meso-, and exosystems. The macrosystem encompasses the broad age stereotypes and values assigned to "being old," which are unconsciously adopted and widely held by members of a particular culture (sociocultural perspective on age stereotypes; Hummert, 2011), and also includes cultural structures and social policies. Such stereotypes and values about aging are apparent within the broader culture. Throughout this chapter, we will focus mainly on processes at the micro- and macrosystems because we assume that these are particularly critical from an intervention and practical perspective related to subjective aging. However, elements anchored in mesosystems and exosystems will also be mentioned throughout.

Of course, research and theory indicate that individual and societal views on aging are interdependent, and this interdependence fits perfectly with Bronfenbrenner's (1994) model that all ecological levels deserve consideration in understanding human development. For example, according to Levy's (2009) stereotype embodiment theory, age stereotypes become increasingly self-salient with age and, in turn, are directed inward and incorporated into a person's own self-directed age stereotypes. Therefore, although we consider subjective aging at different ecological levels, the dynamic interplay among all levels is an underlying assumption. In addition, Bronfenbrenner added the concept of a *chronosystem* to his original model. The term "chronosystem" refers to a time component indicating that the micro-, meso-, exo-, and macrosystems and their interactions are constantly changing. Changing views on aging and indeed of the concept of "old age" may be an important element of future ecologies in which older adults operate and develop.

Across all bioecological levels, negative views on aging represent a potential risk factor for individual development, whereas positive views on aging can be seen as a resource for successful aging. The next logical question to ask is whether views on aging can be made more positive (both on the societal level and on the level of the individual) and, if so, whether changing them in a targeted way does in fact result in tangible developmental outcomes, such as improved mental and physical health or more "aging-friendly" environments.

In this context, the thought-provoking sociological work by Matilda White Riley and John W. Riley (1994) emphasizes a societal problem that requires attention: the structural lag. The term "structural lag" (Riley & Riley, 1994) refers to the inability of society to keep up with rapid biological and life span changes that have emerged during the past century of a drastically extended human life span that includes more healthy years than ever. The lag comes into play when considering that the additional years that many individuals experience are not necessarily matched by opportunities to engage in meaningful and productive work that is recognized or valued by society (Riley & Riley, 1994). Therefore, we can conclude that what we know is possible for older adults is often not expected or encouraged by the larger society or those who interact with older adults (e.g., health care professionals). This failure to capitalize on the capabilities and desires of older adults can be interpreted as a missed opportunity on several levels—economic, productive, familial, and emotional.

To this end, we use the following sections to consider the role of subjective aging from different ecological levels. Such a conceptualization proves useful because subjective aging variables, such as age stereotypes and self-perceptions of aging, are held, influenced, and perpetuated by individuals, interactions between individuals, and by societies. The first sections of this chapter will focus on the micro- and macrolevels of developmental ecologies, exploring the ways in which views on aging are present in different life contexts. We then turn to the question of how views on aging may become subject to change both at micro- and macroecologies. Based on these considerations, we develop a life-span oriented intervention model of subjective aging, which we would like to propose for future research and practice. We close with a discussion of some of the persisting fundamental ethical issues.

RELEVANCE OF SUBJECTIVE AGING ISSUES WITHIN MICROSYSTEMS

Clearly, subjective aging is relevant across many life contexts, such as within the family, the living environment, and so on. In this section, we concentrate on two key ecologies for aging societies to illustrate this point: the work environment and the health care system. Given that Bronfenbrenner (1994) specified that proximal processes within microsystems depend on characteristics of both the person and the environment, we organize these sections accordingly. First, we explore the role of views on aging regarding person characteristics of the aging individual (i.e., the employee, the health care recipient) and then go on to explore the relevant environment characteristics, namely those people who interact with the aging individual (i.e., the employer and workplace culture; the health care provider and health care system).

The Workplace

Person Characteristics

Self-directed views on aging held by older workers exert influence on workplace factors, such as opportunities for workplace engagement, and decisions about retirement. For example, self-directed negative self-perceptions of aging are likely to discourage older workers from seeking out opportunities for growth, interfere with performance, and result in lowered expectations for their own job-related performance (Hedge, Borman, & Lammlein, 2006). In addition, a study of European employees aged 50–59 years found that individuals who identified more strongly as an "older worker" were more likely to want to retire as soon as possible, compared to those who did not hold a strong age-group identity (Desmette & Gaillard, 2008). Not only do views on aging affect workplace successes, but there is also evidence for a bidirectional relationship in which workplace experiences naturally influence how individuals perceive their own aging process. A German study showed that individuals who were not employed (e.g., retired, unemployed, or housewife) in the preretirement years (ages 45–57 years) had poorer perceptions of their own aging process, as well as a lower sense of productivity and responsibility, compared to same-age peers who were employed. This finding held even after controlling for sociodemographic and health variables (Schmitt, 2001). A primary implication from this study is that productive engagement in the workforce can be seen as an important contributor to a more positive subjective experience of aging, at least in the 40s and 50s.

Environment Characteristics

Negative evaluations of older adults are perhaps more common in the workplace than in any other context, perhaps because the workplace emphasizes standards of performance and productivity, and it is often assumed that these standards cannot be met by older workers. It is important to keep in mind that the age at which a person is deemed to be "old" is younger in the work domain than in other domains of life, given that age 65 years is typically the upper limit for employee age. In contrast, other domains of life, such as leisure or family may be evaluated with a different reference point because the upper age limit would be around 100 years old or higher, in line with what is possible regarding human longevity. However, there is a stark contrast between stereotypes of older workers and empirical evidence regarding workers' performance and reliability. Contrary to stereotypical beliefs, work performance does not systematically decline with age and may even improve in some areas (Ng & Feldman, 2008). For example, older adults tend to prioritize accuracy in their tasks (Czaja, 2001) and are able to compensate for age-related declines in speed with their accumulated expertise (Salthouse, 1984). Furthermore, age differences in speed and amount of work completed may be explained by declines in visuomotor and memory performance rather than age per se (Czaja & Sharit, 1998). Despite widespread stereotypes of older workers, evidence suggests that the age group of 55- to 64-year-olds exhibit substantially less turnover (Adler & Hilber, 2009), engage in fewer counterproductive work behaviors such as aggression and substance abuse, and miss fewer days of work (Ng & Feldman, 2008) compared to workers of other ages.

Nonetheless, a long list of stereotypes are directed at older workers, an ambiguous term applied to employees sometimes as young as age 35 years but more commonly to those older than age 50 years (Hedge et al., 2006). This subset of employees is commonly thought to be resistant to change, inflexible, and uninterested or unable to learn new technologies (Hedge et al., 2006). Consistent with the stereotype content model (Cuddy, Norton, & Fiske, 2005), lower perceptions of competence but higher ratings of warmth are commonly found toward older adults (Hummert, 2011) and toward older employees specifically (Krings, Sczesny, & Kluge, 2011). Although "warm" attributes of an older employee's character seem harmless on the surface, they can nonetheless be detrimental because they are associated with less favorable perceptions by hiring personnel and work colleagues (Krings et al., 2011), and higher ratings of warmth for older adults are often accompanied by lower ratings of competence (Cuddy et al., 2005). To summarize the long tradition of research on stereotypes about older adult workers, the presence of overgeneralized, simplified beliefs about older employees simply based on their apparent age is pervasive and poses detrimental consequences for today's and tomorrow's aging workforce, including discrimination, loss of historical company knowledge, and missed opportunities for productivity.

Attitudes toward older workers at the level of the workplace culture play an important role in the experience of work and retirement. The importance of colleagues' attitudes toward older workers is also evident in a recent study of German employees aged 19–64 years who were surveyed about how employees older than age 45 years were regarded by other members of their work team (Bowen & Staudinger, 2013). Although in general, higher age was associated with a decrease in the desire to seek out successes and opportunities for promotion and growth ("promotion orientation"), this association was not evident among employees who sensed that their own team members held positive views of older workers. These findings suggest that a work environment in which older adults are held in high esteem can have protective effects for older workers and can keep them engaged in seeking out new opportunities (Bowen & Staudinger, 2013).

The Health Care System

Person Characteristics

Given that older age is oftentimes equated with poorer health (Ory, Hoffman, Hawkins, Sanner, & Mockenhaupt, 2003), individuals' experiences of health declines and physical functioning are likely to influence their subjective aging experiences. Generally speaking, poorer physical health tends to be associated with feeling older than one's chronological age (Hubley & Russell, 2009). The relationship between more negative subjective aging and poorer physical health is also apparent regarding various specific health conditions. For instance, negative subjective aging experiences are predictive of cardiovascular disease, including heightened physiological stress response, poorer recovery from heart attack, and higher likelihood of experiencing a cardiac event (Levy et al., 2008; Levy, Slade, May, & Caracciolo, 2006; Levy, Zonderman, Slade, & Ferrucci, 2009). More negative subjective aging is also associated with impaired sensory functioning, such as hearing impairment (Levy, Slade, & Gill, 2006). These few selected examples illustrate the persistent themes in the literature in which views on aging and physical health are interrelated across many different conditions and types of situations (see Levy, 2009, for a more extensive review).

Positive views on aging appear to be important for preserving physical function in later life, above and beyond a host of other demographic and health-related variables (Sargent-Cox, Anstey, & Luszcz, 2012). There are many ways in which subjective aging influences physical health, and one important proposed mechanism involves the role of health-promoting behaviors. For example, positive views on aging are associated with the active promotion of one's own health for behaviors such as physical activity, regular physical examinations, eating a balanced diet, and adherence to medication regimes (Levy & Myers, 2004; Wurm, Tomasik, & Tesch-Römer, 2010). Similarly, negative expectations related to aging are associated with a more sedentary lifestyle (Sarkisian, Prohaska, Wong, Hirsch, & Mangione, 2005).

In addition to physical health, subjective aging also has important associations with mental health (Kessler, Kruse, & Wahl, in press), and the relationship appears to be bidirectional. More positive views on aging are thought to serve as protective factors for adverse outcomes. For example, one study found that individuals who felt younger than their chronological age (e.g., had a lower subjective age) were less likely to experience a major depressive episode and also more likely to exhibit signs of flourishing mental health (Keyes & Westerhof, 2012). From the opposite direction, evidence suggests that symptoms of depression predict poorer self-perceptions of aging, even if the depressive symptoms are at a very mild, subclinical level (Chachamovich, Fleck, Laidlaw, & Power, 2008).

Environment Characteristics

Health care providers' views on aging have been shown to influence the quality and amount of care which is provided to older adults. For example, providers' negative attitudes toward older adults have been linked to poorer quality of patient–physician communication, decreased provision of medical information and counseling, failure to recommend certain medical procedures, and limited access to participation in clinical trials, which significantly limits the evidence available for many drugs regularly prescribed to older adults (for more detailed reviews, see Golub & Langer, 2007; Meisner, 2012; Robb, Chen, & Haley, 2002). Because older adults use health care services more than any other age group (U.S. Census Bureau, 2012), their providers' attitudes have a greater likelihood of shaping the ways in which they view their own aging process.

Although evidence of ageist beliefs among health care professionals has been documented for many decades (Golub & Langer, 2007), a recent systematic review (Meisner, 2012) suggests a more complex picture. For example, recent research showed that family care providers' ERA were, on average, more positive than those held by nonphysicians; however, this happened in a rather unrealistic manner (Davis, Bond, Howard, & Sarkisian, 2011). Specifically, more than 70% of providers reported believing that as people grow older, they do *not* need to adjust their expectations regarding physical health. The authors note that this unrealistically positive view of aging is not helpful for patients and may even lead to a process of blaming older individuals for their declines in physical health. On the other hand, a small but not negligible 15% of the surveyed family care providers agreed with the statement that depression is a normal part of aging—a finding that contradicts a large body of literature and that creates unnecessary barriers to mental health treatment for older adults (Davis et al., 2011).

Of course, providers' attitudes toward older adults depend on a myriad of contextual factors. Certain behaviors of the patient such as noncompliance or symptoms of depression were associated with more negative provider attitudes for older patients but not for younger patients (Rybarczyk, Haut, Lacey, Fogg, & Nicholas, 2001). Providers' experiences of *personal* relationships with older adults as well as *professional* experience in treating older adults both seem to be important facets for fostering more positive views on aging (Meisner, 2012). Theoretical reasoning suggests that health care providers specializing in geriatric practice have a somewhat disproportionate exposure to older adults who are in poorer health, which may contribute to more negative attitudes toward older adults in general (Kearney, Miller, Paul, & Smith, 2000), but more gerontological cal *education* is associated with more positive views toward older adults among nurses (Liu, Norman, & While, 2013). These findings emphasize the importance of helping professionals in gerontological practice to counteract their tendency to associate being older with being frail and in poor health.

There are obvious perils of basing decisions about medical care solely on a patient's *chronological* age because of the large degree of heterogeneity that characterizes individuals in the later part of the life span. As Pasupathi and Löckenhoff (2002) explained, "Older adults tend to be more different from one another than are younger adults, making age in later life a poor indicator of an individual's competence or functional ability" (p. 204). Heterogeneity in older ages holds for almost every aspect of functioning, including physical health, sensory functioning, independence, language skills, and social and emotional development. In each of these behavioral domains, older adults show the highest percentage of impairment compared to other age groups; however, still most older adults show little or no impairment in many of these behavioral domains (Pasupathi & Löckenhoff, 2002). So which patients do health care providers then perceive as being old? When making judgments about whether or not a patient is old, physicians and nurses report using both objective (chronological age, functional status) as well as subjective factors (such as disengagement from the world, loss of interest in living, unproductivity, and inflexibility; Fineman, 1994). Interestingly, when asked to talk about the criteria used for perceiving someone as old, physician and nurse participants listed only characteristics with a negative valence, such as being frail, being dependent, not being able to adapt, not being interested in living, and not wanting to be physically active (Fineman, 1994). On the other hand, it is likely that health care providers sometimes do revert to using chronological age as the sole basis when providing care. In fact, most adults older than age 50 years in one study reported that a health care provider had assumed an ailment was because of the patient's age (Palmore, 2004).

Ageism within the health care system is considered to be a primary mechanism by which negative age stereotypes increase older adults' "psychological vulnerability to ill health" (Golub & Langer, 2007, p. 13). Although some have described explicit prejudice and discrimination within the health care system, "characterized by negativism, defeatism, and professional antipathy regarding the provision of care to older patients" (Meisner, 2012, p. 67), implicit prejudice and discrimination are also present and perhaps even more prevalent. For example, there is generally a low degree of interest among medical students to specialize in geriatrics or internal medicine, those specialties that treat the largest numbers of older adults. Moreover, this lack of interest may even be perpetuated during the medical training years (Hauer et al., 2008). Furthermore, medical training among family practitioners may be lacking in gerontological content because physician residents exhibit difficulties in distinguishing signs of normal aging from signs of disease (Beall, Baumhover, Maxwell, & Pieroni, 1996). Discrimination is also apparent regarding the reluctance of many providers to accept older adults into their medical practice (Adams et al., 2002) and by a general perception among nurses that caring for older adults in the hospital is a burden (Liu et al., 2013). One point of caution to consider is that negative attitudes of providers toward the *health care system* itself may have an equally or perhaps even stronger influence on the care which is provided to older adults (Meisner, 2012). For example, in the United States, the most common health care plan for older adults is Medicare, which pays a substantially lower reimbursement rate to providers compared to private insurance companies and also requires more extensive paperwork from physicians' offices (Adams et al., 2002). Therefore, considering the financial and time ramifications, it is common practice for a provider or group of providers to limit the percentage of patients they accept who are covered by Medicare, which directly affects the number of accepted older adult patients. However, despite the presence of negative perceptions toward older adults within the health care system, it is interesting to note that geriatric internist physicians report higher job satisfaction than physicians in other specialties (Leigh, Kravitz, Schembri, Samuels, & Mobley, 2002). This finding might be important to capitalize on to encourage more medical students to consider a career in geriatrics.

Summary

Although a largely negative perception of aging is pervasive across many life contexts, including the workforce and the health care system, this "deficit model of aging" is an outdated and inaccurate organizing principle for the contexts within which older adults live their daily lives. Certainly, failing to recognize individuals' potential for growth and gains in various life contexts even in later life is troublesome and is one reason that negative stereotypes about aging are perpetuated.

RELEVANCE OF SUBJECTIVE AGING ISSUES WITHIN MACROSYSTEMS

As discussed at the outset of this chapter, individual views on aging are not only shaped through social interactions at the microsystem level but also at the macrolevel of ecologies. The aim of this section is to disentangle potential consequences of current trends at the macrolevel, that is, the level of the society and its interaction with views on aging at the microsystem level.

Current Societal Structures of Aging

The demographic change which developed countries have been facing over the past century (Christensen, Doblhammer, Rau, & Vaupel, 2009) has major consequences for subjective aging. For example, the third age (Baltes & Smith, 1999; James & Wink, 2006) represents a historically new life stage with its own characteristics. That is, people have retired from their primary profession and career but do not feel old at all and indeed start new life projects in areas such as partnership, intergenerational engagement, volunteering, housing, or leisure (James & Wink, 2006). At the same time, the age group of people aged 85 years and older, frequently referred to as the fourth age (Baltes & Smith, 1999), has been the fastest growing demographic segment in the developed countries. Although this life stage has been characterized as vulnerable and represents a period with a high risk of multiple losses, there is also now evidence for a postponement of disabilities among very old individuals of more recent cohorts (Christensen et al., 2009). To summarize these changing societal structures of aging, historically speaking, the phenomenon of an extended human life span as a result of ongoing biological and cultural evolution is a rather recent phenomenon, and hence, "old age is young" (Baltes, 1997, p. 367). Consequently, countries faced with an aging society seem to still be in search of new and adequate images of aging.

Indications of Changing Images of Aging

In contrast to older cohorts, who were among the first to experience longevity without having "role models" from previous generations, current generations of young-old adults were the first to realize what it means to live until advanced old age and to plan and prepare for a new life stage of old age. As a consequence of restructured life courses, changing opportunity structures, and major advances in the medical sciences and technology, current generations of older adults might have developed a different understanding of the adult years and old age, including the recognition that old age is characterized not only by losses but also by its own potentials and opportunities. Preliminary evidence for this assumption comes from the German Aging Survey. Cohort comparisons between three subsequent measurement waves reveal that self-perceptions of aging became more positive over time. Across age groups, aging was viewed more in terms of ongoing development and less as a process of physical decline in 2002 as compared to 1996. Data from 2008 indicate a stabilizing trend of this development (Wurm & Huxhold, 2010). Furthermore, comparisons of studies from different historical times indicate a shift in people's perceptions of appropriate age norms for certain social roles (Hagestad & Neugarten, 1985). Overall, however, empirical research on historical changes in subjective aging remains scarce.

At the same time, there is increasing public awareness of the difficulties that go along with longer life expectancies (e.g., increasing number of individuals with dementia, increasing need for long-term care). Such societal views of aging that focus on the problems of the fourth age and picture old age as a life phase in which morbidity and frailty prevail might likewise have implications for subjective aging. First, vulnerabilities of the fourth age are very much driven by biology and neurophysiology and, hence, confront individuals with the limits of the human condition. Therefore, mastery and perceived competence might gain importance for preserving positive perceptions of aging in advanced old age (Infurna, Gerstorf, Robertson, Berg, & Zarit, 2010). Second, age-related losses of the fourth age are highly undesirable, and more frequent encounters with the problems of the fourth age in an aging society might fuel aging anxiety or disease-specific concerns, such as dementia worries (Kessler, Bowen, Baer, Froelich, & Wahl, 2012). Concerns or even fears about one's own aging process might, in turn, increase attention for the experience of age-related loss (Diehl & Wahl, 2010). At the same time, individuals will strive to delay or avoid the period of old-old age as long as possible. Such notions of individual responsibility for health and successful aging are being emphasized in public discourse (Galvin, 2002), albeit some intercultural differences concerning individual versus public/governmental responsibility for health care do exist (Westerhof & Barrett, 2005). The effect of individual factors on healthy aging should not be underestimated, and the subjective perception of taking and being in control of one's health might counteract aging anxiety (Pond, Stephens, & Alpass, 2010). However, there are also drawbacks to this moral imperative. That is, if health status is out of individual control (e.g., because of genetic makeup or socioeconomic resources), poor health might be interpreted as a sign of individual failure, resulting in feelings of guilt and anxiety (Pond et al., 2010) with potentially negative consequences for self-perceptions of aging. The close association between socioeconomic position and health might thus predispose individuals from lower socioeconomic positions to have more negative aging attitudes and self-perceptions of aging (Barrett, 2003). Overall, it should be acknowledged in public discourse that a person's health results from the interplay of social, environmental, and individual factors. But the question remains how individuals can be motivated and empowered to exploit their full scope of individual influence, in a way that taking responsibility and ownership for one's own health and aging fosters individual feelings of control.

Persisting Societal Age Norms and Subjective Aging

Another way in which society might impact subjective aging is in terms of the formal and informal age norms related to the timing and sequencing of certain life events, such as obligatory retirement age or eligibility age for Social Security benefits. Such formal and informal age norms, although standing in stark contrast to the desires and ways of living of today's older adults, persist in modern society and exhibit considerable staying power (Riley, Kahn, & Foner, 1994). The case of transitions into retirement may serve as an illustrative example of how age norms and societal constraints govern individual lives (Moen, Fields, Meador, & Rosenblatt, 2000). Today's changing nature of retirement (e.g., retirees being younger, healthier, and spending more years in retirement) results in the construction of a new life phase, with effective social opportunities and roles for this population still needing to be defined (Moen et al., 2000). Furthermore, nationally held attitudes and norms are important for shaping how older workers are perceived. In a study including data from 28 countries, older adults were perceived as more competent in countries that have a greater number of opportunities for paid and volunteer work, (e.g., Netherlands, Norway) even after taking into account variables such as gender, education, and country-specific life expectancy (Bowen & Skirbekk, 2013). Greater flexibility instead of a rigid age patterning of the life course would thus not only be beneficial for maximizing individual choice and opportunities but could also have tremendous implications for subjective aging. Formal and informal age norms are often intended to protect society or the older person from harm caused by declining abilities and diminishing opportunities. These norms often overgeneralize age-related decline and are therefore inconsistent with the increasing number of healthy and longer living older adults. A lack of differentiation between individuals in the third and the fourth age, as implied by in the application of negative age stereotypes and frailty perceptions to both middle-old and old-old individuals (Hummert, 1993), might be one cause for the persistence of such a structural lag. This structural lag between the need and competencies of an individual and the opportunities provided by society (Riley et al., 1994) might reinforce loss-oriented experiences of aging and, in turn, limit access to meaningful roles which could provide individuals with the opportunity to have experiences of mastery and competence.

Summary

Societal transitions, including demographic changes, necessitate a shift in views on aging. With increasing numbers of individuals growing old in a relatively healthy way and with many resources preserved up until old age, views on aging might become more positive or at least more differentiated. Yet other trends observable at the macrolevel, such as an increasing visibility of the vulnerabilities of the fourth age, represent a threat to positive self-perceptions of aging that incorporate notions of individual responsibility.

MAKING USE OF THE PLASTICITY OF SUBJECTIVE AGING: INTERVENTIONS NEEDED AT THE MICRO- AND MACROLEVEL OF ECOLOGIES

Given the linkages between subjective aging and psychophysical functioning and the influence of micro- and macrolevel factors on subjective aging discussed earlier, sufficient justification exists for designing and evaluating interventions targeted at improving individual views on aging. In this section, we will discuss certain challenges which exist at each of the bioecological levels and also explore some possible approaches.

Changing Views on Aging Within Microsystems: Challenges and Approaches

Tailoring Interventions to the Population

One challenge for the development of interventions at the microsystem level rests on the question of who should be the ideal recipient of such an intervention. Given the abundance of negative, unidimensional, and inaccurate stereotypes of aging that persist in daily life, many people of all ages hold negative views on aging, but certain subgroups of individuals are even more susceptible than others to developing such views. For instance, research findings point to several variables that are associated with more negative evaluations of one's own aging process, such as higher tendencies toward neuroticism (Moor, Zimprich, Schmitt, & Kliegel, 2006), living in socioeconomically disadvantaged conditions (Barrett, 2003), a higher number of television viewing hours (Donlon, Ashman, & Levy, 2005), and a family history of Alzheimer's disease (Suhr & Kinkela, 2007). In addition, health care professionals who work with the sickest older adults are limited in the opportunities they might have to interact with healthy older adults and are therefore at risk of developing more negative views on aging (Meisner, 2012). One approach to intervention design would be to focus on subgroups with the highest risk of holding negative views on aging, whereas another approach would be to target the general public. Another approach would be to design interventions targeting professionals who work with older adults, especially given the pervasive culture of negative stereotypes in the medical community in particular (Samra, Griffiths, Cox, Conroy, & Knight, 2013). Whether promoting attitude change at an individual or professional level, the targeted recipients should be considered carefully in intervention design to maximally combat inaccurate age stereotypes.

Designing Effective Intervention Components

A second challenge of changing views on aging is that little evidence is available regarding the best strategies for how such change can be achieved in a reliable way. The task of changing attitudes toward aging, which have been developed over the course of many years and have been reinforced in many ways, requires a nuanced program design. For instance, a program for older adults that includes activities in which participants are supported in successful completion of a meaningful task may help reinforce feelings of competence and control, thereby resulting in improved views on aging. One effective example of this is an exercise intervention for older women that resulted in improved views on aging (Klusmann, Evers, Schwarzer, & Heuser, 2012). Regarding health care professionals, evidence from a systematic review found that providing education to medical students and physicians was important but not sufficient alone to result in attitudinal change toward older patients (Samra et al., 2013). Instead, interventions that included experiential components, such as simulations and activities designed to promote empathy, were more successful in subsequent attitude change of the participating medical professionals (Samra et al., 2013). Advanced methodological approaches within prevention science, such as the Multiphase Optimization Strategy (MOST), may be useful for determining which intervention components offer the greatest potential benefit to participants (Collins et al., 2011; Dziak, Nahum-Shani, & Collins, 2012).

Contributions of Subjective Aging Research

Subjective aging research provides useful insights for developing interventions within microsystem ecologies to promote more positive outcomes related to health and well-being. In particular, theory and research have begun to shed light on potential mechanisms by which subjective aging influences physical health outcomes, and these mechanisms are prime targets for intervention work. Stereotype embodiment theory highlights three particular pathways: psychological, behavioral, and physiological (Levy, 2009). Empirical research has begun to examine psychological links between subjective aging and health. For instance, self-regulation strategies (e.g., selection, optimization, and compensation) appear to be important, particularly among individuals facing a serious health condition. In such a case, individuals are less likely to use adaptive self-regulation strategies if they hold negative self-perceptions of aging, thereby experiencing poorer health outcomes (Wurm, Warner, Ziegelmann, Wolff, & Schuz, 2013). In addition, the process of misattributing symptoms of illness or disability as signs of pathological aging as opposed to normal aging has detrimental consequences for physical health. For example, a recent study found that adults aged 80 years and older who attributed a chronic health condition to old age tended to report more bothersome symptoms, engaged in fewer health behaviors, and were also twice as likely to have died by the 2-year follow-up (Stewart, Chipperfield, Perry, & Weiner, 2012). Similarly, adults who attributed symptoms of arthritis, heart disease, and sleeping problems to normal aging rather than chronic disease were significantly less likely to have sought preventive medical services in the previous year (Goodwin, Black, & Satish, 1999). Therefore, when individuals interpret the subjective experience of aging as being undistinguishable from declining health, more negative health outcomes are likely to follow. Hence, intervention efforts that target expectancies and attributions of aging may be particularly effective for promoting positive health, and there is some preliminary work to support this (Sarkisian, Prohaska, Davis, & Weiner, 2007; Wolff, Warner, Ziegelmann, & Wurm, 2014). Because more empirical evidence emerges regarding associations between subjective aging and health, the list of potential mechanisms to target in intervention work will grow. Those mechanisms with strong empirical support should be explicitly tested for their effectiveness in helping individuals and professionals consciously combat the influences of age stereotypes.

Although stereotype embodiment theory specifically explains how subjective aging influences physical health, the same mechanisms might also be applied to the benefit of other (non–health-related) developmental outcomes. For instance, workplace performance among older adults might plausibly improve after an intervention which helps individuals become aware of age stereotypes and change their expectations, aging attributions, self-efficacy, or control beliefs. To the knowledge of the authors, theoretical and empirical work promoting other facets of well-being has not yet been published and represents an important area of future research.

In summary, intervening to promote more realistic views on aging at the individual and professional level is not without its challenges but is a logical next step given the body of evidence pointing to the importance of views on aging. Interventions designed for individuals and professionals should target key psychological, behavioral, and physiological pathways by which negative self-views and age stereotypes influence health and well-being. A thorough discussion of implications of subjective aging research for intervention is presented in Chapter 9, this volume.

Changing Views on Aging at the Macrolevel: Challenges and Approaches

The Role of Social and Health Care Policy

In several Western countries, such as Germany, the United Kingdom, and the United States, there has been a vivid debate about how subjective aging might be changed at the societal level. To date, this debate has focused on three aspects (e.g., German Federal Ministry for Family Affairs, Senior Citizens, Women and Youth, 2010). First, there has been an appeal for a more balanced and differentiated view of both the virtues and the risks of the aging process and societal aging in general. Increasing public awareness for the potentials of old age is important to activate and take advantage of the developmental plasticity of older adults and to encourage individuals to recognize and seize opportunities for growth and development also in the later phases of the life span. The second challenge is to move away from considering old age as a static phase of life with clear-cut and unmovable boundaries (e.g., determined by functional status) and to establish a more dynamic conceptualization of aging as a lifelong developmental process. For the individual, this view could imply to regard later adulthood as a "project" for which he or she holds responsibility rather than as a static phase in which little change and improvement is possible. A third endeavor in the public debate is to dissociate aging and disease in individual and societal conceptions of the aging process. Falsely attributing health conditions to the aging process goes along with the belief that such age-related decline is inevitable, uncontrollable, and irreversible and, therefore, undermines decisions for otherwise effective treatment or rehabilitation plans. In addition to health care, social policies regarding retirement age are also implicated in the endeavor to disentangle aging from disease. Some European countries mandate retirement at age 65 years, whereas this practice is prohibited in other countries for most professions and for age discrimination purposes (see the Age Discrimination in Employment Act in the United States). Basing retirement policies strictly on chronological age assumes that disability and functional decline go hand in hand with getting older—an implicit assumption that reinforces and perpetuates negative perceptions toward older adults. The intentions behind such policies must be examined to evaluate whether they contribute to successful aging or whether they interfere with it. In addition, such policies are also completely counterproductive in some industries where a shortage of skilled younger workers exists who can replace the older and experienced workers if they retire. Particularly in such cases, companies and policies need to find ways to address the needs of older workers to maintain and support their ability to work and to enable them to make the most of their skills and experience.

The Role of the Mass Media

Besides social and health care policies, the mass media and the internet play an important role in conveying societal views on aging. In particular, portrayals of older adults in the media create reference points for the future selves of younger adults and influence older adults' self-evaluations of their resources and limitations (Vasil & Wass, 1993). Empirical studies find that older people, especially old-old adults and women, are underrepresented in several television formats, such as advertisements, talk shows, and movies, and that the roles which are ascribed to older adults in the media represent only a limited and stereotypical range of the various roles occupied by older adults in real life (Kessler, Rakoczy, & Staudinger, 2004; Robinson & Skill, 1995; Vasil & Wass, 1993). Social networking sites, such as Facebook, represent another and increasingly used platform to propagate negative stereotypes of old age (Levy, Chung, Bedford, & Navrazhina, 2013). Vasil and Wass (1993) describe two approaches to counter such stereotypical portrayals of older adults in the mass media. The first approach is to develop instructional formats providing accurate knowledge to the public, both young and old, and promoting constructive attitudes toward older adults. The second approach is to influence the mass media directly through monitoring and lobbying against ageism. The importance of this approach is not negligible given empirical evidence that older adults with greater television exposure hold more negative views on aging (Donlon et al., 2005).

Contributions of Subjective Aging Research

Two essential findings of subjective aging research lay the foundation of interventions targeting views on aging at the macrolevel of ecologies. First, societal age stereotypes are being internalized by the members of a society starting in the early years of life and continuing throughout the life span (Levy, 2009). Second, these internalized age stereotypes become increasingly self-relevant as individuals age and have tremendous implications for psychophysical functioning in later adulthood (e.g., Levy, Slade, & Kasl, 2002; Sargent-Cox, Anstey, & Luszcz, 2014; Wurm et al., 2010). Furthermore, subjective aging research has provided first evidence that certain developmental contexts, such as different socioeconomic strata (Barrett, 2003), provide opportunities and constraints for positive views on aging. Overall, subjective aging research has recognized the role and importance of macrolevel ecologies for individuals' views on aging by examining the intricate processes through which broad societal age stereotypes are being internalized by individuals (Kornadt & Rothermund, 2012; Levy, 2009). This recognition is, however, not widely shared yet, and we are still lacking knowledge about subjective aging in specific developmental and environmental contexts. Consequently, important potential for interventions at the macrolevels of society might be overlooked.

Despite the solid foundation of research on subjective aging, we are currently not yet in a position to provide a strong empirical basis for societal interventions. Thus, additional work needs to be done to build a broad, solid, and evidence-based foundation for such envisioned initiatives. First, a systematic review of the subjective aging literature that investigates changes in views on aging across historical periods could inform the discussion about the role of societal change as an influencing factor for subjective aging. A second open question for subjective aging research is whether solely positive or solely negative views on aging exert an influence on developmental outcomes. To date, subjective aging research has provided evidence that late life developmental outcomes benefit from positive (as compared to risks associated with negative) views on aging. Alternative perspectives, as implied in the public debate about interventions for subjective aging, could be that it is the balance between positive and negative views on aging that matters or that a realistic evaluation of one's own limits and potentials (i.e., being aware of the positive and negative aspects of growing older) is optimal in terms of successful aging. Third, to date, subjective aging research has identified some subgroups of society that are relatively disadvantaged in terms of their views on aging, such as individuals of lower socioeconomic strata or racial or ethnic minority groups. However, it seems that more effort needs to be put into this area of subjective aging research. For example, we know relatively little about the influencing factors of subjective aging in different contexts and environments, such as individuals of ethnic minorities; the gay, lesbian, bisexual, transgender (GLBT) community; or nursing home residents. Moreover, subjective aging research has generalized its findings to a wide age range including individuals from midlife to old-old age. In contrast, predictors, outcomes, and trajectories of subjective aging for specific age groups have been widely neglected (Miche, Elsässer, & Wahl, 2014). More research on similarities and differences between age groups is necessary to draw solid conclusions about the strength of the relationship between subjective aging and developmental outcomes, such as health and well-being, from mid-adulthood to old age. Studying age-group differences in the predictors and plasticity of subjective aging could also provide valuable insights regarding the optimal timing and target groups of subjective aging interventions. Finally, a vital area for future research that could shed light on the interplay between societal age norms and subjective aging on the microlevel will be to examine the subjective aging experiences among individuals in various stages of retirement (e.g., planning for, entering, and living in retirement as well as reentering the workforce).

A LIFE-SPAN ORIENTED FRAMEWORK FOR CHANGING VIEWS ON AGING

Based on our review of subjective aging phenomena in different life contexts and their potential for change, we propose a framework for intervention and future research that targets views on aging across the entire life span. This framework takes into account subjective aging phenomena at different bioecological levels and suggests that effective micro- and macrolevel interventions must be tailored to the respective life phase. Figure 10.1 gives an overview of such a life-span oriented framework.

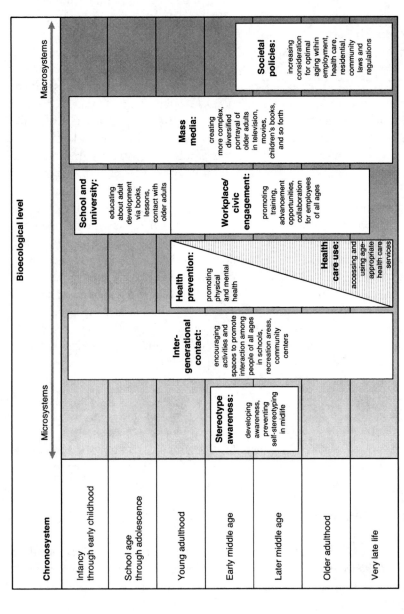

FIGURE 10.1 A bioecological framework to guide subjective aging interventions in research and practice. Although we use the term *chrono-system* in this figure predominantly as reflecting individual developmental stages, it is also meant to address changes at the systems level. For example, the period of old age itself undergoes historical cultural changes and this may also impact on views on aging.

The Early Years of Life: Interventions from Infancy Through Young Adulthood

Internalization processes of age stereotypes begin early in life. Children as young as age 4 years hold stereotypes about salient social groups, including the group of older adults (Bigler & Liben, 2007). Thus, in our framework, we begin with the earliest developmental contexts of infancy and early childhood. Children develop stereotypes based on explicit and implicit information from their environment: "When groups are labeled, treated, or sorted differently, children come to conceptualize groups as different in meaningful ways" (p. 166). In such a way, children's literature, TV programs, and cartoons are sources in which stereotypic beliefs about older adults are communicated to children (Hollis-Sawyer & Cuevas, 2013; Vasil & Wass, 1993). Recurrent connections between a social group and attributes as presented in the media (e.g., older adults being characterized as fragile and dependent) are likely to be detected and internalized by children, even without explicit reference (Bigler & Liben, 2007). Portrayals of older adults in the media thus need to reflect the broad spectrum of social roles, resources, and contributions of older adults as well as their vulnerabilities or impairments.

Furthermore, children internalize stereotypes from nonverbal behavior that adults direct to members of a social group (Bigler & Liben, 2007). Intergenerational contact may be effective for reducing prejudice especially for children (Allport, 1954), provided that older adults who participate in intergenerational contact are particularly sensitive to their unconscious nonverbal behavior. In adolescence and young adulthood, other aspects of intergenerational contact might become more important, such as equal status between group members, common goals, intergroup cooperation, and support of relevant institutions and authorities, according to a meta-analytic review of 515 studies on intergroup contact (Pettigrew & Tropp, 2006). Additional evidence for the benefits of intergenerational contact comes from research on the Experience Corps program, an inner city school–based volunteering program for older adults which has been implemented in several U.S. cities. Older adult volunteers benefit from the program regarding improved physical and cognitive health, whereas at-risk youth in the program see academic and educational improvements (Fried et al., 2004). Although the effects of age stereotypes held by students and volunteers have not been explicitly assessed as part of the program, benefits have been documented regarding improved social capital and school climate (Glass et al., 2004).

Finally, beginning at school age and even throughout higher education, when cultural knowledge is conveyed through explicit means of education, current gerontological knowledge of adult development needs to find better reflection in text books and teaching materials. The overall goal here consists of incorporating notions of differential aging, the plasticity of cognitive and physical functioning, and the role of lifestyle factors for successful late life development into the general knowledge of societal education. Aging societies could profit from such knowledge in two ways. First, because attention to aging education is still lacking in schools today, many people "are less socially, emotionally or physically prepared for old age than they could be if they had knowledge about aging and an understanding of how early life decisions have later life consequences" (McGuire, Klein, & Couper, 2005, p. 444). Second, because the demand for products and services designed to meet the needs of an aging population is increasing, higher education must provide professionals and paraprofessionals with accurate knowledge about aging to enable them to develop adequate solutions for older adults (Karcher & Whittlesey, 2007).

Mid-Adulthood: Prime Time for Subjective Aging Interventions

Further along the life course, mid-adulthood might constitute a "prime time" to address topics of subjective aging. In this life phase, individuals face multiple challenges and role demands with pronounced interindividual variability (Heckhausen, 2001), which might be reflected in a wide range of subjective aging experiences among middle-aged adults. For example, challenges in the workforce (e.g., rebalancing the intensity of one's job involvement) might co-occur with shifting time perspectives (e.g., remaining lifetime instead of time since birth) and a complex constellation of gains and losses (e.g., signs of emerging physical and cognitive constraints may occur at the same time as the new pleasures of grandparenthood). Midlife is also a time when physical changes relevant to subjective aging start to surface (Lachman, 2004). In summary, midlife may be characterized as the life phase when age stereotypes start to become self-relevant. This, however, tends to happen with pronounced interindividual variation. For example, a 55-year-old person who is completing a 6-day bike race on a mountainous course is very likely to hold different age stereotypes and different views on aging than another 55-year-old who is suffering from major emphysema and leads a mostly sedentary life. Because of the important preparatory role of midlife for health and psychosocial adjustment in old age (Lachman, 2004), subjective aging interventions that encourage and support individuals in taking up healthy lifestyles might be most effective in midlife.

Thus, in addition to microlevel interventions that educate individuals about the aging process, the strengths and vulnerabilities of older adults, and the ways in which older adults can counteract or cope with the challenges of later life, interventions that target views on aging held by professionals working with middle-aged adults (e.g., physicians, employers) are also indicated. An important first step in such interventions is to raise awareness for the often unconscious attitudes and misconceptions about old age and aging. Being aware of such implicit biases and of their influence on behavior is a prerequisite for questioning and eventually overcoming the widely held stereotypes and misconceptions. In a survey about ERA administered to 374 primary care clinicians, Davis and colleagues (2011) found great variation in terms of realistic expectations about the aging process. Although attitudes toward aging have become more positive in younger cohorts, there still seems to be a great proportion of health care professionals having overly positive or negative expectations about aging. Commonly held misconceptions about the aging process (Sarkisian, Steers, Hays, & Mangione, 2005) concern the view that aging is characterized by declines, not only in the domain of physical functioning but also in terms of cognitive functioning and mental health. Furthermore, many people believe that once age-related declines set in, there is nothing they can do about it: Age-related losses are often viewed as inevitable, uncontrollable, and irreversible. These misconceptions, however, have detrimental effects on objective performance measures on the one hand (Lachman, 2006; Plaks & Chasteen, 2013) and are strongly refuted by a solid body of research findings on the other hand. Therefore, professionals whose primary focus is to help older adults to maintain or improve functioning can exert important influences on delaying or minimizing any trajectory of decline and on motivating older adults to work toward the maintenance of their abilities as much as possible.

Subjective Aging Interventions in the Later Years of Life

Although we argue that the best timing for education about adult development is probably mid-adulthood, we believe that this issue requires continued efforts across the entire second half of life because there is growing evidence that subjective aging affects developmental outcomes at all stages of adulthood (Kotter-Grühn, Kleinspehn-Ammerlahn, Gerstorf, & Smith, 2009; Levy, 2003; Spuling, Miche, Wurm, & Wahl, 2013). It is important to note that in the group of old-old adults, functional status is more strongly linked to negative views of one's own aging in everyday life than chronological age (Miche, Wahl, et al., 2014). The subgroup of functionally impaired old-old adults thus represents an at-risk group, which should receive particular attention in subjective aging interventions. Thus, in very late life, the challenge for subjective aging interventions is to promote a positive view of aging despite the increasing risks for illnesses, disability, and dependency. Research indicates that self-regulation competencies represent a key resource for preserving positive views on aging among old-old adults (Infurna et al., 2010). Consequently, subjective aging interventions in the later years of life should equip individuals with the ability to make a realistic evaluation of their own strengths and vulnerabilities. Such a realistic self-assessment that is untainted by age stereotypes can be seen as a prerequisite for old-old individuals to counter developmental losses with adequate compensatory self-regulation strategies.

Although the role of health prevention in advanced old age declines at the expense of an increasing focus on restorative health care and long-term care, there is ample support for the beneficial effects of geriatric rehabilitation even in old-old age. For example, a systematic review and meta-analysis including 4,780 individuals with mean sample ages ranging from 74 to 86 years found that inpatient rehabilitation intervention programs fared better on a range of outcomes, such as functional improvement, admissions to nursing homes, and mortality, as compared to usual care (Bachmann et al., 2010). Physicians, nursing staff, relatives, and older adults themselves thus need to be sensitized to the fact that maintenance of mobility and everyday competence (e.g., competence in instrumental activities of daily living) can be achieved through rehabilitation, prevention, and (technical) assistive equipment.

Besides adequate health prevention and health care in very late life, another important task for promoting more realistic views on aging is to create opportunities for *social participation*. The period of very late life is still often viewed solely in terms of loss and decline. A reconsideration of societal age norms and policies is necessary to develop opportunities that enable the oldest old to take part in the social and cultural life of society. Such opportunities for social participation can be created at the microlevel (e.g., involvement in enjoyable social activities, intergenerational contact) as well as at the macrolevel (e.g., with communities' attention to the availability of opportunities for productive work and social engagement).

DISCUSSION AND FUTURE DIRECTIONS

Throughout this chapter, Bronfenbrenner's (1994) bioecological framework has proven particularly useful for summarizing subjective aging issues across different levels and ecologies of development. From the perspective of this model, it becomes evident that views on aging are established, communicated, and perpetuated at the level of the individual, in interactions among individuals, and at the level of society as a whole. Distinguishing between subjective aging issues at the micro- and macrolevels of ecologies while at the same time considering the interconnections between these levels provides a useful basis to derive potential avenues for subjective aging interventions. Moreover, the concept of a chronosystem emphasizes that the views on aging held by individuals, professionals, and society are constantly changing both as a result of historical as well as life span developmental change. To be effective, subjective aging interventions therefore must be tailored to the respective life phase as proposed in our life-span oriented framework for changing views on aging.

Although age norms and age expectations have become blurred because of a more fluid life cycle in today's society as evidenced by an increasing variety of older adults' socials roles, behavior, and functioning across the adult life span (Freund, Nikitin, & Ritter, 2009), chronological age is still used as a marker for behavioral competencies and social privileges and has not become completely irrelevant in the various settings of social life. To summarize, in our review of the literature on subjective aging issues across micro- and macrolevels of society, we observe a structural lag between the needs and competencies of aging individuals and the opportunities provided by society (Riley et al., 1994). On the other hand, the appraisal of individuals merely based on their chronological age may be starting to give way to a more differentiated consideration of a person's functional status and objective need for care (Neugarten, 1996), as can be seen in the distinction between the third and the fourth age. However, without also considering the strengths and competencies of older adults, this shift involves the danger that age is determined by functional status alone, which would result in an overgeneralized loss-oriented focus in the subjective perceptions of older adults themselves and in professionals working with older adult populations. This failure to capitalize on the capabilities and desires of older adults results in unexploited potential—economic, productive, familial, and emotional. We have argued that effective subjective aging interventions could release this potential both for the benefit of older adults themselves and for society as a whole.

When it comes to subjective aging interventions, an important question has to do with the extent to which views on aging can, in fact, be changed at the individual level, given the degree to which views on aging are societally determined. The sociocultural perspective on age stereotypes holds that with age, most members of a given society will become increasingly exposed to these negative views and will encounter some psychological pressure toward adopting at least some of them. This raises the question whether there is little escape from negative views on aging. Throughout this chapter, several implications of subjective aging research for developing interventions were discussed. Among these, education was suggested as a means to refute commonly held misconceptions about aging and to increase awareness for the potentials of old age. We have proposed specific mindsets about age and aging that need to become common practice at the microlevel as well as at the macrolevel. In particular, we have argued that (a) developmental gains represent an important but mostly neglected aspect of growing older; (b) individuals can, within certain parameters, exert control to delay or prevent many age-related declines; and (c) there are many effective ways to halt, slow, or even reverse physical and cognitive decline and to optimize quality of life. To increase public awareness for the many possibilities of old age, to establish a more dynamic conceptualization of aging as a lifelong developmental process, and to dissociate aging and disease in the mind of the public should thus become major goals of subjective aging interventions. Furthermore, traditional age norms that do not fit the real lives of today's older adults need to be over-come. Instead of a rigid age patterning of the life course, new and enriched opportunity structures for older adults need to be created by society as a whole to maximize individual choices and opportunities for development.

To summarize, the evaluation that we have not (yet) achieved an age-irrelevant (Neugarten, 1996) or age-integrated society (Riley & Riley, 2000) still holds. As Maddox (1996) stated, "The age-irrelevant society has not arrived. But age certainly has more varied, flexible, and changing meanings today than two decades ago when Bernice Neugarten forecast the age-irrelevant society" (p. 20). Yet the question remains whether an age-irrelevant society, from the perspective of subjective aging research, is or is not a desirable or even ethical goal. On the one hand, chronological age is a meaningful variable in certain respects and for certain parts of the life span. On the other hand, age norms have become a more fluid entity and, hence, should be revisited in terms of their use when broader cultural and societal changes indicate that a revision might be warranted. We would thus argue that a society that embraces the earlier mentioned mindsets would go beyond the age-irrelevant society, namely to a society where the allocation of services and the communication with and about older adults is truly *age-sensitive* rather than age-blind. Such a society, in our opinion, would be aware of the limitations that a "blind age orientation" can entail and thus would distinguish between chronological age and neediness or frailty (e.g., lack of physical functioning) while at the same time also recognize the potential and capacities of the aging individual.

We are also keenly aware that the idea of intervening to change views on aging raises several ethical issues. An overly simplistic approach, in which negative, deficit-oriented views on aging are only replaced by an unrealistic positive view of aging that negates any age-related loss, entails a moral imperative that can be achieved only by few individuals. As a consequence, age-related decline would be interpreted as individual failure and accompanied by feelings of guilt and anxiety (Pond et al., 2010). However, the negative views on aging that are prevalent in today's society hinder older adults from realizing their full potential of resources and capacities. We therefore argue that the challenge for intervention programs will be to foster *realistic views on aging* that motivate individuals and equip them with coping strategies to face the vulnerabilities of old age. At the same time, new challenges arise for an aging society that abandons traditional age norms. As Freund and colleagues (2009) have argued, it is important to recognize that "age-related expectations may not only guide the selection and timing of personal goals, but may also directly influence behavior that requires little or no self-regulation" (p. 6). Thus, individuals will have to compensate for vanishing age norms and conceptions of a normative life course—not only in old age but also at all stages of the adult life span—by taking an active and responsible role in engaging and disengaging in personal goals. In other words, the concept of an *age-sensitive society* might imply a greater focus on self-regulation competencies across the adult life span and will definitely put greater emphasis on the self-directedness of the individual. Again, there are large interindividual differences in self-regulation competencies, which relate to successful development and aging (Freund et al., 2009). Developing ways to teach such self-regulation strategies, thus, seems to be the next challenge lying ahead.

Certainly, the demographic change within developed countries confronts aging societies with new public health challenges. Lifelong prevention measures that target views on aging represent a promising means to empower individuals to take control of their health and aging. Therefore, developing, testing, and implementing creative approaches at the individual and societal level will be an essential next step for the field.

ACKNOWLEDGMENTS

The preparation of this work was supported by a grant from the Alexander von Humboldt Foundation awarded to Manfred Diehl and Hans-Werner Wahl. Martina Miche's work on this chapter was supported by a fellowship from the German National Academic foundation. Manfred Diehl and Allyson Brothers's work was supported in part by grant R21 AG041379 from the National Institute of Aging, National Institutes of Health.

REFERENCES

Adams, W. L., McIlvain, H. E., Lacy, N. L., Magsi, H., Crabtree, B. F., Yenny, S. K., & Sitorius, M. A. (2002). Primary care for elderly people: Why do doctors find it so hard? *The Gerontologist, 42*, 835–842. http://dx.doi.org/10.1093/geront/42.6.835

Adler, G., & Hilber, D. (2009). Industry hiring patterns of older workers. *Research on Aging, 31*, 69–88. http://dx.doi.org/10.1177/0164027508324635

Allport, G. W. (1954). *The nature of prejudice.* Cambridge, MA: Addison-Wesley.

Bachmann, S., Finger, C., Huss, A., Egger, M., Stuck, A. E., & Clough-Gorr, K. M. (2010). Inpatient rehabilitation specifically designed for geriatric patients: Systematic review and meta-analysis of randomised controlled trials. *British Medical Journal, 340*, c1718. http://dx.doi.org/10.1136/bmj.c1718

Baltes, P. B. (1997). On the incomplete architecture of human ontogeny. Selection, optimization, and compensation as foundation of developmental theory. *American Psychologist, 52*, 366–380. http://dx.doi.org/10.1037//0003-066x.52.4.366

Baltes, P. B., & Smith, J. (1999). Multilevel and systemic analyses of old age: Theoretical and empirical evidence for a fourth age. In V. L. Bengtson & K. W. Schaie (Eds.), *Handbook of theories of aging* (pp. 153–173). New York, NY: Springer Publishing.

Barrett, A. E. (2003). Socioeconomic status and age identity: The role of dimensions of health in the subjective construction of age. *The Journals of Gerontology. Series B, Psychological Sciences and Social Sciences, 58B*, 101–109. http://dx.doi.org/10.1093/geronb/58.2.S101

Beall, S. C., Baumhover, L. A., Maxwell, A. J., & Pieroni, R. E. (1996). Normal versus pathological aging: Knowledge of family practice residents. *The Gerontologist, 36*, 113–117. http://dx.doi.org/10.1093/geront/36.1.113

Bigler, R. S., & Liben, L. S. (2007). Developmental intergroup theory: Explaining and reducing children's social stereotyping and prejudice. *Current Directions in Psychological Science, 16*, 162–166. http://dx.doi.org/10.1111/j.1467-8721.2007.00496.x

Bowen, C., & Skirbekk, V. (2013). National stereotypes of older people's competence are related to older adults' participation in paid and volunteer work. *The Journals of Gerontology. Series B, Psychological Sciences and Social Sciences, 68*, 974–983. http://dx.doi.org/10.1093/geronb/gbt101

Bowen, C., & Staudinger, U. (2013). Relationship between age and promotion orientation depends on perceived older worker stereotypes. *The Journals of Gerontology. Series B, Psychological Sciences and Social Sciences, 68*, 59–63. http://dx.doi.org/10.1093/geronb/gbs060

Bronfenbrenner, U. (1994). Ecological models of human development. In T. Husen & T. N. Postlethwaite (Eds.), *International encyclopedia of education* (2nd ed., Vol. 3, pp. 1643–1647). Oxford, United Kingdom: Pergamon Press/Elsevier Science.

Chachamovich, E., Fleck, M., Laidlaw, K., & Power, M. (2008). Impact of major depression and subsyndromal symptoms on quality of life and attitudes toward aging in an international sample of older adults. *The Gerontologist, 48*, 593–602. http://dx.doi.org/10.1093/geront/48.5.593

Christensen, K., Doblhammer, G., Rau, R., & Vaupel, J. W. (2009). Ageing populations: The challenges ahead. *The Lancet, 374*, 1196–1208. http://dx.doi.org/10.1016/S0140-6736(09)61460-4

Collins, L., Baker, T., Mermelstein, R., Piper, M., Jorenby, D., Smith, S., . . . Fiore, M. (2011). The multiphase optimization strategy for engineering effective tobacco use interventions. *Annals of Behavioral Medicine, 41*(2), 208–226. http://dx.doi.org/10.1007/s12160-010-9253-x

Cuddy, A. J. C., Norton, M. I., & Fiske, S. T. (2005). This old stereotype: The pervasiveness and persistence of the elderly stereotype. *Journal of Social Issues, 61*, 267–285. http://dx.doi.org/10.1111/j.1540-4560.2005.00405.x

Czaja, S. J. (2001). Technological change and the older worker. In J. E. Birren & K. W. Schaie (Eds.), *Handbook of the psychology of aging* (5th ed., pp. 547–568). San Diego, CA: Academic Press.

Czaja, S. J., & Sharit, J. (1998). Ability–performance relationships as a function of age and task experience for a data entry task. *Journal of Experimental Psychology: Applied, 4*, 332–351. http://dx.doi.org/10.1037/1076-898x.4.4.332

Davis, M. M., Bond, L. A., Howard, A., & Sarkisian, C. A. (2011). Primary care clinician expectations regarding aging. *The Gerontologist, 51*, 856–866. http://dx.doi.org/10.1093/geront/gnr017

Desmette, D., & Gaillard, M. (2008). When a "worker" becomes an "old worker": The effects of age-related social identity on attitudes towards retirement and work. *The Career Development International, 13*, 168–185. http://dx.doi.org/10.1108/13620430810860567

Diehl, M., & Wahl, H. W. (2010). Awareness of age-related change: Examination of a (mostly) unexplored concept. *The Journals of Gerontology. Series B, Psychological Sciences and Social Sciences, 65*, 340–350. http://dx.doi.org/10.1093/geronb/gbp110

Diehl, M., Wahl, H. W., Barrett, A. E., Brothers, A. F., Miche, M., Montepare, J. M., . . . Wurm, S. (2014). Awareness of aging: Theoretical considerations on an emerging concept. *Developmental Review, 34*, 93–113. http://dx.doi.org/10.1016/j.dr.2014.01.001

Donlon, M. M., Ashman, O., & Levy, B. R. (2005). Re-vision of older television characters: A stereotype-awareness intervention. *Journal of Social Issues, 61*, 307–319. http://dx.doi.org/10.1111/j.1540-4560.2005.00407.x

Dziak, J. J., Nahum-Shani, I., & Collins, L. M. (2012). Multilevel factorial experiments for developing behavioral interventions: Power, sample size, and resource considerations. *Psychological Methods, 17*(2), 153–175. http://dx.doi.org/10.1037/a0026972

Fineman, N. (1994). Health care providers' subjective understandings of old age: Implications for threatened status in late life. *Journal of Aging Studies, 8*, 255–270. http://dx.doi.org/10.1016/0890-4065(94)90003-5

Freund, A. M., Nikitin, J., & Ritter, J. O. (2009). Psychological consequences of longevity. *Human Development, 52*, 1–37. http://dx.doi.org/10.1159/000189213

Fried, L. P., Carlson, M. C., Freedman, M., Frick, K. D., Glass, T. A., Hill, J., . . . Zeger, S. (2004). A social model for health promotion for an aging population: Initial evidence on the Experience Corps model. *Journal of Urban Health-Bulletin of the New York Academy of Medicine, 81*(1), 64–78.

Galvin, R. (2002). Disturbing notions of chronic illness and individual responsibility: Towards a genealogy of morals. *Health, 6*, 107–137. http://dx.doi.org/10.1177/136345930200600201

German Federal Ministry for Family Affairs, Senior Citizens, Women and Youth. (Ed.). (2010). *A new culture of ageing. Images of ageing in society.* Berlin, Germany: Bundesanzeiger.

Glass, T. A., Freedman, M., Carlson, M. C., Hill, J., Frick, K. D., Ialongo, N., . . . Fried, L. (2004). Experience Corps: Design of an intergenerational program to boost social capital and promote the health of an aging society. *Journal of Urban Health-Bulletin of the New York Academy of Medicine, 81*(1), 94–105. http://dx.doi.org/10.1093/jurban/jth096

Golub, S. A., & Langer, E. J. (2007). Challenging assumptions about adult development: Implications for the health of older adults. In C. A. Aldwin, C. L. Park, & A. Spiro, III (Eds.), *Handbook of health psychology and aging* (pp. 9–29). New York, NY: Guilford Press.

Goodwin, J. S., Black, S. A., & Satish, S. (1999). Aging versus disease: The opinions of older black, Hispanic, and non-Hispanic white Americans about the causes and treatment of common medical conditions. *Journal of the American Geriatrics Society, 47*, 973–979.

Hagestad, G. O., & Neugarten, B. L. (1985). Age and the life course. In R. H. Binstock & E. Shanas (Eds.), *Handbook of aging and the social sciences* (pp. 35–61). New York, NY: Van Nostrand Reinhold.

Hauer, K. E., Durning, S. J., Kernan, W. N., Fagan, M. J., Mintz, M., O'Sullivan, P. S., . . . Schwartz, M. D. (2008). Factors associated with medical students' career choices regarding internal medicine. *Journal of the American Medical Association, 300,* 1154–1164. http://dx.doi.org/10.1001/jama.300.10.1154

Heckhausen, J. (2001). Adaptation and resilience in midlife. In M. E. Lachman (Ed.), *Handbook of midlife development* (pp. 345–394). Hoboken, NJ: Wiley.

Hedge, J. W., Borman, W. C., & Lammlein, S. E. (2006). Age stereotyping and age discrimination. In J. W. Hedge, W. C. Borman, & S. E. Lammlein (Eds.), *The aging workforce: Realities, myths, and implications for organizations* (pp. 27–48). Washington, DC: American Psychological Association.

Hollis-Sawyer, L., & Cuevas, L. (2013). Mirror, mirror on the wall: Ageist and sexist double jeopardy portrayals in children's picture books. *Educational Gerontology, 39*(12), 902–914. http://dx.doi.org/10.1080/03601277.2013.767650

Hubley, A. M., & Russell, L. B. (2009). Prediction of subjective age, desired age, and age satisfaction in older adults: Do some health dimensions contribute more than others? *International Journal of Behavioral Development, 33,* 12–21. http://dx.doi.org/10.1177/0165025408099486

Hummert, M. L. (1993). Age and typicality judgments of stereotypes of the elderly: Perceptions of elderly vs. young adults. *The International Journal of Aging & Human Development, 37*(3), 217–226. http://dx.doi.org/10.2190/L01P-V960-8P17-PL56

Hummert, M. L. (2011). Age stereotypes and aging. In K. W. Schaie & S. L. Willis (Eds.), *Handbook of the psychology of aging* (7th ed., pp. 249–262). San Diego, CA: Elsevier Academic Press.

Infurna, F. J., Gerstorf, D., Robertson, S., Berg, S., & Zarit, S. H. (2010). The nature and cross-domain correlates of subjective age in the oldest old: Evidence from the OCTO Study. *Psychology and Aging, 25,* 470–476. http://dx.doi.org/10.1037/a0017979

James, J. B., & Wink, P. (2006). The third age: A rationale for research. In J. B. James, P. Wink, & K. W. Schaie (Eds.), *Annual Review of Gerontology and Geriatrics* (Vol. 26, pp. xix–xxxii). New York, NY: Springer Publishing.

Karcher, B. C., & Whittlesey, V. (2007). Bridging the gap between academic gerontology and the educational needs of the aging network. *Educational Gerontology, 33,* 209–220. http://dx.doi.org/10.1080/03601270600894055

Kearney, N., Miller, M., Paul, J., & Smith, K. (2000). Oncology healthcare professionals' attitudes toward elderly people. *Annals of Oncology, 11,* 599–601. http://dx.doi.org/10.1023/a:1008327129699

Kessler, E. M., Bowen, C., Baer, M., Froelich, L., & Wahl, H. W. (2012). Dementia worry: A psychological examination of an unexplored phenomenon. *European Journal of Ageing,* 1–10. http://dx.doi.org/10.1007/s10433-012-0242-8

Kessler, E. M., Kruse, A., & Wahl, H. W. (in press). Clinical gero-psychology: A lifespan perspective. In N. A. Pachana & K. Laidlaw (Eds.), *The Oxford handbook of clinical geropsychology: International perspectives.* London, England: Oxford University Press.

Kessler, E. M., Rakoczy, K., & Staudinger, U. M. (2004). The portrayal of older people in prime time television series: The match with gerontological evidence. *Ageing & Society*, 24, 531–552. http://dx.doi.org/10.1017/S0144686X04002338

Keyes, C. L. M., & Westerhof, G. J. (2012). Chronological and subjective age differences in flourishing mental health and major depressive episode. *Aging & Mental Health*, 16, 67–74. http://dx.doi.org/10.1080/13607863.2011.596811

Klusmann, V., Evers, A., Schwarzer, R., & Heuser, I. (2012). Views on aging and emotional benefits of physical activity: Effects of an exercise intervention in older women. *Psychology of Sport and Exercise*, 13(2), 236–242. http://dx.doi.org/10.1016/j.psychsport.2011.11.001

Kornadt, A. E., & Rothermund, K. (2012). Internalization of age stereotypes into the self-concept via future self-views: A general model and domain-specific differences. *Psychology and Aging*, 27, 164–172. http://dx.doi.org/10.1037/a0025110

Kotter-Grühn, D., Kleinspehn-Ammerlahn, A., Gerstorf, D., & Smith, J. (2009). Self-perceptions of aging predict mortality and change with approaching death: 16-year longitudinal results from the Berlin Aging Study. *Psychology and Aging*, 24, 654–667. http://dx.doi.org/10.1037/a0016510

Krings, F., Sczesny, S., & Kluge, A. (2011). Stereotypical inferences as mediators of age discrimination: The role of competence and warmth. *British Journal of Management*, 22, 187–201. http://dx.doi.org/10.1111/j.1467-8551.2010.00721.x

Lachman, M. E. (2004). Development in midlife. *Annual Review of Psychology*, 55, 305–331. http://dx.doi.org/10.1146/annurev.psych.55.090902.141521

Lachman, M. E. (2006). Perceived control over aging-related declines: Adaptive beliefs and behaviors. *Current Directions in Psychological Science*, 15, 282–286. http://dx.doi.org/10.1111/j.1467-8721.2006.00453.x

Leigh, J. P., Kravitz, R. L., Schembri, M., Samuels, S. J., & Mobley, S. (2002). Physician career satisfaction across specialties. *Archives of Internal Medicine*, 162, 1577–1584. http://dx.doi.org/10.1001/archinte.162.14.1577

Levy, B. R. (2003). Mind matters: Cognitive and physical effects of aging self-stereotypes. *The Journals of Gerontology. Series B, Psychological Sciences and Social Sciences*, 58(4), 203–211. http://dx.doi.org/10.1093/geronb/58.4.P203

Levy, B. R. (2009). Stereotype embodiment: A psychosocial approach to aging. *Current Directions in Psychological Science*, 18, 332–336. http://dx.doi.org/10.1111/j.1467-8721.2009.01662.x

Levy, B. R., Chung, P. H., Bedford, T., & Navrazhina, K. (2013). Facebook as a site for negative age stereotypes. *The Gerontologist*, 54, 172–176. http://dx.doi.org/10.1093/geront/gns194

Levy, B. R., & Myers, L. M. (2004). Preventive health behaviors influenced by self-perceptions of aging. *Preventive Medicine*, 39, 625–629. http://dx.doi.org/10.1016/j.ypmed.2004.02.029

Levy, B. R., Ryall, A. L., Pilver, C. E., Sheridan, P. L., Wei, J. Y., & Hausdorff, J. M. (2008). Influence of African American elders' age stereotypes on their cardiovascular response to stress. *Anxiety, Stress, & Coping*, 21, 85–93. http://dx.doi.org/10.1080/10615800701727793

Levy, B. R., Slade, M. D., & Gill, T. M. (2006). Hearing decline predicted by elders' stereotypes. *Journals of Gerontology. Series B, Psychological Sciences and Social Sciences*, *61*(2), P82–P87. http://dx.doi.org/10.1093/geronb/61.2.P82

Levy, B. R., Slade, M. D., & Kasl, S. V. (2002). Longitudinal benefit of positive self-perceptions of aging on functional health. *The Journals of Gerontology. Series B, Psychological Sciences and Social Sciences*, *57*, 409–417. http://dx.doi.org/10.1093/geronb/57.5.P409

Levy, B. R., Slade, M. D., May, J., & Caracciolo, E. A. (2006). Physical recovery after acute myocardial infarction: Positive age self-stereotypes as a resource. *The International Journal of Aging & Human Development*, *62*, 285–301. http://dx.doi.org/10.2190/ejk1-1q0d-lhge-7a35

Levy, B. R., Zonderman, A. B., Slade, M. D., & Ferrucci, L. (2009). Age stereotypes held earlier in life predict cardiovascular events in later life. *Psychological Science*, *20*, 296–298. http://dx.doi.org/10.1111/j.1467-9280.2009.02298.x

Liu, Y. E., Norman, I. J., & While, A. E. (2013). Nurses' attitudes towards older people: A systematic review. *International Journal of Nursing Studies*, *50*, 1271–1282. http://dx.doi.org/10.1016/j.ijnurstu.2012.11.021

Maddox, G. L. (1996). Definitions and descriptions of age. In D. A. Neugarten (Ed.), *The meanings of age: Selected papers of Bernice L. Neugarten* (pp. 19–23). Chicago, IL: The University of Chicago Press.

McGuire, S., Klein, D., & Couper, D. (2005). Aging education: A national imperative. *Educational Gerontology*, *31*, 443–460. http://dx.doi.org/10.1080/03601270590928170

Meisner, B. A. (2012). Physicians' attitudes toward aging, the aged, and the provision of geriatric care: A systematic narrative review. *Critical Public Health*, *22*, 61–72. http://dx.doi.org/10.1080/09581596.2010.539592

Miche, M., Elsässer, V., & Wahl, H. W. (2014). *Attitude toward own aging in midlife and early old age over a 12-year period: Examination of measurement equivalence and developmental trajectories*. Manuscript submitted for publication.

Miche, M., Wahl, H. W., Diehl, M., Oswald, F., Kaspar, R., & Kolb, M. (2014). Natural occurrence of subjective aging experiences in community-dwelling older adults. *The Journals of Gerontology. Series B, Psychological Sciences and Social Sciences*, *69*, 174–187. http://dx.doi.org/10.1093/geronb/gbs164

Moen, P., Fields, V., Meador, R., & Rosenblatt, H. (2000). Fostering integration: A case study of the Cornell Retirees Volunteering in Service (CRVIS) program. In K. Pillemer, P. Moen, E. Wethington, & N. Glasgow (Eds.), *Social integration in the second half of life* (pp. 247–264). Baltimore, MD: Johns Hopkins University Press.

Moor, C., Zimprich, D., Schmitt, M., & Kliegel, M. (2006). Personality, aging self-perceptions, and subjective health: A mediation model. *International Journal of Aging & Human Development*, *63*(3), 241–257. http://dx.doi.org/10.2190/Akry-Um4k-Pb1v-Pbhf

Neugarten, B. L. (1996). The young-old and the age-irrelevant society. In D. A. Neugarten (Ed.), *The meanings of age: Selected papers of Bernice L. Neugarten* (pp. 47–55). Chicago, IL: The University of Chicago Press.

Ng, T. W. H., & Feldman, D. C. (2008). The relationship of age to ten dimensions of job performance. *Journal of Applied Psychology, 93*, 392–423. http://dx.doi .org/10.1037/0021-9010.93.2.392

Ory, M., Hoffman, M. K., Hawkins, M., Sanner, B., & Mockenhaupt, R. (2003). Challenging aging stereotypes: Strategies for creating a more active society. *American Journal of Preventive Medicine, 25*(3), 164–171. http://dx.doi.org/10.1016/ S0749-3797(03)00181-8

Palmore, E. (2004). Research note: Ageism in Canada and the United States. *Journal of Cross-Cultural Gerontology, 19*, 41–46. http://dx.doi.org/10.1023/ B:JCCG.0000015098.62691.ab

Pasupathi, M., & Löckenhoff, C. E. (2002). Ageist behavior. In T. D. Nelson (Ed.), *Ageism: Stereotyping and prejudice against older persons* (pp. 201–246). Cambridge, MA: The MIT Press.

Pettigrew, T. F., & Tropp, L. R. (2006). A meta-analytic test of intergroup contact theory. *Journal of Personality and Social Psychology, 90*, 751–783. http://dx.doi .org/10.1037/0022-3514.90.5.751

Plaks, J. E., & Chasteen, A. L. (2013). Entity versus incremental theories predict older adults' memory performance. *Psychology and Aging, 28*, 948–957. http://dx.doi .org/10.1037/a0034348

Pond, R., Stephens, C., & Alpass, F. (2010). Virtuously watching one's health. *Journal of Health Psychology, 15*, 734–743. http://dx.doi.org/10.1177/1359105310368068

Riley, M. W., Kahn, R. L., & Foner, A. (1994). *Age and structural lag: Society's failure to provide meaningful opportunities in work, family, and leisure.* New York, NY: Wiley.

Riley, M. W., & Riley, J. W., Jr. (1994). Structural lag: Past and future. In M. W. Riley, R. L. Kahn, & A. Foner (Eds.), *Age and structural lag: Society's failure to provide meaningful opportunities in work, family, and leisure* (pp. 15–36). Oxford, United Kingdom: Wiley.

Riley, M. W., & Riley, J. W., Jr. (2000). Age integration: Conceptual and historical background. *The Gerontologist, 40*, 266. http://dx.doi.org/10.1093/geront/40.3.266

Robb, C., Chen, H., & Haley, W. (2002). Ageism in mental health and health care: A critical review. *Journal of Clinical Geropsychology, 8*(1), 1–12. http://dx.doi .org/10.1023/a:1013013322947

Robinson, J. D., & Skill, T. (1995). Media usage patterns and portrayals of the elderly. In J. F. Nussbaum & J. Coupland (Eds.), *Handbook of communication and aging research* (pp. 359–391). Hillsdale, NJ: Lawrence Erlbaum Associates.

Rybarczyk, B., Haut, A., Lacey, R. F., Fogg, L. F., & Nicholas, J. J. (2001). A multifactorial study of age bias among rehabilitation professionals. *Archives of Physical Medicine and Rehabilitation, 82*, 625–632. http://dx.doi.org/10.1053/apmr.2001.20834

Salthouse, T. A. (1984). Effects of age and skill in typing. *Journal of Experimental Psychology: General, 113*, 345–371. http://dx.doi.org/10.1037/0096-3445.113.3.345

Samra, R., Griffiths, A., Cox, T., Conroy, S., & Knight, A. (2013). Changes in medical student and doctor attitudes toward older adults after an intervention: A systematic review. *Journal of the American Geriatrics Society, 61*(7), 1188–1196. http://dx.doi .org/10.1111/jgs.12312

Sargent-Cox, K. A., Anstey, K. J., & Luszcz, M. A. (2012). The relationship between change in self-perceptions of aging and physical functioning in older adults. *Psychology and Aging, 27*(3), 750–760. http://dx.doi.org/10.1037/A0027578

Sargent-Cox, K. A., Anstey, K. J., & Luszcz, M. A. (2014). Longitudinal change of self-perceptions of aging and mortality. *The Journals of Gerontology. Series B, Psychological Sciences and Social Sciences, 69,* 168–173. http://dx.doi.org/10.1093/geronb/gbt005

Sarkisian, C. A., Prohaska, T. R., Davis, C., & Weiner, B. (2007). Pilot test of an attribution retraining intervention to raise walking levels in sedentary older adults. *Journal of the American Geriatrics Society, 55,* 1842–1846. http://dx.doi .org/10.1111/j.1532-5415.2007.01427.x

Sarkisian, C. A., Prohaska, T. R., Wong, M. D., Hirsch, S., & Mangione, C. M. (2005). The relationship between expectations for aging and physical activity among older adults. *Journal of General Internal Medicine, 20,* 911–915. http://dx.doi .org/10.1111/j.1525-1497.2005.0204.x

Sarkisian, C. A., Steers, W. N., Hays, R. D., & Mangione, C. M. (2005). Development of the 12-item Expectations Regarding Aging Survey. *The Gerontologist, 45,* 240–248. http://dx.doi.org/10.1093/geront/45.2.240

Schmitt, E. (2001). The impact of employment and unemployment in middle and upper adulthood on subjective perceptions of ones' own aging process, potentials and barriers of leading a productive and responsible life. *Zeitschrift Fur Gerontologie Und Geriatrie, 34*(3), 218–231. http://dx.doi.org/10.1007/s003910170066

Spuling, S. M., Miche, M., Wurm, S., & Wahl, H. W. (2013). Exploring the causal inter-play of subjective age and health dimensions in the second half of life. A cross-lagged panel analysis. *Zeitschrift für Gesundheitspsychologie, 21,* 5–15. http://dx.doi .org/10.1026/0943-8149/a000084

Stewart, T. L., Chipperfield, J. G., Perry, R. P., & Weiner, B. (2012). Attributing illness to 'old age:' Consequences of a self-directed stereotype for health and mortality. *Psychology & Health, 27,* 881–897. http://dx.doi.org/10.1080/08870446.2011.630735

Suhr, J. A., & Kinkela, J. H. (2007). Perceived threat of Alzheimer disease (AD): The role of personal experience with AD. *Alzheimer Disease and Associated Disorders, 21*(3), 225–231. http://dx.doi.org/10.1097/WAD.0b013e31813e6683

U.S. Census Bureau. (2012). Table 166. Percent distribution of number of visits to health care professionals by selected characteristics: 2000 and 2009. *Health & Nutrition: Health Care Utilization.* Retrieved from http://www.census.gov/compendia/statab/2012/tables/12s0166.pdf

Vasil, L., & Wass, H. (1993). Portrayal of the elderly in the media: A literature review and implications for educational gerontologists. *Educational Gerontology, 19,* 71–85. http://dx.doi.org/10.1080/0360127930190107

Westerhof, G. J., & Barrett, A. E. (2005). Age identity and subjective well-being: A com-parison of the United States and Germany. *The Journals of Gerontology. Series B, Psychological Sciences and Social Sciences, 60,* 129–136. http://dx.doi.org/10.1093/geronb/60.3.S129

Wolff, J. K., Warner, L. M., Ziegelmann, J. P., & Wurm, S. (2014). What does targeting positive views on ageing add to a physical activity intervention in older adults? Results from a randomized controlled trial. *Psychology & Health, 29*, 915–932.

Wurm, S., & Huxhold, O. (2010). Individuelle Altersbilder [Individual views on aging]. In A. Motel-Klingebiel, S. Wurm, & C. Tesch-Römer (Eds.), *Altern im Wandel: Befunde des Deutschen Alterssurveys (DEAS)* (pp. 246–262). Stuttgart, Germany: Kohlhammer.

Wurm, S., Tomasik, M. J., & Tesch-Römer, C. (2010). On the importance of a positive view on ageing for physical exercise among middle-aged and older adults: Cross-sectional and longitudinal findings. *Psychology & Health, 25*, 25–42. http://dx.doi.org/10.1080/08870440802311314

Wurm, S., Warner, L. M., Ziegelmann, J. P., Wolff, J. K., & Schuz, B. (2013). How do negative self-perceptions of aging become a self-fulfilling prophecy? *Psychology and Aging, 28*(4), 1088–1097. http://dx.doi.org/10.1037/a0032845

Index

Note: Page references followed by "*f*" and "*t*" denote figures and tables